To my friends, the Ben-Bassats
with affection

Bethesda, 'China Village' Dec 25, 2000.

CONTEMPORARY ISSUES IN MODELING PSYCHOPATHOLOGY

NEUROBIOLOGICAL FOUNDATION OF ABERRANT BEHAVIORS

CONTEMPORARY ISSUES IN MODELING PSYCHOPATHOLOGY

edited by

Michael S. Myslobodsky
Tel Aviv University &
Howard University

Ina Weiner
Tel Aviv University

KLUWER ACADEMIC PUBLISHERS
Boston / Dordrecht / London

Distributors for North, Central and South America:
Kluwer Academic Publishers
101 Philip Drive
Assinippi Park
Norwell, Massachusetts 02061 USA
Telephone (781) 871-6600
Fax (781) 681-9045
E-Mail <kluwer@wkap.com>

Distributors for all other countries:
Kluwer Academic Publishers Group
Distribution Centre
Post Office Box 322
3300 AH Dordrecht, THE NETHERLANDS
Telephone 31 78 6392 392
Fax 31 78 6546 474
E-Mail <services@wkap.nl>

 Electronic Services <http://www.wkap.nl>

Library of Congress Cataloging-in-Publication Data

Contemporary issues in modeling psychopathology / edited by Michael S. Myslobodsky,
and Ina Weiner.
    p. cm. – (Neurobiological foundation of aberrant behaviors ; 1)
    Includes bibliographical references and index.
    ISBN 0-7923-7942-X (alk. paper)
  1. Psychology, pathological. 2. Biological models. 3. Biological psychiatry. 4. Mental
disorders.
  I. Myslobodsky, Michael. II Weiner, Ina, 1949-. III Series.
[DNLM: WM 102 C761 2000]
RC465 .C65 2000
616.89 – dc21   00-059275

Printed on acid-free paper. Printed in the United States of America

***The Publisher offers discounts on this book for course use and bulk purchases.
For further information, send email to <michael.williams@wkap.com> .***

TABLE OF CONTENTS

LIST OF CONTRIBUTORS

Hymie Anisman, Institute of Neuroscience, Department of Psychology, Carleton University, 1125 Colonel By Drive Ottawa, Ontario, Canada K1S 5B6. e-mail: hanisman@cc.carleton.ca

Robert H. Belmaker, Beer Sheva Mental Health Center, Faculty of Health Sciences, Ben-Gurion University of The Negev, Beer Sheva, Israel.

Jeffrey N. Carlson, Department of Pharmacology and Neuroscience, Albany Medical College, MC-136, Albany, NY 12208, USA. e-mail: CarlsoJ@mail.amc.edu

Marc G. Caron, Howard Hughes Medical Institute, Departments of Cell Biology and Medicine, Duke University Medical Center, Durham, NC, USA.

Jacqueline N. Crawley, Section of Behavioral Neuropharmacology, Experimental Therapeutics Branch, National Institute of Mental Health, Bethesda, MD, 20892-1375, USA. e-mail: jncrawle@codon.nih.gov

Michael Davis, Department of Psychiatry and Behavioral Sciences, Emory University School of Medicine, Atlanta, GA, USA. e-mail: mdavis4@emory.edu

Haim Einat, Beer Sheva Mental Health Center, Faculty of Health Sciences, Ben-Gurion University of The Negev, Beer Sheva, Israel.

Joram Feldon, Laboratory of Behavioural Neurobiology, Swiss Federal Institute of Technology, Zürich, Switzerland. e-mail: feldon@toxi1.ethz.ch

William A. Falls, Department of Psychology, University of Vermont, Burlington, VT, USA.

Raul R. Gainetdinov, Howard Hughes Medical Institute, Departments of Cell Biology and Medicine, Duke University Medical Center, Durham, NC, USA.

Jonathan Gewirtz, Department of Psychology, University of Minnesota, Elliot Hall, 75 East River Road, Minneapolis, MN, USA.

Mark A. Geyer, Department of Psychiatry University of California at San Diego, 9500 Gilman Dr., 0804 La Jolla, CA 92093-0804, USA. e-mail: mgeyer@ucsd.edu

Stanley D. Glick, Department of Pharmacology and Neuroscience, Albany Medical College, MC-136, Albany, NY 12208, USA. e-mail: sglick@ccgateway.amc.edu

Andrew Holmes, Section of Behavioral Neuropharmacology, Experimental Therapeutics Branch, National Institute of Mental Health, Bethesda, MD 20892-1375, USA.

Loring J. Ingraham, Center for Professional Psychology, George Washington University, Washington, DC 20037, USA. e-mail: Loring_ingraham@nih.gov

Ora Kofman, Department of Behavioral Sciences, Ben-Gurion University of The Negev, Beer Sheva, Israel. e-mail: kofman@bgumail.bgu.ac.il

Julia Lehmann, Laboratory of Behavioural Neurobiology, Swiss Federal Institute of Technology, Zürich, Switzerland. email: lehmann@ toxi.biol.ethz.ch

Barbara K. Lipska, Clinical Brain Disorders Branch, Intramural Research Program, National Institute of Mental Health, Bethesda, MD 20892, USA. e-mail: lipskab@intra.nimh.nih.gov

Isabelle M. Maisonneuve, Department of Pharmacology and Neuroscience, Albany Medical College, MC-136 Albany, NY 12208, USA.

Dan C. McIntyre, Institute of Neuroscience, Department of Psychology, Carleton University, 1125 Colonel By Drive, Ottawa, Ontario, Canada K1S 5B6. e-mail: dmcintyr@ccs.carleton.ca

Gary W. Miller, Division of Pharmacology and Toxicology, College of Pharmacy, University of Texas at Austin, Austin, USA. e-mail: gwmiller@mail.utexas.edu

Matti Mintz, Psychobiology Research Unit, Department of Psychology, Tel-Aviv University, Tel-Aviv 69978, Israel. e-mail: mintz@freud.tau.ac.il

Michael Myslobodsky, Psychobiology Research Unit, Department of Psychology, Tel-Aviv University, Tel-Aviv 69978, Israel. e-mail: michael2@freud.tau.ac.il

Bradley D. Pearce, Emory University School of Medicine, Department of Psychiatry and Behavioral Sciences, Atlanta, GA, USA. e-mail: bpearce@learnlink.emory.edu

Christopher Pryce, Laboratory of Behavioural Neurobiology, Swiss Federal Institute of Technology, Zürich, Switzerland. e-mail: pryce@toxi.biol.ethz.ch

Trevor W. Robbins, Department of Experimental Psychology, University of Cambridge, UK. e-mail: twr2@cus.cam.ac.uk

Terry E. Robinson, Department of Psychology (Biopsychology Program), The University of Michigan, 525 E. University Street, Ann Arbor, MI 48109, USA. e-mail: ter@umich.edu

Daniel R. Weinberger, Clinical Brain Disorders Branch, Intramural Research Program, National Institute of Mental Health, Bethesda, MD 20892, USA. e-mail: weinberd@intra.nimh.nih.gov

Ina Weiner, Department of Psychology, Tel-Aviv University, Tel-Aviv 69978, Israel. e-mail: weiner@post.tau.ac.il

Marta Weinstock, Department of Pharmacology, Hebrew University, Hadassah Medical Center, Jerusalem 91120, Israel. e-mail: martar@cc.huji.ac.il

Isabelle Weiss, Laboratory of Behavioural Neurobiology, Swiss Federal Institute of Technology Zürich, Switzerland. email: weiss@toxi.biol.ethz.ch

PREFACE

In the Hans Christian Andersen story, 'The Nightingale', a royal court was treated with disdain for judging a mechanical model superior to a live bird. One might wonder why? After all, the analogue model did sing. The number of songs was certainly limited, but they were predictable, replicable, and easy to trigger. Their 'preprogrammed' character would have even offered certain advantages for planning some experiments with the real birds, if needed. Those who have been humbled by the efforts to produce animal models of psychopathology may understand the sentiment of the royal court.

Despite considerable progress in clinical and basic neurosciences the cure of psychiatric disorders is still remote, little is known about their prevention, and the etiology and molecular mechanisms of mental disorders are still obscure. Psychiatry is not high on signs and markers, so that diagnoses are still guided by the patients' stories. The mission of animal models is to bridge the gap between "the story and the synapse". The questions to this approach are, What good might come from such a model? Are we wasting our time? How far can we carry results from model animals, like rats or mice without practicing what Dennett (1995) called "greedy reductionism" and causing a highly distorted view of the field and its goals? The answers are not easy to come by. As Susan Iversen wrote in 1987, "A decade ago it was a satisfying experience to prepare a review chapter relating to animal models of schizophrenia. At that time it seemed that everything was beginning to fit together and that the answers to the remaining problems would fall into place quite soon. This situation is rather different now" (p. 171)...

Actually, in 1987 life was still easy. The Diagnostic and Statistical Manual of Mental Disorders (DSM) included then 272 disorders. The DSM-IV, published in 1994 had already 297 disorders and still counting. Assuming that the Wernicke-Kleist contribution to psychiatric nosology will finally regain its scientific respectability, the number of psychiatric diseases would easily go well over 300 items. That does not mean that our taxonomic order would be identical to the realities of nature or that mental disease would be promptly identified according to its anatomy and cause. As the 'library' of mental disorders keeps expanding, their diversity will never be matched by that of the 'library' of models. Clearly, our models are not intended to teach us much about rebellious adolescents, deficiency of moral judgment, altered insight or rationality, delayed identity formation, traumatic flashbacks, concentration on depressive ideas, and rumination of past faults, and much more of all that is neatly packaged in DSM. Psychiatry has yet to acquire the power of neurology, where the nosological borders are more solid and are determined by a cluster of signs or markers which converge on specific brain sites, mechanisms, or genes so that even *Drosophila's* locomotion becomes a key to Parkinson's disease (Feany & Bender, 2000). That is why the library of animal psychopathology models has to be written in the language of orienting responses and startle, deficient memory, aberrant drives, sleep disturbances, fear, or changes in some acquired or innate behavioral patterns.

Should then the nosological labels so liberally applied to the experimentally reproduced phenomena be taken seriously? Are we generalizing too far from our models?

The present book is a sampler of some themes that reflected explicitly or implicitly these concerns and questions during a meeting on psychopathology modeling in Tel-Aviv in 1998. Collectively, they provide various perspectives on psychopathology suggested by targeted neurotransmitter changes, brain lesions, developmental manipulations, selective breeding, transgenic and knockout techniques, and experimental behavioral aberrations. Its contributors are active neuroscientists of the US, Canada, UK, and Israel. The list was limited due to space considerations and our ability to identify appropriate contributors able to complete the chapters within a narrow time window. The book provides, however, adequate evidence that animal models have become an integral part of psychiatry research. This reflects an irreversible turn to the biological bases of mental illness which psychiatry was nudged to take since the early 1950's. It was initiated and lead by Dr. Seymour Kety, then the first scientific director of the National Institute of Mental Health. Among many other things, we owe it to him that not many psychiatry purists throw hands up in mock display of dismay at the limitations imposed by the method of scrutiny of mental disorders. This great scientist and a unique man died in May 2000. My sad privilege is writing these lines to a book that we were hoping he would be able to introduce.

Before closing, I have several debts to acknowledge. My thanks and recognition goes to Dr. Doug Jones from NIMH who designed the cover for the book which alone will certainly prod many to thumb it. I am extremely grateful to Mary Panarelli at Kluwer Academic who gave valuable assistance at a number of crossroads, when we were about to run a red light. Last, but not the least, Mike Williams' enthusiasm and vision makes this book an opening volume for a series, *Neurobiological Foundations of Aberrant Behavior*. The aim of the series is to serve the growing community of neuroscientists and research psychiatrists who are engaged in the study of aberrant behavior and psychopathology. We hope that it will provide a crossroad where readers from every discipline can find something of value.

Michael Myslobodsky
Tel-Aviv - Washington, DC

Dennett, D.C. (1995) *Darwin's dangerous idea: Evolution and the meaning of life.* New York: Touchstone, (p. 82-83).

Feany, M.B. & Bender, W.W. (2000) A Drosophila model of Parkinson's disease. *Nature,* 404: 394-398.

Iversen, S.D. (1987) Is it possible to model psychotic state in animals? *J. Psychopharmacol.* 1:154-176.

ACKNOWLEDGMENTS

This book grew out of Bat-Sheva Seminar on Contemporary Issues in Modeling Psychopathology held at Tel-Aviv University in June 1998 under the auspices of the Adams Super Center for Brain Research and the Gershon H. Gordon Faculty of Social Sciences. The support by the Bat-Sheva de Rothschild Fund as well as grants from AGIS (Israel), Eli Lilly (USA), Marmot Family, and Adams Super Center are gratefully acknowledged. We wish to acknowledge personally Mr. Moshe Arkin, (AGIS) for his support of the project. The invaluable cooperation of Prof. David Horn, the Head of Adams Super Center, and Ms. Michal Finkelman, who assisted in the planning arrangements deserve a special mention. Our thanks and recognition go to Dr. Doug Jones from NIMH who designed the cover for the book.

1 INVOLVEMENT OF DOPAMINE TRANSPORTERS IN PSYCHIATRIC DISORDERS

Gary W. Miller, Raul R. Gainetdinov and Marc G. Caron

INTRODUCTION

The plasma membrane dopamine transporter (DAT) and the vesicular monoamine transporter (VMAT2) are key regulators of dopamine neurotransmission. DAT acts to terminate the actions of dopamine by rapidly removing dopamine from the synapse, while VMAT2 mediates loading of dopamine from the cytoplasm to vesicles for storage and subsequent release. Recent data from our laboratories and others' suggest that perturbation of the tightly regulated balance between these two transporters alters dopamine function and may predispose the neuron to damage by a variety of insults. While the selective degeneration of DAT- and VMAT2- expressing dopamine nerve terminals in the striatum that leads to Parkinson's disease is the most well known example, several other disorders may result or be exacerbated by the altered transporter function. Data from cell culture, knockout models, and human studies reveal that DAT and VMAT2 expression can predict the selective vulnerability of neuronal populations. Here, we review the role of DAT and VMAT2 in neurodegenerative disease and suggest how these findings can be applied to our understanding of psychiatric disorders.

FUNCTIONAL IMPORTANCE OF DOPAMINE TRANSPORTERS

In the synapse dopamine exerts its effects through activation of postsynaptic and presynaptic dopamine receptors (D_{1-5})(Sibley, 1999). The action of dopamine is terminated by rapid reuptake into the presynaptic terminal by the plasma membrane dopamine transporter (DAT). DAT is a member of the Na^+/Cl^- coupled neurotransmitter gene family, which includes plasma membrane serotonin and norepinephrine transporters (Blakely et al., 1991; Bruss et al., 1997; Fritz et al., 1998; Giros and Caron, 1993; Giros et al., 1992; Miller et al., 1999; Shimada et al., 1991). Inhibition of dopamine reuptake leads to elevated and prolonged extracellular and synaptic concentrations of dopamine. This, in turn, produces prolonged stimulation of the dopamine receptors. Cocaine is known to effectively block DAT and the resultant increase in extracellular dopamine is thought to be responsible for the euphoria that results after its administration (Kuhar, 1992). In addition, the expression of DAT appears to be the defining molecule of the dopamine neuron. Other markers of dopamine neurons, such as the rate limiting dopamine synthetic enzyme tyrosine hydroxylase, are also present in non-dopaminergic catecholaminergic cell groups. In contrast, DAT is exclusively expressed in dopamine neurons.

Dopamine present in the cytoplasm of the presynaptic nerve terminal is quickly transported into small synaptic and dense core vesicles by the vesicular monoamine transporter (VMAT2) (Erickson et al., 1992; Liu et al., 1992). Repackaged dopamine can then be released, which completes the recycling of the neurotransmitter. VMAT2 is also responsible for packaging serotonin, norepinephrine, epinephrine, and histamine in their respective neurons, suggesting that the selectivity of monoaminergic neurotransmission is determined by the specific plasma membrane transporters. VMAT2 is a member of the toxin-extruding antiporter (TEXAN) gene family, which includes some bacterial antibiotic resistance genes (Schuldiner et al., 1995; Yelin and Schuldiner, 1995). The function of VMAT2 is coupled to a proton ATP'ase in the vesicular membrane. In bacteria the transporters act to extrude potentially toxic substances from the cell. It has been hypothesized that VMAT2 has evolved to serve a parallel function in eukaryotes. However, in higher life forms it appears that this function has been adapted to provide a mechanism to remove potentially toxic substances from the cytoplasm. By sequestering the toxic substances into vesicles, VMAT2 prevents interaction of the toxin with cellular machinery without exposing neighboring cells to the toxin. For a multicellular organism, this process of sequestration may be the most effective way to prevent damage to individual cells without compromising the entire organism. Indeed, the cloning of the VMAT1 (formerly CGAT (Liu et al., 1992a; Liu et al., 1992b)) and VMAT2 (formerly SVAT; MAT (Erickson et al., 1992)) was actually the result of a series of elegant experiments that focused on the ability to genetically transfer the resistance to the neurotoxin MPP+ from chromaffin cells to cells that were sensitive to MPP+ (Liu et al., 1992). VMAT1 has since been shown to be present in peripheral tissues and developing neurons, while VMAT2 is found in dopaminergic, serotonergic, noradrenergic, adrenergic, and histaminergic neurons (Erickson et al., 1996; Peter et al., 1995). While VMAT2 appears to provide a level of protection, several exogenous and endogenous toxins appear to target or gain access to the dopamine neuron by DAT. Thus, the interaction of these transporters with potentially toxic compounds may impact the function and ultimate survival of the dopamine neuron.

DAT IS MOLECULAR GATEWAY FOR DOPAMINERGIC TOXINS

While DAT expression is crucial for normal dopamine neurotransmission, it also renders the dopamine neuron susceptible to damage by toxic substances that can be transported by DAT. Since many potential neurotoxins resemble dopamine and are thus substrates for DAT, they are accumulated in the dopamine neuron by selective uptake mediated by DAT (See Figure 1, upper panel). Inside the neuron, these compounds are able to disrupt mitochondrial function or react with other vulnerable targets within the cell. A prime example is 1-methyl-4-phenyl-1,2,3,6-tetrahydropyridine (MPTP) whose selective neurotoxic properties were discovered by its inadvertent administration by several heroin addicts in the early 1980's (Langston et al., 1983). Individuals exposed to the compound developed an acute form of parkinsonism with slowed movement, gait problems, and other features of idiopathic Parkinson's disease, most of which were relieved the administration of L-DOPA. It was later determined that the specific death of the dopamine neurons in the substantia nigra pars compacta was responsible for the clinical manifestations. MPTP is now routinely used to produce an experimental condition in monkeys that closely resembles the clinical symptomology of Parkinson's disease. Specifically, it has been determined that MPTP is metabolized by monoamine oxidase B in the central nervous system to MPP+ (Chiba et al., 1985; Heikkila et al., 1984; Markey et al., 1984). MPP+, whose chemical structure resembles that of dopamine, can be actively transported into the dopamine neuron by DAT (Chiba et al., 1985; Javitch et al., 1985). Indeed, it appears that neurons that express higher levels of DAT are more susceptible to the neurotoxic effects of MPP+ (Sanghera et al., 1997; Shimada et al., 1992). DAT expression has also been shown to correlate with the extent of cellular damage in transfected cells expressing different levels of the transporter (Kitayama et al., 1992; Pifl et al., 1993; Pifl et al., 1996a; Pifl et al., 1996b). In addition to exogenous toxins, like MPTP, there are several putative endogenous toxins. These include reactive metabolites of dopamine, such as 6-hydroxydopamine, and the isoquinoline derivatives and their metabolites, many of which have been shown to be transported by DAT (Ben-Shachar et al., 1995; Hastings et al., 1996; Jellinger et al., 1995; Kawai et al., 1998; McNaught et al., 1998; Naoi et al., 1998). The metabolism of these compounds can lead to the production of free radicals and cause oxidative damage to cellular constituents. While DAT appears to confer susceptibility to dopaminergic toxins, it appears as if VMAT2 functions to oppose this potentially harmful process.

VMAT2 PROVIDES INTRACELLULAR PROTECTION FROM DOPAMINERGIC TOXINS

Several lines of evidence support the notion that VMAT2 serves a neuroprotective role in dopamine neurons. By removing endogenous and exogenous toxins from the cytoplasm and sequestering them into intracellular vesicles, VMAT2 can minimize the cellular damage produced by these compounds when they are free in the cytoplasm to act upon vital cellular components (Liu et al., 1992a; Liu et al., 1992b) (Figure 1. Upper panel). The presence of a vesicular uptake system that protected catecholaminergic cells from MPP+ was first demonstrated by Reinhard and colleagues (Daniels and Reinhard, 1988; Reinhard et al., 1987). The protective effect could be prevented by treatment with reserpine or tetrabenazine, compounds known to block vesicular storage. It had long been known that the administration of reserpine, a drug once used to treat hypertension (and still is in some countries), sharply increases the incidence of depression. Thus, the perturbation of vesicular storage of monoamines by reserpine is thought to be responsible for the resultant depression. Recent studies suggest that VMAT1 and VMAT2 are responsible for the vesicular-mediated cytoprotection previously seen in various cells and represented primary targets of reserpine.

VMAT2 helps maintain normal function of the cell by keeping cytosolic levels of dopamine low. High levels of cytosolic dopamine have been shown to

4

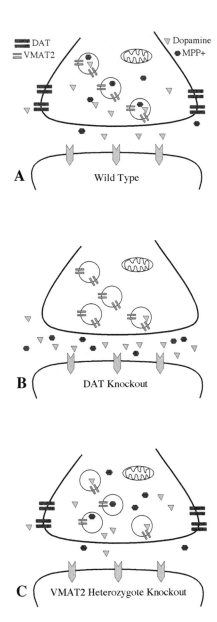

Figure 1. **Effects of genetic manipulation of transporter expression on dopamine compartmentalization**. Upper panel. Wild type. In the normal animal DAT and VMAT2 act to transport dopamine and MPP+ into different cellular compartments. MPP+ can interact with mitochondria and cause cellular damage. Middle panel. DAT Knockout. In the animal lacking DAT, MPP+ does not enter the nerve terminal and dopamine levels are reduced in the vesicles and cytosol, but increased in the extracellular space. The increase in extracellular dopamine is thought to lead to hyperactivity. Since MPP+ does not enter the nerve terminal there is no toxicity. Lower panel. VMAT2 Heterozygote Knockout. In the animal expressing 50% of normal VMAT2, dopamine and MPP+ is reduced in the vesicle and extracellular space, but increased in the cytosol, where it is more likely to interact with intracellular components such as mitochondria. In these animals there is increased neurotoxicity due to MPTP administration.

inhibit mitochondrial respiration and lead to autooxidation of dopamine, which can result in free radical formation (Ben-Shachar et al., 1995; Hastings et al., 1996). As mentioned above, VMAT2 has been demonstrated to suppress MPP+ toxicity in a similar fashion by sequestering the metabolite into vesicles, thereby preventing it from reaching its putative site of action in the mitochondria (Erickson et al., 1992; Liu et al., 1992). Since VMAT2 mRNA is present in all the major cell groups damaged in PD (dopaminergic, and to lessor degrees noradrenergic and serotonergic neurons), it has been suggested that VMAT2 may help prevent neuronal damage in neurological diseases. While the mere presence of this transporter obviously does not appear to protect the monoaminergic neurons from damage, we (Miller et al., 1999) and others (Edwards, 1993; Uhl, 1998) believe that among these cell populations, those with relatively low levels of VMAT2 expression, due to environmental or genetic factors, may be more susceptible to damage by a putative neurotoxic agent or monoamine autooxidation. We have hypothesized that the ratio of DAT to VMAT2 dictates a neuron's sensitivity to dopaminergic toxins (Miller et al., 1999). A high DAT to VMAT2 ratio increases a cell's susceptibility, while a low DAT to VMAT2 ratio decreases it. One could actually view VMAT2 as a contributor to neurotoxicity in the long term. Although VMAT2 allows for the sequestration of MPP+ and monoamines and neuroprotection in the short term, it is possible that maintaining a cellular presence of the potentially toxic substances in the long term may be harmful to the cell (Del Zompo et al., 1993). That is to say the neurons that have the highest level of VMAT2 will accumulate the highest levels of toxin (Speciale et al., 1998). Challenge to the vesicular system (reserpine, metabolic, drugs of abuse, etc.) or simple neuronal activity could cause the vesicles to release their contents and injure the cell. In addition, there may be other cellular factors involved in the susceptibility of the neuron. Either way, it appears that the carefully controlled compartmentalization of dopamine and other potentially toxic substances is necessary to prevent undue internal cellular damage. While our hypothesis has focused on neuronal injury, one could view the damage to the dopamine neuron as a step in the pathogenesis of neuropsychiatric disorders. Thus, the ratio of DAT to VMAT2 may be predictive of an individual's vulnerability not only to neuronal damage, but psychiatric disorders, as well.

ANIMAL MODELS OF DOPAMINERGIC TOXICITY

Specific lesioning of components of the dopamine system in animals has provided a wealth of information regarding Parkinson's disease and related conditions. One of the most studied models is the degeneration of the nigrostriatal dopamine neurons induced by systemic administration of MPTP (Graybiel et al., 1993). Several strains of mice and non-human primates are sensitive to the destructive effects of MPTP. While some of the characteristic neuropatholgical features, such as Lewy bodies, are not observed after MPTP, the neuroanatomical lesions and resulting motor deficits resemble that seen in idiopathic PD (Forno et al., 1993). Surprisingly, rats are insensitive to the neurotoxic actions of MPTP. The reason for this has been the subject of considerable debate. Some have suggested levels of DAT and VMAT2 may vary among strains and species, however, this does not appear to be able to account for the drastic differences seem among species (Giovanni et al., 1994a; Giovanni et al., 1994b). The fact that rats and mice are equally sensitive to intrastriatal injections of 6-hydroxydopamine suggests that the difference may be due to uptake and disposition; however, MPP+ has been shown to reach concentrations in rat brain that are neurotoxic in mouse brain (Zuddas et al., 1994). Thus, the resistance of rats to MPTP remains a mystery. This also suggests that there may be key differences in the monoaminergic systems of mice and rats, which should be considered when trying to compare findings between the two species.

The administration of MPTP to monkeys provides one of the best correlates to human Parkinson's disease (Fischman et al., 1997; Graybiel et al., 1993; Irwin et al., 1990; Moratalla et al., 1992; Morris et al., 1996). Specifically, the unilateral administration of MPTP via the intracarotid artery produces a nigrostriatal lesion in only one hemisphere, providing an internal control on the contralateral side. We have examined the effects of unilateral MPTP on the expression of DAT (Miller et al., 1998) and VMAT2 (Miller et al., 1999) and have observed an association between the level of DAT expression and the extent of injury. The caudate and the putamen, which have the highest levels of DAT expression are the most severely affected, while the nucleus accumbens is partially spared. Monoaminergic regions in the hypothalamus and amygdala are unaffected (Miller et al., 1999). These regions have relatively high expression of VMAT2, but relatively low levels of DAT. Given the high incidence of depression in Parkinson's disease (Cummings, 1992) and the fact that norepinephrine and sertonin neurons are susceptible to MPTP, this model may be of use in exploring the underlying mechanisms of neuropsychiatric conditions in Parkinson's disease.

GENETIC KNOCKOUT OF DOPAMINE TRANSPORTERS

One of the most useful tools for understanding the function of a particular protein is the deletion of the encoding gene, commonly known as a knockout or null mutant. By inserting or deleting key sequences of DNA that disrupt normal transcription of the gene (typically encoding antibiotic resistance to aid in the selection of mutant gene), expression of the particular protein is effectively blocked. Since a given protein is encoded by two copies of a gene it is necessary to have the gene on both alleles knocked out. When only one allele is modified the animal is referred to as heterozygote, while an animal with both alleles affected is termed homozygote. A homozygote knockout animal is produced through breeding two heterozygotes. The resulting offspring will be a mix of wild type, heterozygote, and homozygote at a 1:2:1 ratio.

The importance of DAT in terminating the actions of dopamine is exemplified in animals in which DAT has been genetically deleted (DAT KO)(Giros et al., 1996). In the homozygote DAT KO mice, dopamine remains in the extracellular space up to 300 times longer than normal. As expected, these animals display the expected hyperdopaminergia that occurs from the continued excitation of dopamine receptors, similar to that observed following cocaine administration (Figure 1, middle panel). Given the fact that these animals do not express the primary target of cocaine, it is remarkable that the animals still self-administer the drug (Rocha et al., 1998), suggesting other actions of cocaine. Several possible explanations have been put forth including involvement of serotonergic and noradrenergic systems, among others. Furthermore, the DAT KO mice reveal that DAT is a major controller of presynaptic dopamine function, including the storage of dopamine (Jones et al., 1998). These animals cannot recycle any dopamine and are thus reliant on newly synthesized dopamine. While the overall tissue levels of dopamine are low, the enzymatic activity of tyrosine hydroxylase is doubled. Thus, deletion of DAT highlights its essential role in maintaining dopamine homeostasis.

The genetic deletion of VMAT2 reveals a more profound role of vesicular storage and release of monoamines (Fon et al., 1997; Takahashi et al., 1997; Wang et al., 1997). The homozygote VMAT2 knockout mice do not survive past postnatal day 3 (P3), although administration of amphetamine can increase survival for several weeks (Fon et al., 1997). Studies performed in homozygote pups and heterozygote adults demonstrate that the level of VMAT2 expression calibrates the vesicular filling of dopamine. Heterozygote animals, which only have 50% of normal VMAT2, have reduced vesicular filling and release (Figure 1., lower panel). These alterations in presynaptic monoamine function in the heterozygotes are thought to be responsible for the observed sensitization to the psychostimulants, cocaine and amphetamine, and to ethanol (Wang et al., 1997). While wild type mice take several days to attain maximal locomotor sensitization, the naïve heterozygote knockouts display locomotor activity in response to cocaine that is the same as the sensitized wild type animal. Furthermore, repeated exposure to the psychostimulants does not produce any further increase of activity. Thus, heterozygote knockout mice exhibit a phenotype of a sensitized animal and may be very useful in studying the adaptations that occur following drug exposure. The knockout animals also appear to parallel the changes that occur in reserpinized animals, suggesting that the adverse actions of this drug are exclusively due to the direct interaction with VMAT2.

According to the above hypothesis, one would predict that animals with low DAT expression would be less susceptible to MPTP, while those with low VMAT2 expression would be more susceptible to MPTP. Studies in the transporter knockout animals yield the expected results. DAT knockout mice are completely resistant to MPTP-induced nigrostriatal damage (Gainetdinov et al., 1997) (Figure 1). These findings support the notion that DAT is the molecular gateway by which MPP+ enters the nigrostriatal neuron. Heterozygote DAT knockout mice, which express approximately 50% of normal DAT, display nigrostriatal damage that is approximately half of that seen in wild type mice.

Genetic deletion of VMAT2 is lethal to the neonate precluding MPTP toxicity studies, but raises the question of whether auto-oxidized monoamines may contribute in some way to the lethality. However, the VMAT2 heterozygote mice survive and provide an opportunity to determine if reduced VMAT2 levels increase susceptibility to neuronal damage (Figure 1). Indeed, VMAT2 heterozygote mice display increased vulnerability to MPTP as evidenced by reductions in nigral dopamine cell counts, striatal dopamine, and dopamine transporter and increases in GFAP expression (Gainetdinov et al., 1998; Takahashi et al., 1997). Using data from the knockout mice, Figure 2 reveals the relationship between the ratio of DAT to VMAT2 and susceptibility to MPTP.

Similar results have been observed after the administration of methamphetamine. Methamphetamine also targets the dopamine transporter but through a different mechanism of action. The illegal use of methamphetamine has skyrocketed over the past several years. This form of amphetamine has a longer half-life and has been proposed to injure neurons either by increasing the cytoplasmic levels or through excessive elevation of extracellular dopamine levels (Wilson et al., 1996a). Animals that did not express DAT were immune to damage

8

to the dopamine system, but not the serotonin system, while those that expressed half the amount of DAT displayed partial damage (Fumagalli et al., 1998). The lack of dopaminergic neurotoxicity in DAT-KO animals correlated with the absence of alterations in extracellular DA as well as indices of free radical formation after methamphetamine. Nevertheless there are indications that methamphetamine can still enter the neuron, even without DAT. Thus, even with the data from the DAT-KO animals it was still unclear whether remarkably altered intraneuronal DA homeostatsis (particularly dramatically diminished storage of DA) or lack of extracellular elevation of DA is responsible for the lack of neurotoxicity. Further insight into the mechanisms of methamphetamine neurotoxicity was gained in mice with reduced VMAT2 expression. These animals showed a significant increase in damage to the dopamine system in response to methamphetamine. This exaggerated toxicity was most likely due to altered intracellular compartmentalization of dopamine in VMAT2 mutant mice since the effect of the drug on extracellular DA dynamics and indices of free radical formation were actually attenuated in these animals (Fumagalli et al., 1999). Taken together these findings not only emphasize the role of transporters in vulnerability to methamphetamine toxicity, but also strongly suggest a role of intraneuronal processes as primary mediators of this type of injury.

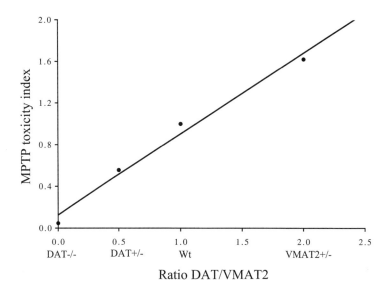

Figure 2. Ratio of DAT/VMAT2 as a predictor of dopaminergic susceptibility to MPTP. Data from wildtype (Wt), DAT heterozygote (DAT+/-) and homozygote (DAT-/-) knockout mice, and VMAT2 heterozygote (VMAT+/-) knockout mice, reveal a correlation between DAT/VMAT2 ratios and sensitivity to MPTP. Toxicity index is expressed as relative decrease in striatal dopamine 2 days after administration of MPTP compared to untreated animals of same genotype. Data taken with permission from (Gainetdinov et al., 1997; Gainetdinov et al., 1998).

To date only one manuscript has reported the generation of animals that overexpress DAT or VMAT (Donovan, 1999). In this paper, a small increase (30%) in DAT was seen using the tyrosine hydroxylase promoter with a concomitant increase in MPTP susceptibility. One of the problems in developing mice that overexpress these transporters is identifying and utilizing a promoter that is selective and robust enough to increase the expression of these transporters to higher levels. Development of mice with a more robust increase in transporter expression (>%50) increased expression of these transporters would be quite valuable and hopefully such animals will become available in the near future.

DOPAMINE TRANSPORTERS IN NEURODEGENERATIVE DISEASE

The production of specific antibodies and radiolabeled ligands for DAT (Ciliax et al., 1995; Hersch et al., 1997; Miller et al., 1997; Wilson et al., 1996c) and VMAT2 (Erickson et al., 1996; Miller et al., 1999) has greatly facilitated the direct visualization of the protein. Since the expression of these transporters appears to provide an accurate marker of the nigrostriatal dopamine terminals, their visualization in vivo has the potential to monitor their status in human brain. Several laboratories have developed techniques to monitor the expression of the dopamine transporters in human brain using PET and SPECT imaging (Fischman et al., 1998; Frey et al., 1996; Kazumata et al., 1998; Laakso et al., 1998; Madras et al., 1998). The results from these *in vivo* studies correspond very well with more invasive *in vitro* studies performed on post mortem human brain tissue. We have performed detailed neuroanatomical analyses on brains from control and Parkinson's diseased brain and found that the regions that express the highest levels of DAT protein, caudate and putamen, are the most sensitive to damage in Parkinson's disease (Miller et al., 1997). These regions also have high levels of VMAT2 (Miller et al., 1999) (Figure 3). However, the putamen, which is the most severely affected region in PD, has a higher ratio of DAT to VMAT2 than the caudate in control populations. The ratios of the striatal proteins correspond to the differences in mRNA expression by the respective cell groups where these nerve terminals originate (Uhl, 1998). Thus, it does appear that the ratio of DAT to VMAT2 may help predict those areas that are most susceptible to damage.

It is also important to note that Parkinson's disease is not purely a motor disorder. Many patients suffer from dementia or depression (Cummings, 1992; McKeith et al., 1999). While an increased rate of depression would seem likely in a debilitating disease state, the incidence of depression in Parkinson's disease is higher than would be expected (40-50%). It has been proposed that the increased incidence of depression in Parkinson's disease is a manifestation of the neuropathological features of the disease. In addition, dementia with Lewy bodies shares some of the pathological feature of Parkinson's disease, but patients exhibit profound cognitive impairment. It is not clear what role dopamine and its transport may play in this disorder, but dopamine function is known to be impaired.

Despite recent progress in understanding of the genetic basis of Huntington's disease (Wellington et al., 1997), much less is known about particular mechanisms underlying the hyperkinesis and dopaminergic pathogenesis of this disorder. DAT is an obvious candidate mediator of dopamine damage and, in fact, significant decrease in DAT levels have been reported (Backman et al., 1997; Chinaglia et al., 1992; Ginovart et al., 1997).

If DAT and VMAT2 do mediate susceptibility to neurodegenerative disease, it is possible that pharmacological intervention aimed at these transporters may be beneficial to the obvious motor symptoms as well as the associated psychiatric problems. In patients in the early stages of Parkinson's disease, decreasing dopamine uptake may not only increase synaptic and decrease intracellular dopamine concentrations, but may also slow the progression of the disease if an endogenous or exogenous toxin is involved. The drug may also be useful in later stages where side effects, such as dyskinesias, often limit conventional dopaminergic therapies. VMAT2 is another potentially useful target, particularly for neuroprotective agents. For example, therapies resulting in increased vesicular uptake by VMAT2 may act to decrease cytosolic dopamine and perhaps prevent oxidation. The above studies supports the use of DAT and VMAT2 as targets of *in vivo* monitoring of the viability of monoaminergic terminals and perhaps the pharmacological treatment of various neurodegenerative disorders.

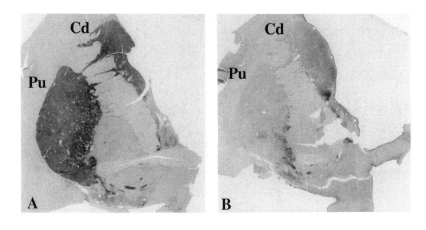

Figure 3. Loss of vesicular monoamine transporter (VMAT2)-immunoreactive fibers in Parkinson's disease striatum. A. Age-matched control case. B. Parkinson's disease. Note significant depletion of VMAT2-immunoreactive fibers in caudate (Cd) and putamen (Pu). While dopaminergic terminals are obviously afffected, it is likely that this depletion also includes serotonergic and noradrenergic terminals as well, which may contribute to psychiatric symptoms seen in some cases of Parkinson's disease.

DAT AND VMAT2 AS TARGETS OF ENVIRONMENTAL CONTAMINANTS

A recent study of twin pairs demonstrated that idiopathic Parkinson's disease with an age of onset of 50 or greater has no genetic component (Tanner et al., 1999). This raises the question of what environmental agent(s) may be involved in this disease. Several epidemiological studies have indicated that pesticide exposure is a risk factor for Parkinson's disease (Gorell et al., 1998). In addition, one study has identified that in patients with Parkinson's disease there was an increase in the brain levels of dieldrin, a banned organochlorine pesticide that was widely used and persists in the environment (Fleming et al., 1994). However, no mechanism for the increased incidence of Parkinson's disease has been identified.

Recent data from our laboratory (Miller et al., 1999) and others' (Vaccari and Saba, 1995) suggest that some classes of pesticides, especially organochlorines, increase the expression of DAT. Not only does this provide a possible explanation of increased vulnerability to Parkinson's disease, but suggests that environmental factors may contribute to other disorders that involve dopamine impairment. It is possible that an environmental toxin does not need to be overtly toxic, but rather just slightly to disrupt the homeostasis that exists within the dopamine neuron. By altering the functional ratio of DAT to VMAT2, an environmental toxin may disrupt dopamine homeostasis and increase the likelihood of psychiatric disorders.

DOPAMINE TRANSPORTERS AND NEUROPSYCHIATRIC DISORDERS

Since dopamine neurotransmission is intimately involved in the control of motor and emotional behaviors, alterations in dopamine homeostasis are likely to be involved in a variety of pathological conditions. Disruptions in the functional states of vesicular and plasma membrane transporters, which are key players in maintaining this homeostasis, might be important contributors to these disease states. The pioneering work with reserpine, a potent inhibitor of VMAT2, strongly suggested that disruption of vesicular loading has a significant impact on the pathogenesis of depressive disorders (Carlsson, 1987). However, despite over four decades of research definitive evidence of this link is still elusive (Lesch et al., 1994). Numerous studies have shown that alterations of vesicular dopamine release may lead to postsynaptic receptor supersenstivity (Wang et al., 1997). Increased dopamine receptor responsiveness has been suggested to be involved in either the pathogenesis /or aversive side effects of drug treatment of several disorders, such as drug or alcohol abuse, schizophrenia, and Tourette Syndrome. Therefore, the role of VMAT2 dysfunction in these conditions represents an important avenue of future research.

There is substantially more evidence that DAT is involved in pathologic conditions. This is consistent with the more profound changes in extracellular dopamine dynamics produced by modification of DAT versus VMAT2 (Gainetdinov et al., 1998; Jones et al., 1998). It is well known that elevated extracellular dopamine translates into hyperactivity, compulsive and erratic behavior, and even psychosis (Carlsson, 1987; Wang et al., 1997). Intuitively, many conditions believed to have a basis in hyperdopaminergia, such as drug abuse, schizophrenia, Huntington's Disease, Tourette Syndrome, and ADHD, have been connected to DAT dysfunction. In fact, the role of DAT as a primary, but not exclusive, target of drugs of abuse (Rocha et al., 1998), such as cocaine and amphetamine, strongly suggest that alterations in DAT – mediated functions may have a serious impact on addictive behaviors. In addition, it is known that DAT can be regulated by intrinsic cellular mechanisms and it is possibly that this regulation of monoamine transporters can be directly affected by pharmacological drugs such as psychostimulants (Daniels, 1999; Ramamoorthy and Blakely, 1999). Indeed, recent reports in chronic methamphetamine and cocaine abusers demonstrated a down-regulation of striatal dopaminergic parameters consistent with the observed reduction in DAT protein levels in these subjects and the findings in DAT-KO mice (Wilson et al., 1996a; Wilson et al., 1996b). To explore, whether these DAT mediated alterations in DA neurotransmission can account for the dysphoric effects of the drugs (Koob et al., 1998; Markou et al., 1998) and/or serve as a basis for drug-seeking behavior during withdrawal represent a major challenge for future research. It is interesting to note also, that association of cocaine–induced paranoia and DAT polymorphism was recently noted (Gelernter et al., 1998; Gelernter et al., 1994).

The dopaminergic hypothesis of schizophrenia and well known psychoto-mimetic action of amphetamine (Carlsson, 1987; Kokkinidis and Anisman, 1980) provided the basis for the expectations that DAT can contribute to this disorder. In fact, several groups tested for association of DAT polymorphism in schizophrenia, however no evidence for allelic association was found (Bodeau-Pean et al., 1995; Inada et al., 1996; King et al., 1997; Persico and Macciardi, 1997). Although it is unlikely that DAT alterations can be a primary reason for this disorder, the possibility certainly exist that diminished DAT function can amplify the disturbances in other neuronal components (Persico and Macciardi, 1997). DAT abnormalities has been recently reported also in violent alcoholic offenders (Kuikka et al., 1998), and association was found with alcoholism (Ueno et al., 1999) and schizoid/avoidant behaviors (Blum et al., 1997) but more studies are required to confirm these observations. Another condition that is suspected to be associated with altered DAT function is Tourette Syndrome (Comings et al., 1996). Although it is highly likely that this disorder is polygenic (Sibley et al., 1992) and many other factors can contribute significantly to this disorder as well, there are some indications that abnormalities in dopamine uptake can be involved (Rabey et al., 1998).

The paradoxical ability of psychostimulants, which exert their psychotropic action primarily through the blockade of the DAT, to ameliorate symptoms of ADHD has provided the basis for the hypodopaminergic hypothesis of the disorder and the possible connection between DAT and ADHD. Indeed, Cook et al. (1995) reported a significant association between DAT polymorphism and ADHD. The haplotype-based haplotype relative risk (HHRR) method was used to test the association between variable number of tandem repeats (VNTR) polymorphism at the dopamine transporter locus and DSM-III-R -diagnosed ADHD in trios composed of father, mother, and affected offspring revealed a significant association between ADHD and the 480-bp DAT1 allele. Gill and coworkers (Gill et al., 1997) using the same approach confirmed these observations in another cohort of patients and also concluded that 480-bp allele of DAT1 preferentially transmitted to ADHD probands. More recently Waldman and associates (Waldman et al., 1998) used four different analytical strategies to examine the association and linkage of the DAT gene and ADHD in children. The authors replicated previous findings (Cook et al., 1995; Gill et al., 1997) demonstrating the 480-bp allele as the high risk allele. Moreover the relation of DAT1 to ADHD was found to be increased monotonically, from low to medium to high levels of symptom severity, with some specificity for the hyperactive-impulsive spectrum of symptoms. Taken together these molecular genetic studies provide a solid basis to expect that alterations in DAT -mediated processes could significantly contribute to the pathogenesis of this disorder. However the functional consequences of this association still remain unclear. Hyperactivity is classically considered to be a behavior of increased, not decreased dopaminergic tone (Carlsson, 1987). Numerous pharmacological studies in a variety of experimental models with the drugs enhancing or reducing dopaminergic transmission support this notion. Recent data showed also that the dopamine transporter knockout mice display several key characteristics of ADHD, including hyperactivity, cognitive impairments and paradoxical calming responses to psychostimulants (Gainetdinov et al., 1999). In contrast, mice with increased DAT expression show hypoactivity (Donovan, 1999). Thus there is more reason to believe that ADHD represents a hyperdopaminergic condition and the calming effect of psychostimulants is most likely mediated through targets other than DAT. Particularly, interaction of psychostimulants with the serotonin transporter (another well-known, but largely ignored target of psychostimulants), may provide enhanced serotonergic tone, sufficient enough to exert inhibitory influence on behavior (Lucki, 1998; Gainetdinov et al., 1999). While there are conflicting preliminary reports as to whether serotonergic drugs are beneficial in ADHD patients (Barrickman et al., 1991; Popper, 1997), the same drugs were clearly effective in DAT-KO animals (Gainetdinov et al., 1999). Future controlled clinical studies warranted to test this hypothesis.

It should be noted however, that it is premature to claim that DAT dysfunction is a core underlying mechanism of ADHD, and further in depth studies, particularly on human subjects, are required. It is worth mentioning that DAT is a substrate of substantial postnatal structural and functional modification (Jones et al., 1996; Patel et al., 1994). Thus, the possibility exists that genetically or environmentally determined dysregulation of DAT maturation may be involved in pathogenesis of this developmental disorder. For example, childhood lead exposure has also been linked to attention deficit hyperactivity disorder (Brockel, 1998). It is not clear where lead is acting, but it is plausible that dopamine transport may be involved (Boykin et al., 1991). Thus, it may be prudent to explore these transporters as targets of environmental contaminants in respect of this disorder as well.

In conclusion, recent animal studies, particularly those involving genetic approaches, have provided several new lines of research on the role of transporters in the pathogenesis of neuropsychiatric disease. Furthermore, given the growing feasibility of *in vivo* human research on transporter function and genetic linkage approaches, the associations between transporter function and these disorders should be forthcoming.

REFERENCES

Backman, L., Robins-Wahlin, T. B., Lundin, A., Ginovart, N., Farde, L. (1997). Cognitive deficits in Huntington's disease are predicted by dopaminergic PET markers and brain volumes. Brain *120*, 2207-17.

Barrickman, L., Noyes, R., Kuperman, S., Schumacher, E., Verda, M. (1991). Treatment of ADHD with fluoxetine: a preliminary trial. J Am Acad Child Adolesc Psychiatry *30*, 762-7.

Ben-Shachar, D., Zuk, R., Glinka, Y. (1995). Dopamine neurotoxicity: inhibition of mitochondrial respiration. J Neurochem *64*, 718-23.

Blakely, R. D., Berson, H. E., Fremeau, R. T., Jr., Caron, M. G., Peek, M. M., Prince, H. K., Bradley, C. C. (1991). Cloning and expression of a functional serotonin transporter from rat brain. Nature *354*, 66-70.

Blum, K., Braverman, E. R., Wu, S., Cull, J. G., Chen, T. J., Gill, J., Wood, R., Eisenberg, A., Sherman, M., Davis, K. R., Matthews, D., Fischer, L., Schnautz, N., Walsh, W., Pontius, A. A., Zedar, M., Kaats, G., Comings, D. E. (1997). Association of polymorphisms of dopamine D2 receptor (DRD2), and dopamine transporter (DAT1) genes with schizoid/avoidant behaviors (SAB). Mol Psychiatry *2*, 239-46.

Bodeau-Pean, S., Laurent, C., Campion, D., Jay, M., Thibaut, F., Dollfus, S., Petit, M., Samolyk, D., d'Amato, T., Martinez, M. et al. (1995). No evidence for linkage or association between the dopamine transporter gene and schizophrenia in a French population. Psychiatry Res *59*, 1-6.

Boykin, M. J., Chetty, C. S., Rajanna, B. (1991). Effects of lead on kinetics of 3H-dopamine uptake by rat brain synaptosomes. Ecotoxicol Environ Saf *22*, 88-93.

Brockel, B. J., Cory-Slechta, D.A. (1998). Lead, attention, and impulsive behavior: changes in a fixed-ratio waiting-for-reward paradigm. Pharmacol Biochem Behav 60, 545-552.

Bruss, M., Porzgen, P., Bryan-Lluka, L. J, Bonisch, H. (1997). The rat norepinephrine transporter: molecular cloning from PC12 cells and functional expression. Brain Res Mol Brain Res 52, 257-62.

Carlsson, A. (1987). Perspectives on the discovery of central monoaminergic neurotransmission. Annu Rev Neurosci 10, 19-40.

Chiba, K., Trevor, A. J, Castagnoli, N., Jr. (1985). Active uptake of MPP+, a metabolite of MPTP, by brain synaptosomes. Biochem Biophys Res Commun 128, 1228-32.

Chinaglia, G., Alvarez, F. J., Probst, A, Palacios, J. M. (1992). Mesostriatal and mesolimbic dopamine uptake binding sites are reduced in Parkinson's disease and progressive supranuclear palsy: a quantitative autoradiographic study using [3H]mazindol. Neuroscience 49, 317-27.

Ciliax, B. J., Heilman, C., Demchyshyn, L. L., Pristupa, Z. B., Ince, E., Hersch, S. M., Niznik, H. B, Levey, A. I. (1995). The dopamine transporter: immunochemical characterization and localization in brain. J Neurosci 15, 1714-23.

Comings, D. E., Wu, S., Chiu, C., Ring, R. H., Gade, R., Ahn, C., MacMurray, J. P., Dietz, G, Muhleman, D. (1996). Polygenic inheritance of Tourette syndrome, stuttering, attention deficit hyperactivity, conduct, and oppositional defiant disorder: the additive and subtractive effect of the three dopaminergic genes--DRD2, D beta H, and DAT1. Am J Med Genet 67, 264-88.

Cook, E. H., Jr., Stein, M. A., Krasowski, M. D., Cox, N. J., Olkon, D. M., Kieffer, J. E, Leventhal, B. L. (1995). Association of attention-deficit disorder and the dopamine transporter gene. Am J Hum Genet 56, 993-8.

Cummings, J. L. (1992). Depression in Parkinson's disease: a review. American Journal of Psychiatry 149, 443-454.

Daniels, A. J. and Reinhard, J. F., Jr. (1988). Energy-driven uptake of the neurotoxin 1-methyl-4-phenylpyridinium into chromaffin granules via the catecholamine transporter. J Biol Chem 263, 5034-6.

Daniels, G. M. and Amara, S.G. (1999). Regulated Trafficking of the Human Dopamine Transporter. Clatherin-mediated internalization and lysosomal degradation in response to phorbol esters. J. Biol. Chem. 274, 35794-35801.

Del Zompo, M., Piccardi, M. P., Ruiu, S., Quartu, M., Gessa, G. L, Vaccari, A. (1993). Selective MPP+ uptake into synaptic dopamine vesicles: possible involvement in MPTP neurotoxicity. Br J Pharmacol 109, 411-4.

Donovan, D. M., Miner, L.L., Perry, M.P., Revay, R.S., Sharpe, L.G., Przedborski, S., Kostic, V., Philpot, R.M., Kirstein, C.L., Rothman, R.B., Schindler, C.W, Uhl, G.R. (1999). Cocaine reward and MPTP toxicity: alteration by regional variant dopamine transporter overexpression. Molecular Brain Research 73, 37-49.

Edwards, R. H. (1993). Neural degeneration and the transport of neurotransmitters. Ann Neurol 34, 638-45.

Erickson, J. D., Eiden, L. E, Hoffman, B. J. (1992). Expression cloning of a reserpine-sensitive vesicular monoamine transporter. Proc Natl Acad Sci U S A 89, 10993-7.

Erickson, J. D., Schafer, M. K., Bonner, T. I., Eiden, L. E, Weihe, E. (1996). Distinct pharmacological properties and distribution in neurons and endocrine cells of two isoforms of the human vesicular monoamine transporter. Proc Natl Acad Sci U S A 93, 5166-71.

Fischman, A. J., Babich, J. W., Elmaleh, D. R., Barrow, S. A., Meltzer, P., Hanson, R. N, Madras, B. K. (1997). SPECT imaging of dopamine transporter sites in normal and MPTP-Treated rhesus monkeys. J Nucl Med 38, 144-50.

Fischman, A. J., Bonab, A. A., Babich, J. W., Palmer, E. P., Alpert, N. M., Elmaleh, D. R., Callahan, R. J., Barrow, S. A., Graham, W., Meltzer, P. C., Hanson, R. N, Madras, B. K. (1998). Rapid detection of Parkinson's disease by SPECT with altropane: a selective ligand for dopamine transporters. Synapse 29, 128-41.

Fleming, L., Mann, J. B., Bean, J., Briggle, T, Sanchez-Ramos, J. R. (1994). Parkinson's disease and brain levels of organochlorine pesticides. Ann Neurol 36, 100-3.

Fon, E. A., Pothos, E. N., Sun, B. C., Killeen, N., Sulzer, D, Edwards, R. H. (1997). Vesicular transport regulates monoamine storage and release but is not essential for amphetamine action. Neuron 19, 1271-83.

Forno, L. S., DeLanney, L. E., Irwin, I, Langston, J. W. (1993). Similarities and differences between MPTP-induced parkinsonsim and Parkinson's disease. Neuropathologic considerations. Adv Neurol 60, 600-8.

Frey, K. A., Koeppe, R. A., Kilbourn, M. R., Vander Borght, T. M., Albin, R. L., Gilman, S, Kuhl, D. E. (1996). Presynaptic monoaminergic vesicles in Parkinson's disease and normal aging. Ann Neurol 40, 873-84.

Fritz, J. D., Jayanthi, L. D., Thoreson, M. A, Blakely, R. D. (1998). Cloning and chromosomal mapping of the murine norepinephrine transporter. J Neurochem 70, 2241-51.

Fumagalli, F., Gainetdinov, R. R., Valenzano, K., Wang, Y. M., Miller, G. W, Caron, M. G. (1999). Increased methamphetamine toxicity in heterozygote VMAT2 knockout mice. J Neuroscience 19, 2424-2431.

Fumagalli, F., Gainetdinov, R. R., Valenzano, K. J, Caron, M. G. (1998). Role of dopamine transporter in methamphetamine-induced neurotoxicity: evidence from mice lacking the transporter. J Neurosci 18, 4861-9.

Gainetdinov, R. R., Fumagalli, F., Jones, S. R, Caron, M. G. (1997). Dopamine transporter is required for in vivo MPTP neurotoxicity: evidence from mice lacking the transporter. J Neurochem 69, 1322-5.

Gainetdinov, R. R., Fumagalli, F., Wang, Y. M., Jones, S. R., Levey, A. I., Miller, G. W, Caron, M. G. (1998). Increased MPTP neurotoxicity in vesicular monoamine transporter 2 heterozygote knockout mice. J Neurochem 70, 1973-8.

Gainetdinov, R. R., Jones, S. R., Fumagalli, F., Wightman, R. M, Caron, M. G. (1998). Re-evaluation of the role of the dopamine transporter in dopamine system homeostasis. Brain Res Brain Res Rev 26, 148-53.

Gainetdinov, R. R., Wetsel, W. C., Jones, S. R., Levin, E. D., Jaber, M, Caron, M. G. (1999). Role of serotonin in the paradoxical calming effect of psychostimulants on hyperactivity. Science 283, 397-401.

Gelernter, J., Kranzler, H, Lacobelle, J. (1998). Population studies of polymorphisms at loci of neuropsychiatric interest (tryptophan hydroxylase (TPH), dopamine transporter protein (SLC6A3), D3 dopamine receptor (DRD3), apolipoprotein E (APOE), mu opioid receptor (OPRM1), and ciliary neurotrophic factor (CNTF)). Genomics 52, 289-97.

Gelernter, J., Kranzler, H. R., Satel, S. L, Rao, P. A. (1994). Genetic association between dopamine transporter protein alleles and cocaine-induced paranoia. Neuropsychopharmacology 11, 195-200.

Gill, M., Daly, G., Heron, S., Hawi, Z, Fitzgerald, M. (1997). Confirmation of association between attention deficit hyperactivity disorder and a dopamine transporter polymorphism. Mol Psychiatry 2, 311-313.

Ginovart, N., Lundin, A., Farde, L., Halldin, C., Backman, L., Swahn, C. G., Pauli, S, Sedvall, G. (1997). PET study of the pre- and post-synaptic dopaminergic markers for the neurodegenerative process in Huntington's disease. Brain 120, 503-14.

Giovanni, A., Sieber, B. A., Heikkila, R. E, Sonsalla, P. K. (1994a). Studies on species sensitivity to the dopaminergic neurotoxin 1-methyl- 4-phenyl-1,2,3,6-tetrahydropyridine. Part 1: Systemic administration. J Pharmacol Exp Ther 270, 1000-7.

Giovanni, A., Sonsalla, P. K, Heikkila, R. E. (1994b). Studies on species sensitivity to the dopaminergic neurotoxin 1-methyl- 4-phenyl-1,2,3,6-tetrahydropyridine. Part 2: Central administration of 1-methyl-4-phenylpyridinium. J Pharmacol Exp Ther 270, 1008-14.

Giros, B. and Caron, M. G. (1993). Molecular characterization of the dopamine transporter. Trends Pharmacol Sci 14, 43-9.

Giros, B., el Mestikawy, S., Godinot, N., Zheng, K., Han, H., Yang-Feng, T, Caron, M. G. (1992). Cloning, pharmacological characterization, and chromosome assignment of the human dopamine transporter. Mol Pharmacol 42, 383-90.

Giros, B., Jaber, M., Jones, S. R., Wightman, R. M, Caron, M. G. (1996). Hyperlocomotion and indifference to cocaine and amphetamine in mice lacking the dopamine transporter. Nature 379, 606-12.

Gorell, J. M., Johnson, C. C., Rybicki, B. A., Peterson, E. L, Richardson, R. J. (1998). The risk of Parkinson's disease with exposure to pesticides, farming, well water, and rural living. Neurology 50, 1346-50.

Graybiel, A. M., Moratalla, R., Quinn, B., DeLanney, L. E., Irwin, I, Langston, J. W. (1993). Early-stage loss of dopamine uptake-site binding in MPTP-treated monkeys. Adv Neurol 60, 34-9.

Hastings, T. G., Lewis, D. A, Zigmond, M. J. (1996). Reactive dopamine metabolites and neurotoxicity: implications for Parkinson's disease. Adv Exp Med Biol 387, 97-106.

Heikkila, R. E., Hess, A, Duvoisin, R. C. (1984). Dopaminergic neurotoxicity of 1-methyl-4-phenyl-1,2,5,6- tetrahydropyridine in mice. Science 224, 1451-3.

Hersch, S. M., Yi, H., Heilman, C. J., Edwards, R. H, Levey, A. I. (1997). Subcellular localization and molecular topology of the dopamine transporter in the striatum and substantia nigra. J Comp Neurol 388, 211-27.

Inada, T., Sugita, T., Dobashi, I., Inagaki, A., Kitao, Y., Matsuda, G., Kato, S., Takano, T., Yagi, G, Asai, M. (1996). Dopamine transporter gene polymorphism and psychiatric symptoms seen in schizophrenic patients at their first episode. Am J Med Genet 67, 406-8.

16

Irwin, I., DeLanney, L. E., Forno, L. S., Finnegan, K. T., Di Monte, D. A, Langston, J. W. (1990). The evolution of nigrostriatal neurochemical changes in the MPTP- treated squirrel monkey. Brain Res *531*, 242-52.

Javitch, J. A., D'Amato, R. J., Strittmatter, S. M, Snyder, S. H. (1985). Parkinsonism-inducing neurotoxin, N-methyl-4-phenyl-1,2,3,6 - tetrahydropyridine: uptake of the metabolite N-methyl-4-phenylpyridine by dopamine neurons explains selective toxicity. Proc Natl Acad Sci U S A *82*, 2173-7.

Jellinger, K., Linert, L., Kienzl, E., Herlinger, E, Youdim, M. B. (1995). Chemical evidence for 6-hydroxydopamine to be an endogenous toxic factor in the pathogenesis of Parkinson's disease. J Neural Transm Suppl *46*, 297-314.

Jones, S. R., Bowman, B. P., Kuhn, C. M, Wightman, R. M. (1996). Development of dopamine neurotransmission and uptake inhibition in the caudate nucleus as measured by fast-cyclic voltammetry. Synapse *24*, 305-7.

Jones, S. R., Gainetdinov, R. R., Jaber, M., Giros, B., Wightman, R. M, Caron, M. G. (1998). Profound neuronal plasticity in response to inactivation of the dopamine transporter. Proc Natl Acad Sci U S A *95*, 4029-34.

Kawai, H., Makino, Y., Hirobe, M, Ohta, S. (1998). Novel endogenous 1,2,3,4-tetrahydroisoquinoline derivatives: uptake by dopamine transporter and activity to induce parkinsonism. J Neurochem *70*, 745-51.

Kazumata, K., Dhawan, V., Chaly, T., Antonini, A., Margouleff, C., Belakhlef, A., Neumeyer, J, Eidelberg, D. (1998). Dopamine transporter imaging with fluorine-18-FPCIT and PET. J Nucl Med *39*, 1521-30.

King, N., Bassett, A. S., Honer, W. G., Masellis, M, Kennedy, J. L. (1997). Absence of linkage for schizophrenia on the short arm of chromosome 5 in multiplex Canadian families. Am J Med Genet *74*, 472-4.

Kitayama, S., Shimada, S., Uhl, G. R. (1992). Parkinsonism-inducing neurotoxin MPP+: uptake and toxicity in nonneuronal COS cells expressing dopamine transporter cDNA. Ann Neurol *32*, 109-11.

Kokkinidis, L. and Anisman, H. (1980). Amphetamine models of paranoid schizophrenia: an overview and elaboration of animal experimentation. Psychol Bull *88*, 551-79.

Koob, G. F., Rocio, M., Carrera, A., Gold, L. H., Heyser, C. J., Maldonado-Irizarry, C., Markou, A., Parsons, L. H., Roberts, A. J., Schulteis, G., Stinus, L., Walker, J. R., Weissenborn, R, Weiss, F. (1998). Substance dependence as a compulsive behavior. J Psychopharmacol *12*, 39-48.

Kuhar, M. J. (1992). Molecular pharmacology of cocaine: a dopamine hypothesis and its implications. Ciba Found Symp *166*, 81-9.

Kuikka, J. T., Tiihonen, J., Bergstrom, K. A., Karhu, J., Rasanen, P, Eronen, M. (1998). Abnormal structure of human striatal dopamine re-uptake sites in habitually violent alcoholic offenders: a fractal analysis [In Process Citation]. Neurosci Lett *253*, 195-7.

Laakso, A., Bergman, J., Haaparanta, M., Vilkman, H., Solin, O, Hietala, J. (1998). [18F]CFT [(18F)WIN 35,428], a radioligand to study the dopamine transporter with PET: characterization in human subjects. Synapse *28*, 244-50.

Langston, J. W., Ballard, P., Tetrud, J. W, Irwin, I. (1983). Chronic Parkinsonism in humans due to a product of meperidine-analog synthesis. Science *219*, 979-80.

Lesch, K. P., Gross, J., Wolozin, B. L., Franzck, E., Bengel, D., Riederer, P, Murphy, D. L. (1994). Direct sequencing of the reserpine-sensitive vesicular monoamine transporter complementary DNA in unipolar depression and manic depressive illness. Psychiatr Genet *4*, 153-160.

Liu, Y., Peter, D., Roghani, A., Schuldiner, S., Prive, G. G., Eisenberg, D., Brecha, N, Edwards, R. H. (1992a). A cDNA that suppresses MPP+ toxicity encodes a vesicular amine transporter. Cell *70*, 539-51.

Liu, Y., Roghani, A, Edwards, R. H. (1992b). Gene transfer of a reserpine-sensitive mechanism of resistance to N- methyl-4-phenylpyridinium. Proc Natl Acad Sci U S A *89*, 9074-8.

Lucki, I. (1998). The spectrum of behaviors influenced by serotonin. Biol Psychiatry *44*, 151-62.

Madras, B. K., Meltzer, P. C., Liang, A. Y., Elmaleh, D. R., Babich, J, Fischman, A. J. (1998). Altropane, a SPECT or PET imaging probe for dopamine neurons: I. Dopamine transporter binding in primate brain. Synapse *29*, 93-104.

Markey, S. P., Johannessen, J. N., Chiueh, C. C., Burns, R. S, Herkenham, M. A. (1984). Intraneuronal generation of a pyridinium metabolite may cause drug- induced parkinsonism. Nature *311*, 464-7.

Markou, A., Kosten, T. R. and Koob, G. F. (1998). Neurobiological similarities in depression and drug dependence: a self- medication hypothesis. Neuropsychopharmacology *18*, 135-74.

McKeith, I. G., Perry, E. K, Perry, R. H. (1999). Report of the second dementia with Lewy body international workshop: diagnosis and treatment. Consortium on Dementia with Lewy Bodies. Neurology *53*, 902-5.

McNaught, K. S., Carrupt, P. A., Altomare, C., Cellamare, S., Carotti, A., Testa, B., Jenner, P, Marsden, C. D. (1998). Isoquinoline derivatives as endogenous neurotoxins in the aetiology of Parkinson's disease. Biochem Pharmacol 56, 921-33.

Miller, G. W., Erickson, J. D., Perez, J. T., Penland, S. N., Mash, D. C., Rye, D. B, Levey, A. I. (1999). Immunochemical analysis of vesicular monoamine transporter (VMAT2) protein in Parkinson's disease. Experimental Neurology 154, 138-148.

Miller, G. W., Gainetdinov, R. R., Levey, A. I, Caron, M. G. (1999). Dopamine transporters and neuronal injury. Trends in Pharmacological Sciences 20, 424-429.

Miller, G. W., Gilmor, M. L, Levey, A. I. (1998). Generation of transporter specific antibodies. Methods in Enzymology 296, 407-422.

Miller, G. W., Kirby, M. L., Levey, A. I, Bloomquist, J. R. (1999). Heptachlor alters expression and function of dopamine transporters. Neurotoxicology 20, 631-638.

Miller, G. W., Staley, J. K., Heilman, C. J., Perez, J. T., Mash, D. C., Rye, D. B, Levey, A. I. (1997). Immunochemical analysis of dopamine transporter protein in Parkinson's disease. Ann Neurol 41, 530-9.

Moratalla, R., Quinn, B., DeLanney, L. E., Irwin, I., Langston, J. W, Graybiel, A. M. (1992). Differential vulnerability of primate caudate-putamen and striosome- matrix dopamine systems to the neurotoxic effects of 1-methyl-4-phenyl- 1,2,3,6-tetrahydropyridine. Proc Natl Acad Sci U S A 89, 3859-63.

Morris, E. D., Babich, J. W., Alpert, N. M., Bonab, A. A., Livni, E., Weise, S., Hsu, H., Christian, B. T., Madras, B. K, Fischman, A. J. (1996). Quantification of dopamine transporter density in monkeys by dynamic PET imaging of multiple injections of 11C-CFT. Synapse 24, 262-72.

Naoi, M., Maruyama, W., Kasamatsu, T, Dostert, P. (1998). Oxidation of N-methyl(R)salsolinol: involvement to neurotoxicity and neuroprotection by endogenous catechol isoquinolines. J Neural Transm Suppl 52, 125-38.

Patel, A. P., Cerruti, C., Vaughan, R. A, Kuhar, M. J. (1994). Developmentally regulated glycosylation of dopamine transporter. Brain Res Dev Brain Res 83, 53-8.

Persico, A. M. and Macciardi, F. (1997). Genotypic association between dopamine transporter gene polymorphisms and schizophrenia. Am J Med Genet 74, 53-7.

Peter, D., Liu, Y., Sternini, C., de Giorgio, R., Brecha, N, Edwards, R. H. (1995). Differential expression of two vesicular monoamine transporters. J Neurosci 15, 6179-88.

Pifl, C., Giros, B, Caron, M. G. (1993). Dopamine transporter expression confers cytotoxicity to low doses of the parkinsonism-inducing neurotoxin 1-methyl-4-phenylpyridinium. J Neurosci 13, 4246-53.

Pifl, C., Giros, B, Caron, M. G. (1996a). The dopamine transporter. The cloned target site of parkinsonism- inducing toxins and of drugs of abuse. Adv Neurol 69, 235-8.

Pifl, C., Hornykiewicz, O., Giros, B, Caron, M. G. (1996b). Catecholamine transporters and 1-methyl-4-phenyl-1,2,3,6- tetrahydropyridine neurotoxicity: studies comparing the cloned human noradrenaline and human dopamine transporter. J Pharmacol Exp Ther 277, 1437-43.

Popper, C. W. (1997). Antidepressants in the treatment of attention-deficit/hyperactivity disorder. J Clin Psychiatry 58, 14-29; discussion 30-1.

Rabey, J. M., Amir, I., Treves, T. A., Oberman, Z, Korczyn, A. D. (1998). Dopamine uptake by platelet storage granules in first-degree relatives of Tourette's syndrome patients [In Process Citation]. Biol Psychiatry 44, 1166-70.

Ramamoorthy, S. and Blakely, R. D. (1999). Phosphorylation and sequestration of serotonin transporters differentially modulated by psychostimulants. Science 285, 763-6.

Reinhard, J. F., Jr., Diliberto, E. J., Jr., Viveros, O. H, Daniels, A. J. (1987). Subcellular compartmentalization of 1-methyl-4-phenylpyridinium with catecholamines in adrenal medullary chromaffin vesicles may explain the lack of toxicity to adrenal chromaffin cells. Proc Natl Acad Sci U S A 84, 8160-4.

Rocha, B. A., Fumagalli, F., Gainetdinov, R. R., Jones, S. R., Ator, R., Giros, B., Miller, G. W, Caron, M. G. (1998). Cocaine self-administration in dopamine transporter knockout mice. Nature Neuroscience 1, 132-137.

Sanghera, M. K., Manaye, K., McMahon, A., Sonsalla, P. K, German, D. C. (1997). Dopamine transporter mRNA levels are high in midbrain neurons vulnerable to MPTP. Neuroreport 8, 3327-31.

Schuldiner, S., Shirvan, A, Linial, M. (1995). Vesicular neurotransmitter transporters: from bacteria to humans. Physiol Rev 75, 369-92.

Shimada, S., Kitayama, S., Lin, C. L., Patel, A., Nanthakumar, E., Gregor, P., Kuhar, M, Uhl, G. (1991). Cloning and expression of a cocaine-sensitive dopamine transporter complementary DNA [published erratum appears in Science 1992 Mar 6;255(5049):1195]. Science 254, 576-8.

Shimada, S., Kitayama, S., Walther, D, Uhl, G. (1992). Dopamine transporter mRNA: dense expression in ventral midbrain neurons. Brain Res Mol Brain Res 13, 359-62.

Sibley, D. R. (1999). New insights into dopaminergic receptor function using antisense and genetically altered animals [In Process Citation]. Annu Rev Pharmacol Toxicol *39*, 313-41.

Sibley, D. R., Monsma, F. J., Jr., McVittie, L. D., Gerfen, C. R., Burch, R. M, Mahan, L. C. (1992). Molecular neurobiology of dopamine receptor subtypes. Neurochem Int *20 Suppl*, 17S-22S.

Speciale, S. G., Liang, C. L., Sonsalla, P. K., Edwards, R. H, German, D. C. (1998). The neurotoxin 1-methyl-4-phenylpyridinium is sequestered within neurons that contain the vesicular monoamine transporter. Neuroscience *84*, 1177-85.

Takahashi, N., Miner, L. L., Sora, I., Ujike, H., Revay, R. S., Kostic, V., Jackson-Lewis, V., Przedborski, S, Uhl, G. R. (1997). VMAT2 knockout mice: heterozygotes display reduced amphetamine-conditioned reward, enhanced amphetamine locomotion, and enhanced MPTP toxicity. Proc Natl Acad Sci U S A *94*, 9938-43.

Tanner, C. M., Ottman, R., Goldman, S. M., Ellenberg, J., Chan, P., Mayeux, R, Langston, J. W. (1999). Parkinson Disease in Twins. Journal American Medical Association *281*, 341-346.

Ueno, S., Nakamura, M., Mikami, M., Kondoh, K., Ishiguro, H., Arinami, T., Komiyama, T., Mitsushio, H., Sano, A, Tanabe, H. (1999). Identification of a novel polymorphism of the human dopamine transporter (DAT1) gene and the significant association with alcoholism. Mol Psychiatry *4*, 552-557.

Uhl, G. R. (1998). Hypothesis: the role of dopaminergic transporters in selective vulnerability of cells in Parkinson's disease. Ann Neurol *43*, 555-60.

Vaccari, A. and Saba, P. (1995). The tyramine-labelled vesicular transporter for dopamine: a putative target of pesticides and neurotoxins. Eur J Pharmacol *292*, 309-14.

Waldman, I. D., Rowe, D. C., Abramowitz, A., Kozel, S. T., Mohr, J. H., Sherman, S. L., Cleveland, H. H., Sanders, M. L., Gard, J. M, Stever, C. (1998). Association and Linkage of the Dopamine Transporter Gene and Attention- Deficit Hyperactivity Disorder in Children: Heterogeneity owing to Diagnostic Subtype and Severity. Am J Hum Genet *63*, 1767-1776.

Wang, Y. M., Gainetdinov, R. R., Fumagalli, F., Xu, F., Jones, S. R., Bock, C. B., Miller, G. W., Wightman, R. M, Caron, M. G. (1997). Knockout of the vesicular monoamine transporter 2 gene results in neonatal death and supersensitivity to cocaine and amphetamine. Neuron *19*, 1285-96.

Wellington, C. L., Brinkman, R. R., O'Kusky, J. R, Hayden, M. R. (1997). Toward understanding the molecular pathology of Huntington's disease. Brain Pathol *7*, 979-1002.

Wilson, J. M., Kalasinsky, K. S., Levey, A. I., Bergeron, C., Reiber, G., Anthony, R. M., Schmunk, G. A., Shannak, K., Haycock, J. W, Kish, S. J. (1996a). Striatal dopamine nerve terminal markers in human, chronic methamphetamine users. Nat Med *2*, 699-703.

Wilson, J. M., Levey, A. I., Bergeron, C., Kalasinsky, K., Ang, L., Peretti, F., Adams, V. I., Smialek, J., Anderson, W. R., Shannak, K., Deck, J., Niznik, H. B, Kish, S. J. (1996b). Striatal dopamine, dopamine transporter, and vesicular monoamine transporter in chronic cocaine users. Ann Neurol *40*, 428-39.

Wilson, J. M., Levey, A. I., Rajput, A., Ang, L., Guttman, M., Shannak, K., Niznik, H. B., Hornykiewicz, O., Pifl, C., Kish, S. J. (1996c). Differential changes in neurochemical markers of striatal dopamine nerve terminals in idiopathic Parkinson's disease. Neurology *47*, 718-26.

Yelin, R. and Schuldiner, S. (1995). The pharmacological profile of the vesicular monoamine transporter resembles that of multidrug transporters. FEBS Lett *377*, 201-7.

Zuddas, A., Fascetti, F., Corsini, G. U, Piccardi, M. P. (1994). In brown Norway rats, MPP+ is accumulated in the nigrostriatal dopaminergic terminals but it is not neurotoxic: a model of natural resistance to MPTP toxicity. Exp Neurol *127*, 54-61.

2 THE LONG-TERM BEHAVIORAL AND NEUROBIOLOGICAL CONSEQUENCES OF TREATMENT WITH PSYCHOMOTOR STIMULANT DRUGS: IMPLICATIONS FOR PSYCHOPATHOLOGY

Terry E. Robinson

INTRODUCTION

When psychoactive drugs are administered repeatedly many of their effects change, and these changes take two main forms: tolerance or sensitization. The sensitization produced by the repeated administration of psychostimulant drugs, such as amphetamine or cocaine, has attracted considerable attention recently, for two major reasons. First, psychostimulant sensitization is an interesting example of experience-dependent plasticity, whereby very persistent changes in behavior occur as a function of past experience – in this case, past *drug* experience. Thus, the phenomenon provides an interesting model to explore the nature of neuroplastic adaptations underlying experience-dependent changes in behavior. Second, psychomotor stimulant drug-induced sensitization is thought to provide an animal model for studying some forms of drug-induced psychopathology. These include the development of paranoid schizophrenic-like symptoms often seen with repeated exposure to amphetamine or cocaine (Post, 1975; Segal et al., 1981; Robinson and Becker, 1986), as well as the compulsive patterns of drug-seeking behavior that characterize the development of addiction (Robinson and Berridge, 1993). The purpose of this chapter is to briefly review some recent advances in our understanding of this phenomenon.

PSYCHOMOTOR SENSITIZATION

The phenomenon of drug-induced sensitization refers to an increase in an effect of a drug with repeated drug administration, such that a lower dose of the drug is required to produce a given effect in a drug experienced individual than in a drug naïve subject. It is important to remember that many drug effects do not show sensitization; some effects show tolerance, other effects may not change, and at the same time yet other effects show sensitization. In the case of psychomotor stimulant drugs the two main classes of drug effects that show sensitization are their psychomotor activating effects and their rewarding effects. Thus, the ability of amphetamine or cocaine to produce locomotor hyperactivity, stereotyped behaviors and rotational behavior is increased with repeated drug exposure (Robinson and Becker, 1986). Similarly, prior experience with these drugs facilitates the later acquisition of a drug self-administration habit or a conditioned place preference (Piazza et al., 1991; Robinson and Berridge, 1993; Schenk and Partridge, 1997, for reviews), and increases the "breakpoint" of animals performing on a progressive ratio schedule (Mendrek et al., 1998; Lorrain et al., 2000).

The phenomenon of psychomotor sensitization is very complex and the degree of sensitization is influenced by many variables, including the dose and pattern of drug administration (high doses given intermittently are most effective). There are also large individual differences in susceptibility to sensitization. Individual differences are due to complex (and not well understood) interactions amongst genetic factors, hormonal influences and environmental variables (Robinson, 1988). Once induced, however, sensitization can persist for very long periods of time (months to years) (Paulson et al., 1991). The major characteristics of psychomotor sensitization have been the topic of a number of reviews, and therefore, will not be discussed in detail here (Kalivas and Stewart, 1991; Robinson and Berridge, 1993; Stewart and Badiani, 1993; White and Kalivas, 1998; Wolf, 1998).

There has been considerable research directed at identifying the changes in the nervous system produced by repeated exposure to amphetamine and cocaine that might underlie behavioral sensitization, and much of this work has focussed on the dopamine/accumbens system. Many cellular and systems-level sensitization-related neuroadaptations have been found, and these have been the subject of a number of recent reviews (Pierce and Kalivas, 1997; White and Kalivas, 1998; Wolf, 1998). In the dopamine/accumbens system both presynaptic and postsynaptic adaptations have been described. An example of a presynaptic adaptation is a persistent increase in the ability of psychomotor stimulant drugs to increase dopamine efflux. This has been reported using both in vitro approaches to quantify neurotransmitter release, and in vivo using microdialysis (see reviews above for references). One especially interesting characteristic of the sensitization-related increase in amphetamine-induced dopamine release is that the "sensitized" component is calcium-dependent (Warburton et al., 1996; Pierce and Kalivas, 1997; Kantor et al., 1999). The "normal" component is not, consistent with many reports that amphetamine-stimulated dopamine release is not calcium-dependent (Kuczenski, 1983). These studies suggest, therefore, there is a fundamental change in the mechanism by which amphetamine acts to release dopamine as a function of prior experience with this agent.

In addition to these apparent presynaptic adaptations produced by repeated treatment with psychomotor stimulant drugs, postsynaptic adaptations have also been reported. Probably the best example of these is an increase in the sensitivity of dopamine D1 receptors described by White and his colleagues (Henry and White, 1991; Henry and White, 1995). Finally, the repeated intermittent administration of amphetamine or cocaine not only results in a variety of biochemical adaptations, but in persistent structural modifications in the morphology of output neurons in the nucleus accumbens and prefrontal cortex. Robinson and Kolb (1997, 1999) have reported that a month following the last treatment with amphetamine or cocaine there is an increase in dendritic branching and in the density of dendritic spines on medium spiny neurons in the nucleus accumbens and pyramidal cells in the medial prefrontal cortex. These latter findings suggest that sensitization is associated with alterations in patterns of synaptic connectivity in brain reward systems, a notion that is consistent with increasing evidence that neurotrophic factors play an important role in the induction of sensitization (Flores et al., 1998; Horger et al., 1999; Flores, 2000).

Finally, although much of the research on the neurobiology of sensitization has focussed on the accumbens dopamine system, it is important to keep in mind that sensitization is a very complex phenomenon, and like other forms of experience-dependent plasticity, is presumably associated with systems-level changes in many neural circuits. Consistent with this, sensitization-related neuroadaptations have been described not only in mesotelencephalic dopamine systems (Robinson and Becker, 1986), but in dopaminergic activity in the amygdala (Harmer et al., 1997; Harmer and Phillips, 1999), and in serotonin (Parsons and Justice, 1993), norepinephrine (Camp et al., 1997) and acetylcholine neurotransmission (Bickerdike and Abercrombie, 1997). There is also a wealth of evidence that excitatory amino acid neurotransmission plays a critical role in sensitization processes (Karler et al., 1989; Clark and Overton, 1998; Wolf, 1998). The major challenge for future research on the neurobiology of sensitization will be to determine which neuroadaptations in which neural systems are causally-related to the behavioral phenomenon.

MODULATION BY ENVIRONMENTAL CONTEXT

It is easy to think of psychomotor sensitization as an inevitable consequence of the pharmacological actions of a drug. That is, when a drug interacts with its receptor it initiates a cascade of cellular responses leading to persistent alterations in cell function. However, there is increasing evidence that sensitization is not an inevitable consequence of drug-receptor interactions, but both the induction and expression of psychomotor sensitization can be powerfully modulated by environmental factors, especially the context in which the drug is administered (Robinson et al., 1998). There are at least two ways environmental context may modulate sensitization, and these may represent very different phenomena: modulation of expression versus modulation of induction.

Modulation of Expression

The ability of environmental context to modulate the expression of psychomotor sensitization is best illustrated by a phenomenon usually called context-specific sensitization (Robinson et al., 1998). In such experiments one of animals group (the "paired" group) is transported each day to a distinct test cage, where it receives drug. A second group (the "unpaired" group) is usually transported to the test cage, and given saline, and then later back in it's home cage given drug. Alternatively, this group may receive drug in a third environment, distinct from both the test cage and the home cage (Anagnostaras and Robinson, 1996). On the test day, usually after some withdrawal period, all groups (including saline treated control groups) are given a challenge injection in the test cage. Thus, both the paired and unpaired groups have the same drug history, but only the paired group experienced drug in the challenge test environment. In these experiments only the paired group typically expresses sensitization; the psychomotor response in the unpaired group is often the same as that in saline treated control animals (Tilson and Rech, 1973; Pert et al., 1990; Anagnostaras and Robinson, 1996). Thus, in this situation sensitization is said to be "context-specific". On the other hand, it is also possible to induce sensitization by giving all injections in the animal's home cage (although see below), so that drug injections are not paired with any distinct context (Segal and Schuckit, 1983, for example). The sensitization that is produced in this situation is often referred to as "context-independent" sensitization (although it is impossible, of course, to give a drug "independent" of a context).

So-called context-specific sensitization and context-independent sensitization are frequently discussed as if they represent two different phenomena, and as if they are due to different underlying neuroadaptive processes. This may not be the case. The alternative hypothesis is that both what is called context-specific sensitization and what is called context-independent sensitization represent the same phenomenon, and they are due to the same underlying non-associative drug-induced neuroadaptations (Robinson et al., 1998). There is no doubt that context-specific sensitization represents a powerful example of conditioned stimulus control over the *expression* of sensitization (Stewart and Badiani, 1993; Anagnostaras and Robinson, 1996). However, there are at least two reasons to believe that animals in the "unpaired" groups undergo neural sensitization; that is, their brains are altered by drug exposure in the same manner as in the paired group, even though they may not *express* sensitization in behavior under these specific test conditions.

The first is that animals receiving drug treatments in a distinct environment other than the test environment (e. g., in a "third world") develop normal behavioral sensitization in their drug treatment environment (Anagnostaras and Robinson, 1996). This makes sense because this group is treated in all respects exactly the same as a "paired" group, except on the challenge test day. There is no logical reason to think that there would be any difference between these two groups in the ability of repeated drug treatments to produce whatever drug-induced neuroadaptations underlie sensitization. They just do not *express* this "neural sensitization" in behavior when tested in a unique environment (Anagnostaras and Robinson, 1996). Second, neural sensitization has been described under conditions that preclude the influence of contextual stimuli on the neurobiological expression of the drug response. For example, evidence for neural sensitization to a number of drugs has been reported using striatal tissue slices in vitro and in anaesthetized animals (Robinson and Becker, 1982; Castañeda et al., 1988; Henry and White, 1991; Nestby et al., 1997; Kantor et al., 1999; Vanderschuren et al., 1999).

The most parsimonious hypothesis, therefore, is that repeated exposure to psychostimulant drugs may *induce* neural sensitization non-associatively, and may do so in the same manner in "paired" and "unpaired" groups (although see below for a discussion of how home cage injections can influence the induction of sensitization). That is, these groups may undergo neural sensitization in exactly the same manner; context-specific and context-independent sensitization are not in this respect, distinct phenomena. However, whether the consequences of neural sensitization are expressed in behavior at a particular place or time is determined to a large extent by conditional stimuli (especially contextual stimuli) that have been associatively paired with drug administration (Anagnostaras and Robinson, 1996). It is this "layer" of conditioned stimulus control over the *expression* of neural sensitization that makes it appear as if there are two phenomena. What is not understood is how and under what conditions environmental stimuli can gain control over the sensitized neural substrate. Under what conditions will the expression of sensitization be subject to control by environmental factors ("context-specific") and under what conditions will environmental stimuli exert little control? In discussing this issue Anagnostaras and Robinson, (1996) hypothesized that one way contextual stimuli may modulate the expression of sensitization is by acting as occasion-setters, a class of conditional stimuli that can modulate the response to other stimuli without themselves producing a conditioned response (Rescorla et al., 1985; Holland, 1992; Bouton, 1993), but the actual mechanism(s) involved in the conditioned stimulus control over the expression of sensitization has received very little attention in the literature (Stewart, 1992; Stewart and Badiani, 1993).

Modulation of Induction

Environmental factors may not only modulate whether neural sensitization is expressed in behavior, but whether it is induced in the first place, or at least the rate and degree of sensitization. In the initial studies on this phenomenon Badiani and his colleagues (Badiani et al., 1995a; 1995b; 1997) treated rats with i.p. amphetamine or cocaine either in their home cage (called the HOME group) or in a distinct test chamber that was physically identical to the cage in which the HOME group lived (this group was called the NOVEL group because the test cage was relatively novel). It was found that doses of amphetamine or cocaine that produced robust psychomotor sensitization when given in the NOVEL condition produced only weak sensitization when given in the HOME environment. The influence of environmental context was even greater in subsequent studies in which drug was administered intravenously via a chronic indwelling catheter, eliminated all environmental cues that would otherwise be associated with drug administration (e.g., the appearance of experimenter, handling, the needle prick). Crombag et al. (1996) reported that up to 1.0 mg/kg of i.v. amphetamine induced robust sensitization when given in a NOVEL environment but failed to induce sensitization at all when given at HOME (Robinson et al., 1998, as well). Indeed, on the challenge test day, when both saline and amphetamine treated rats all received an amphetamine challenge, the magnitude of the behavioral response varied 23-fold across groups. This large variation in drug response was due to two factors: (1) whether the animals had experience with drug in the past, and (2) *where* they had that experience. Similar results have been obtained with cocaine (Browman et al., 1998a) and with morphine (Badiani et al., 2000b), and using two different measures of psychomotor activation, rotational behavior (Badiani et al., 1995a; Crombag et al., 1996) and locomotor activity (Badiani et al., 1995a; Fraioli et al., 1999). These results highlight the enormous influence that environmental (and psychological) factors can have on drug responsiveness, and the ability of drugs to induce sensitization-related neuroadaptations, even in a simple animal model.

The effect of environmental context on both acute drug responsiveness and sensitization was so large in the Crombag et al. (1996) experiment we wondered whether it was in fact impossible to induce psychomotor sensitization if amphetamine or cocaine were given intravenously in the absence of any environmental cues predictive of drug administration. The alternative hypothesis, of course, is that the effect of environment is not to gate sensitization in an all-or-none fashion, but to shift the dose-effect curve for the induction of sensitization. This hypothesis was tested by Browman et al., (1998a; 1998b), who found that the effect of environmental context was to shift the dose-effect curve for producing psychomotor sensitization, such that lower doses were needed to induce sensitization when either amphetamine or cocaine were administered in a distinct test environment, relative to when they were administered at home. But when high enough doses were used these drugs induced psychomotor sensitization regardless of the context in which they were given. Furthermore, it appears that the ability of a distinct and relatively novel test environment to promote robust sensitization is not simply because it provides a cue predictive of drug administration. Crombag et al. (1997) have found recently that providing discrete cues (light, tone, odor) in the home cage, which reliably predict drug administration, fail to promote robust sensitization comparable to that seen when drug is administered in a distinct test chamber.

These behavioral studies clearly indicate that the environment (home vs. novel) in which psychostimulants are given must modulate their neurobiological effects in some way, to promote both acute drug responsiveness and the susceptibility to sensitization. How it does so has been the subject of a number of recent studies. The most simple hypothesis is that environmental context determines the amount of drug to reach the brain; i.e., the effect is due to altered pharmacokinetics. This does not seem to be the case for amphetamine because the plasma and striatal levels of amphetamine are not influenced by the context in which it is given (Badiani et al., 1997). A second obvious hypothesis is that environment modulates the primary neuropharmacological effect of amphetamine thought to mediate its psychomotor activating effects, which is to induce dopamine release in the striatal complex. However, in microdialysis studies there was no effect of environmental condition on amphetamine-stimulated dopamine release in the caudate nucleus or in the core or shell of the nucleus accumbens (Badiani et al., 1998; Badiani et al., 2000a). Nevertheless, the neural circuitry engaged by amphetamine and cocaine is powerfully modulated by whether the drug is given in at home or in a novel test environment. This has been shown in recent experiments using the immediate early gene, c-fos, as an indicator of neuronal activation (Badiani et al., 1998).

Badiani et al. (1998) used in situ hybridization to quantify c-fos RNA in animals given amphetamine either at home or in a distinct test chamber, or in control animals. As reported by numerous researchers (Harlan and Garcia, 1998), amphetamine induced c-fos expression in many brain regions, especially throughout the striatal complex. There was, however, a very large effect of environment on the ability of amphetamine to induce c-fos in many brain regions. In nearly every cortical and subcortical region examined amphetamine induced much greater c-fos expression when given in the novel environment than when given at home, although the nature of the drug-environment interaction varied across brain regions. For example, in the neocortex mere exposure to a novel environment (in the absence of drug) produced more robust c-fos expression than did amphetamine given at home, and the effect of amphetamine given in the novel environment was comparable in magnitude to the effect of novelty alone. That is, in much of the neocortex it appears that the increased levels of c-fos mRNA seen after amphetamine was given in a novel environment was due to the effects of novelty alone. In the striatum, however, the interaction was more complex. For example, in the caudate and the core of the nucleus accumbens the effect of amphetamine given in a novel environment was significantly greater than the effect of either amphetamine at home or the effect of mere exposure to the novel environment (Badiani et al., 1998).

Indeed, in the caudate the effect of environment was not only quantitative, but context appeared to modulate *qualitatively* the ability of amphetamine to engage specific cell populations. Using double in situ hybridization Badiani et al. (1999) found that when rats received 2.0 mg/kg of amphetamine at home c-*fos* was induced only in striatal cells also positive for dopamine D1 receptor mRNA (not in cells positive for D2 mRNA). When given in a novel environment, however, amphetamine induced c-*fos* in both D1 and D2 positive cells. Furthermore, the ability to induce c-*fos* in D1 mRNA positive cells was abolished by a 6-OHDA lesion, but this lesion did not abolish the ability of amphetamine to induce c-*fos* in D2 cells. In the caudate cells positive for D1 versus D2 mRNA appear to represent two different populations (Gerfen et al., 1990; Steiner and Gerfen, 1998). The D1 positive cell population (which co-expresses dynorphin) forms the so-called "direct" pathway, projecting directly back to the substantia nigra. The D2 cells on the other hand (which co-express enkephalin) project indirectly back to the substantia nigra, via the pallidum and subthalamic nucleus. It appears, therefore, that when given at home amphetamine engages primarily the direct pathway, and when given in a novel environment amphetamine produces even greater activation of the direct pathway, but now also engages the indirect pathway. Consistent with this notion, Uslaner et al. (1999) have recently reported that amphetamine and cocaine produce the greatest c-*fos* activation in the subthalamic nucleus when given in a novel environment.

In summary, there is now considerable evidence that repeated intermittent exposure to psychostimulant drugs has very persistent consequences for behavior and brain function, as exemplified by the phenomenon of behavioral sensitization. There is no doubt that these drugs alter patterns of neural circuitry and neurotransmission in the very brain regions that mediate their incentive motivational effects. Furthermore, the ability of drugs to induce these neuroplastic adaptations is not a simple function of their pharmacological effects, but is powerfully modulated by environmental context, in ways that are not yet well understood. It seems highly likely that the ability of psychostimulant drugs to produce persistent alterations in the function of the nucleus accumbens, the prefrontal cortex, and related circuitry contribute to the psychopathological consequences of psychostimulant abuse, including the development of amphetamine and cocaine psychosis (Segal and Schuckit, 1983; Robinson and Becker, 1986) and the development of the compulsive drug-seeking and drug-taking behavior that characterize addiction (Robinson and Berridge, 1993). Determining exactly what drug-induced alterations in what neural systems lead to what forms of psychopathology remains a major challenge for future research.

REFERENCES

Anagnostaras S.G. and Robinson T.E. (1996) Sensitization to the psychomotor stimulant effects of amphetamine: modulation by associative learning. Behav Neurosci 110: 1397-1414.

Badiani A., Anagnostaras S.G., Robinson T.E. (1995a) The development of sensitization to the psychomotor stimulant effects of amphetamine is enhanced in a novel environment. Psychopharmacol 117: 443-452.

Badiani A., Browman K.E, Robinson T.E. (1995b) Influence of novel versus home environments on sensitization to the psychomotor stimulant effects of cocaine and amphetamine. Brain Res 674: 291-298.

26

Badiani A., Camp D.M, Robinson T.E. (1997) Enduring enhancement of amphetamine sensitization by drug-associated environmental stimuli. J Pharmacol exp Ther 282: 787-794.

Badiani A, Oates M.M., Day H.E.W., Watson S.J., Akil H., Robinson T.E. (1998) Amphetamine-induced behavior, dopamine release, and c-fos mRNA expression: modulation by environmental novelty. J Neurosci 18: 10579-10593.

Badiani A., Oates M.M., Day H.E.W., Watson S.J., Akil H., Robinson T.E. (1999) Environmental modulation of amphetamine-induced c-fos expression in D1 versus D2 striatal neurons. Behav Brain Res 103: 203-209.

Badiani A., Oates M.M., Fraioli S., Browman K.E., Ostrander M.M., Xue C.-J., Wolf M.E, Robinson T.E. (2000a) Environmental modulation of the response to amphetamine: dissociation between changes in behavior and changes in dopamine and glutamate overflow in the striatal complex. Psychopharmacology (in press).

Badiani A., Oates M.M, Robinson T.E. (2000b) Modulation of morphine sensitization in the rat by contextual stimuli. Psychopharmacology (in press)

Bickerdike M.J. and Abercrombie E.D. (1997) Striatal acetylcholine release correlates with behavioral sensitization in rats withdrawn from chronic amphetamine. J Pharmacol Exp Ther 282: 818-26.

Bouton M.E. (1993) Context, time, and memory retrieval in the interference paradigms of Pavlovian learning. Psychol Bull 114: 80-99.

Browman K.E., Badiani A, Robinson T.E. (1998a) The influence of environment on the induction of sensitization to the psychomotor activating effects of intravenous cocaine in rats is dose-dependent. Psychopharmacology 137: 90-98.

Browman K.E., Badiani A, Robinson T.E. (1998b) Modulatory effect of environmental stimuli on the susceptibility to amphetamine sensitization: a dose-effect study in rats. J Pharmacol exp Ther 287: 1007-1014.

Camp D.M., DeJonghe D.K, Robinson T.E. (1997) Time-dependent effects of repeated amphetamine treatment on norepinephrine in the hypothalamus and hippocampus assessed with in vivo microdialysis. Neuropsychopharmacology 17: 130-140.

Castañeda E., Becker J.B and Robinson T.E. (1988) The long-term effects of repeated amphetamine treatment in vivo on amphetamine, KCl and electrical stimulation evoked striatal dopamine release in vitro. Life Sci 42: 2447-56.

Clark D. and Overton P.G. (1998) Alterations in excitatory amino acid-mediated regulation of midbrain dopa minergic neurones induced by chronic psychostimulant administration and stress: relevance to behavioral sensitization and drug addiction. Addiction Biology 3: 109-135.

Crombag H.S., Badiani A., Robinson T.E. (1996) Signalled versus unsignalled intravenous amphetamine: large differences in the acute psychomotor response and sensitization. Brain Res 722: 227-231.

Crombag H.S., Badiani A, Robinson T.E. (1997) The effects of drug-predictive cues on sensitization to the psychomotor stimulant effects of amphetamine. Soc Neurosci Abst 23: 2404.

Flores C., Samaha, A.-N, Stewart, J. (2000) Requirement of endogenous basic fibroblast growth factor for sensitization to amphetamine. J Neurosci 20 RC55: 1-5.

Flores C., Rodaros D, Stewart J (1998) Long-lasting induction of astrocytic basic fibroblast growth factor by repeated injections of amphetamine: blockade by concurrent treatment with a glutamate antagonist. J Neurosci 18: 9547-55.

Fraioli S., Crombag H.S., Badiani A, Robinson T.E. (1999) Susceptibility to amphetamine-induced locomotor sensitization is modulated by environmental stimuli. Neuropsychopharmacology 20: 533-541.

Gerfen C.R., Engber T.M., Mahan L.C., Susel Z., Chase T.N., Monsma F.J.J, Sibley D.R. (1990) D1 and D2 dopamine receptor-regulated gene expression of striatonigral and striatopallidal neurons. Science 250: 1429-32.

Harlan R.E. and Garcia M.M. (1998) Drugs of abuse and immediate-early genes in the forebrain. Mol Neurobiol 16: 221-67.

Harmer C.J., Hitchcott P.K., Morutto S.L, Phillips G.D. (1997) Repeated d-amphetamine enhances stimulated mesoamygdaloid dopamine transmission. Psychopharmacology 132: 247-54.

Harmer C.J. and Phillips G.D. (1999) Enhanced dopamine efflux in the amygdala by a predictive, but not a non- predictive, stimulus: facilitation by prior repeated D-amphetamine. Neuroscience 90: 119-30.

Henry D.J, White F.J. (1991) Repeated cocaine administration causes persistent enhancement of D1 dopamine receptor sensitivity within the rat nucleus accumbens. J Pharmacol Exp Ther 258: 882-890.

Henry D.J. and White F.J. (1995) The persistence of behavioral sensitization to cocaine parallels enhanced inhibition of nucleus accumbens neurons. J Neurosci 15: 6287-6299.

Holland P.C. (1992) Occasion setting in Pavlovian conditioning. In: P. C. Holland ed. The Psychology of Learning and Motivation, Vol. 28 , 69-125. San Diego: Academic Press.

Horger B.A., Iyasere C.A., Berhow M.T., Messer C.J., Nestler E.J, Taylor J.R. (1999) Enhancement of locomotor activity and conditioned reward to cocaine by brain-derived neurotrophic factor. J Neurosci 19: 4110-22.

Kalivas P.W, Stewart J. (1991) Dopamine transmission in the initiation and expression of drug- and stress-induced sensitization of motor activity. Brain Res Rev 16: 223-244.

Kantor L., Hewlett G.H, Gnegy M.E. (1999) Enhanced amphetamine- and K+-mediated dopamine release in rat striatum after repeated amphetamine: differential requirements for Ca2+- and calmodulin-dependent phosphorylation and synaptic vesicles. J Neurosci 19: 3801-8.

Karler R., Calder L.D., Chaudhry I.A, Turkanis S.A. (1989) Blockade of "reverse tolerance" to cocaine and amphetamine by MK-801. Life Sci 45: 599-606.

Kuczenski R. (1983) Biochemical actions of amphetamine and other stimulants. In: I. Creese, ed. Stimulants: Neurochemical, Behavioral and Clinical Perspectives, 31-61. New York: Raven Press.

Lorrain D.S., Arnold G.M, Vezina P. (2000) Previous exposure to amphetamine increases incentive to obtain the drug: long-lasting effects revealed by the progressive ratio schedule. Behav Brain Res 107: 9-19.

Mendrek A., Blaha C.D, Phillips A.G. (1998) Pre-exposure of rats to amphetamine sensitizes self-administration of this drug under a progressive ratio schedule. Psychopharmacology 135: 416-22.

Nestby P., Vanderschuren L.J., De Vries T.J., Hogenboom F., Wardeh G., Mulder A.H., Schoffelmeer A.N. (1997) Ethanol, like psychostimulants and morphine, causes long-lasting hyperreactivity of dopamine and acetylcholine neurons of rat nucleus accumbens: possible role in behavioural sensitization. Psychopharmacology (Berl) 133: 69-76.

Parsons L.H. and Justice J.B., Jr. (1993) Serotonin and dopamine sensitization in the nucleus accumbens, ventral tegmental area, and dorsal raphe nucleus following repeated cocaine administration. J Neurochem 61: 1611-9.

Paulson P.E., Camp D.M, Robinson T.E. (1991) The time course of transient behavioral depression and persistent behavioral sensitization in relation to regional brain monoamine concentrations during amphetamine withdrawal in rats. Psychopharmacology 103: 480-492.

Pert A., Post R, Weiss S.R. (1990) Conditioning as a critical determinant of sensitization induced by psychomotor stimulants. NIDA Res Monogr 97: 208-41.

Piazza P.V., Deminière J.-M., Maccari S., Le Moal M., Mormède P, Simon H. (1991) Individual vulnerability to drug self-administration: action of corticosterone on dopaminergic systems as a possible pathophysiological mechanism. In: P. Willner and J. Scheel-Kruger, eds. The Mesolimbic Dopamine System: From Motivation to Action, 473-495. New York: John Wiley & Sons Ltd.

Pierce R.C. and Kalivas P.W. (1997) A circuitry model of the expression of behavioral sensitization to amphetamine-like psychostimulants. Brain Res Rev 25: 192-216.

Pierce R.C. and Kalivas P.W. (1997) Repeated cocaine modifies the mechanism by which amphetamine releases dopamine. J Neurosci 17: 3254-61.

Post R.M. (1975) Cocaine psychoses: a continuum model. Am J Psychiatry 132: 225-31.

Rescorla R.A., Durlach P.J, Grau J.W. (1985) Contextual learning in Pavlovian conditioning. In: P. Balsam and A. Tomie, Context and Learning, 23-56. Hillsdale, NJ: Erlbaum.

Robinson T.E. (1988) Stimulant drugs and stress: factors influencing individual differences in the susceptibility to sensitization. In: P. W. Kalivas and C. D. Barnes, eds. CD Sensitization of the Nervous System, 145-173. Caldwell, N. J.: Telford Press.

Robinson T.E. and Becker J.B. (1982) Behavioral sensitization is accompanied by an enhancement in amphetamine-stimulated dopamine release from striatal tissue in vitro. Eur J Pharmacol 85: 253-4.

Robinson T.E. and Becker J.B. (1986) Enduring changes in brain and behavior produced by chronic amphetamine administration: a review and evaluation of animal models of amphetamine psychosis. Brain Res Rev 11: 157-98.

Robinson T.E. and Berridge K.C. (1993) The neural basis of drug craving: An incentive-sensitization theory of addiction. Brain Res Rev 18: 247-291.

Robinson T.E., Browman K.E., Crombag H.S, Badiani A. (1998) Modulation of the induction or expression of psychostimulant sensitization by the circumstances surrounding drug administration. Neurosci Biobehav Rev 22: 347-354.

Robinson T.E. and Kolb B. (1997) Persistent structural modifications in nucleus accumbens and prefrontal cortex neurons produced by previous experience with amphetamine. J Neurosci 17: 8491-8497.

Robinson T.E. and Kolb B. (1999) Alterations in the morphology of dendrites and dendritic spines in the nucleus accumbens and prefrontal cortex following repeated treatment with amphetamine or cocaine. Eur J Neurosci 11: 1598-1604.

Schenk S. and Partridge B. (1997) Sensitization and tolerance in psychostimulant self-administration. Pharmacol Biochem Behav 57: 543-50.

Segal D.S., Geyer M.A, Schuckit M.A. (1981) Stimulant-induced psychosis: an evaluation of animal models. Essays Neurochem Neuropharmacol 5: 95-129.

Segal D.S. and Schuckit M.A. (1983) Animal models of stimulant-induced psychosis. In: I. Creese, ed. Stimulants: Neurochemical, Behavioral and Clinical Perspectives, 131-67. New York: Raven Press.

Steiner H. and Gerfen C.R. (1998) Role of dynorphin and enkephalin in the regulation of striatal output pathways and behavior. Exp Brain Res 123: 60-76.

Stewart J. (1992) Conditioned stimulus control of the expression of sensitization of the behavioral activating effects of opiate and stimulant drugs. In: I. Gormezano and E. A. Wasserman, eds. Learning and Memory: The Behavioral and Biological Substrates, 129-151. Hillsdale, NJ: Erlbaum.

Stewart J. and Badiani A. (1993) Tolerance and sensitization to the behavioral effects of drugs. Behav Pharmacol 4: 289-312.

Tilson H.A. and Rech R.A. (1973) Conditioned drug effects and absence of tolerance to d-amphetamine induced motor activity. Pharmacol Biochem Behav 1: 149-153.

Uslaner J., Badiani A., Day H.E.W., Watson S.E., Akil H, Robinson T.E. (1999) c-fos mRNA expression after acute amphetamine or cocaine: the influence of environmental novelty. Soc Neurosci Abst 25: 310.

Vanderschuren L.J.M.J., Schoffelmeer A.N.M., Mulder A.H, De Vries T.J. (1999) Dopaminergic mechanisms mediating the long-term expression of locomotor sensitization following pre-exposure to morphine or amphetamine. Psychopharmacology 143: 244-253.

Warburton E.C., Mitchell S.N, Joseph M.H. (1996) Calcium dependence of sensitized dopamine release in the rat nucleus accumbens following amphetamine challenge: implications for the disruption of latent inhibition. Behav Pharmacol 7: 119-129.

White F.J. and Kalivas P.W. (1998) Neuroadaptations involved in amphetamine and cocaine addiction. Drug Alcohol Depend 51: 141-53.

Wolf M.E. (1998) The role of excitatory amino acids in behavioral sensitization to psychomotor stimulants. Prog Neurobiol 54: 679-720.

3 ANXIETY AND IMPULSE CONTROL IN RATS SELECTIVELY BRED FOR SEIZURE SUSCEPTIBILITY

Dan C. McIntyre and Hymie Anisman

INTRODUCTION

Behavioral genetic analyses can be a powerful tool in identifying the mechanisms underlying specific pathophysiological states. The most recent approaches in this regard have involved transgenic or knockout mouse models. However, as many pathologies involve multiple gene effects, or an interaction between genes and environment, an alternative approach to assessing pathophysiology involves the use of rat/mouse lines selectively bred to exhibit high or low levels of a given phenotype. These lines can then be used to identify specific neuroanatomical, physiological and/or chemical correlates of the pathology.

In our laboratory, considerable effort has been devoted to the selective breeding of two lines of rats that differ in amygdala excitability, as realized by either their *Fast* or *Slow* kindled seizure development using low-intensity electrical stimulation of the amygdala. The selection procedure for kindling was initially undertaken at McMaster University by Ron Racine. Following the 11th generation of selection, the two rat lines were transferred to Carleton University, where they currently reside. The foundation parent population used to create the two lines consisted of a cross between Long Evans Hooded and Wistar rats (Racine et al., 1999). Following amygdala kindling procedures, the rats with the faster and slower kindling rates were determined. In this determination, kindling rate was the total number of stimulations that were required to develop the first generalized, stage-5 motor convulsion (Racine, 1972). Rats with the faster and slower kindling rates in each generation were subsequently employed as breeders to develop the Fast and Slow kindling lines. Within 6 generations of selection, there was no overlap in the distribution of kindling rates between the two lines. After the 11th generation, selection was relaxed, and random breeding within each line has continued since that time with the provision that only second cousin pairings is allowed. The two lines are now in their 46th generation, and there is no indication of regression towards the mean or random drift. Stage-5 seizures currently are developed in an average of ~45 daily amygdala stimulations in the Slow rats, while only ~10 stimulations produce similar stage-5 seizures in the Fast rats (McIntyre et al., 1999a).

As a first step in identifying the mechanisms underlying the differential seizure susceptibility in the Fast and Slow rats, we have been assessing neurochemical and hormonal differences between the two lines under both basal conditions and in response to various challenges. For example, dramatic differences between the lines exist in their response to GABAergic modulators. Positive modulators, like sodium pentobarbital (McIntyre et al., 1999a) or diazepam (in progress), affect the Slow rats at much lower doses than those that are needed to influence either the Fast rats or Long Evans Hooded control rats. By contrast, negative modulators, like picrotoxin, bicuculline and pentylenetetrazol, have ED50s for producing convulsive seizures in the Fast rats that are significantly lower than control rats and much lower still than Slow rats (in preparation).

Exploration of the GABA receptors that might underwrite these differential pharmacological effects has revealed considerable differences between the two lines in GABA$_A$ subunit expression in several temporal lobe structures. In the amygdala, and adjacent piriform and perirhinal cortices, but not the dorsal hippocampus, the Fast rats overexpress several embryonic subunit forms of the GABA$_A$ receptor, including the $\alpha 2$, $\alpha 3$, $\alpha 5$ forms compared to controls and Slow rats. In stark contrast, the Slow rats underexpress those same embryonic subunits, while they dramatically overexpress the major adult form, $\alpha 1$ (Poulter et al., 1999). Because embryonic GABA$_A$ receptor subunit combinations do not code for adult channel kinetics and are not efficiently assembled into postsynaptic densities, we predicted that the amplitude and time course of inhibitory postsynaptic potentials (IPSPs) in the Fast rats might be different than in controls or Slow rats. Indeed, based on recent physiological experiments, this is the case (McIntyre et al., 1999b).

The functional consequences of these physiological differences, which include reduced amplitude and slower decaying IPSPs in Fast compared to control or Slow rats, is speculative. Recent work on synchronization and oscillatory behavior of synaptic networks has suggested that a powerful role is played by GABAergic mechanisms (Freund and Buzsaki, 1996; Traub et al., 1996). We predict (Poulter et al., 1999) that the embryonic subunit expressions of the Fast rats should result in faulty frequency modulation of network activity, leading to inappropriate timing of inhibitory events and slower oscillations. Because slower oscillations may be more efficient in recruiting synaptic pathways, this should increase the synchrony between interconnected structures and promote faster epileptogenesis. Of course, this precise outcome empirically defines the Fast kindling line (Racine et al., 1999; McIntyre et al., 1999a). In addition, with little oscillatory behavior in the higher frequency range (e.g., gamma), the normal mechanisms of attention associated with learning and memory could be compromised (Traub et al., 1998). This important prediction about the the Fast versus Slow rats is revisited below in our behavioral data sections.

Other mechanisms that could account for the differential epileptogenesis seen in the Fast and Slow lines are numerous. However, we can exclude several possibilities. For example, noradrenaline (NA) is one of the most effective known negative modulators of epileptogenesis (e.g., McIntye et al., 1979; Corcoran and Mason, 1980). Yet, baseline differences were not observed between the Fast and Slow rats in NA concentrations or utilization in either the amygdala, piriform or perirhinal cortices (McIntyre et al., 1999c). Similarly, other systems implicated in epilepsy are not altered in the two lines. Both NMDA and AMPA receptor binding in several temporal lobe structures in the Fast and Slow rats are similar (unpublished data), which agrees with our recent report showing that LTP and LTD in the two lines are not different (Racine et al., 1999). Also, in other unpublished findings, we observed (in collaboration with Z. Kokaia and colleagues) that the two lines do not differ with respect to the number of cholinergic neurons in the basal forebrain, or in their immunoreactivity. Thus, so far, altered $GABA_A$ receptor subunit expression appears to be uniquely related to the Fast and Slow kindling phenotypes.

COMORBIDITY AND EPILEPSY

When a particular phenotype is developed through selective breeding, it is not the case that only this one characteristic will differ between the lines. Pleiotropic effects (i.e., a gene or set of genes having more than a single phenotypic effect) can be expected, and multiple phenotypic differences might be apparent. Indeed, in selecting for amygdala kindling rates, one might be selecting for characteristics in structures distal to the amygdala itself (e.g., resulting in facilitated recruitment of distant structures). Furthermore, in selecting for rate of seizure development, and its associated neural substrate, it needs to be recognized that the substrate(s) and affected brain regions likely have multiple consequences beyond those influencing seizure susceptibility. In doing so, the selected gene(s) could provoke a *serial* cascade of neurochemical changes that leads ultimately to seizure (and other pathologies or phenotypes associated with this cascade), or it (they) may exert parallel cascades, only one of which involves seizure susceptibility. In the first instance, experimental modification of any neurochemical in the serial cascade ought to affect seizure activity. By contrast, where parallel effects occur, the covariates likely would be independent of seizure development, and their manipulation should be ineffective in modifying seizures. Further, it is possible that the gene(s) subserving seizure proneness, and those associated with other pathologies, may be closely located on a chromosome, such that they are inherited as a group (linkage). Thus, a particular phenotype may not be related causally to seizure or its consequences, but is predictive of seizure susceptibility (i.e., a marker gene).

In humans, psychopathology is often associated with comorbid features. Some of these features provide hints as to the processes governing the disorder, while others may be secondary to an associated stress or anxiety reaction. Numerous comorbid features have been identified in epileptic patients. It is not surprising, perhaps, that associated cognitive and memory disturbances have been observed (e.g., Binnie and Marston, 1992; Dodrill, 1992), as well as depression (Kanner and Nieto, 1999; Mendez, Cummings and Benson, 1986; Roberston, Trimble and Townsend, 1987). The memory effects could result from cumulative structural alterations associated with repeated seizures, to neurochemical changes stemming from seizures *per se*, to ongoing interictal discharges and/or other accompanying behavioral alterations, including the stress associated with seizures, a reaction to the psychosocial and economic sequelae of epilepsy, etc.

A role for physiological processes rather than psychosocial factors in comorbid features stems from the finding that epilepsy involving the left temporal lobe is more closely aligned with depression than is epilepsy involving the right hemisphere (Altshuler, Devinsky, Post and Theodore, 1990). Furthermore, it has been reported that temporal lobe epilepsy may be associated with increased impulsivity (and perhaps aggression related to impulsivity), at least within right lateralized patients (McIntyre, Pritchard and Lombroso, 1976). Indeed, impulsivity may account for the increased aggressiveness (frustration) that has been reported to occur in children with epilepsy (Hermann, 1982), although other experiential and psychosocial factors cannot be excluded (Hermann and Whitman, 1984). Finally, fear/anxiety has been reported as a comorbid characteristic of epilepsy in both human studies (de Albuquerque and de Campos, 1993; Ettinger, Weisbrot, Nolan, Gadow, Vitale, Andiola, Lenn, Novak, and Hermann, 1998), as well as in experiments involving rodents (DePaulis, Helfer, Deransart and Marescaux, 1997; Helfer, Deransart, Marescaux, and DePaulis 1996), and panic attacks have frequently been reported in epileptic patients (Alemayehu, Bergey, Barry, Krumholz, Wolf, Fleming and Frear, 1995; Genton, Bartolomei and Guerrini, 1995; Weilburg, Bear and Sachs, 1987). In view of these numerous comorbid features of epilepsy, it should not be surprising to find comorbidity in our rat lines selected for Fast or Slow seizure predispositions to amygdala kindling.

The section that follows provides a description of several behavioral characteristics evident in the Fast and Slow kindling lines of rats that, in some respects, are reminiscent of the diverse features characteristic of certain epileptic patients. It should be kept in mind, however, that our rat lines only have a genetic predisposition for or against epilepsy, and that in the absence of any manipulations (i.e., kindling or pharmacologic), the Fast line is not actually epileptic when behaviorally tested, but may become so 'spontaneously' as they mature into their mid-adult years.

FEAR AND ANXIETY

During the course of conducting kindling experiments with the Fast and Slow rats, one of the most notable characteristics between lines was the difference in ease of handling. Ordinarily, when an experimenter approaches the rats' cage (two per cage), the Fast rats rear up and look out of the cage, whereas the Slow rats retreat to the furthest corner. Moreover, with repeated handling by an experimenter, the Fast rats tend to be active and remain active, while the Slow rats soon become immobile and appeared 'frozen' with fear (if a novice researcher is bitten, it is always by a Slow rat). Thus, in formal experiments, we sought to assess whether the two rat lines could be distinguished from one another in their apparent fear/anxiety characteristics.

Habituation, Open-field Activity and Avoidance Learning

In a series of experiments by Mohapel and McIntyre (1998), marked behavioral differences between the rat lines were observed in several tasks. For instance, in a test of 'anxiety' using the elevated plus-maze, it was observed that the Slow rats tended to venture out on the open arms less readily than did the Fast rats, suggesting greater anxiety. Moreover, following exposure to a mild footshock stressor and later placement into a novel open-field, the Slow rats displayed a more pronounced suppression of motor activity than did the Fast rats. Likewise, the Slow rats exhibited more protracted freezing (immobility) in response to footshock than did Fast rats and, predictably, in an inhibitory avoidance task showed longer step-down latencies than Fast rats. The latter effect, however, was primarily apparent only when contextual cues associated with footshock were weakened, since in the presence of the primary fear cues both strains exhibited similar step-down latencies. In all these experiments, however, freezing behavior was prominent in the Slow rats' profile.

As might be expected from the protracted freezing shown by the Slow rats during inhibitory avoidance conditioning, they performed poorly compared to Fast rats in a simple one-way active avoidance test. In this case, the Slow rats remained immobile until the shock was delivered, rather than anticipating the shock with an active avoidance response as was observed in either control or Fast rats. Associated with this poor avoidance behavior in Slow rats were considerable vocalizations (anticipatory cries) never observed in the Fast rats. Similarly, we recently observed that the *initial* startle response to a loud auditory stimulus in a fear-potentiation paradigm was greater in the Slow than in the Fast rats (in progress). Furthermore, in that situation, as in the active avoidance paradigm, Slow rats consistently emitted vocal signs of distress when the conditioned fear cue was presented, a characteristic not seen in Fast rats. Although, the vocalizations in the Slow rats may simply have reflected the behavioral style of these animals rather than genuine fear expression, these findings are consistent with the suggestion of greater fear/anxiety in the Slow rats.

Taken together, it appears that the Slow rats are inherently more fearful or anxious than the Fast rats, at least with respect to the effects of footshock. However, when the rat lines were evaluated in various open-field tests, the data suggested that there may be factors other than, or in addition to, anxiety that could help account for the differential behaviors. In particular, as shown in Figure 1, when placed in an open field, the Slow rats were initially more active than the Fast rats; however, while habituation progressed readily in the Slow rats, activity levels in the Fast rats remained unchanged. Such an observation could be interpreted in numerous ways. First, the Fast rats might simply be more neophobic than the Slow rats, and thus, initially were less active. As the neophobia diminished, they began to explore the environment more readily than the Slow rats. Alternatively, the Slow rats might initially have been more fearful, leading to a transient motor excitation (as has been known to occur in some stress situations; Anisman, Zalcman, Shanks, and Zacharko, 1991), after which differential rates of habituation eliminated the differences first evident between the lines. A third, and more likely possibility, is that the rat lines initially differed in their anxiety about being placed in a new environment, and also differed with respect to habituation and/or attention associated with the test situation, consequently leading to their differential activity profiles over time.

To obtain further information about the behavioral styles of the rats in open-field situations, we chose to test the rats in an open-field emergence paradigm. In our test, rats were placed in a relatively small (20 x 30 x 20 cm) dark enclosed compartment, which was located within a larger bright white circular arena (120 cm diameter). Initially, Slow rats were found to leave the small compartment fairly quickly (12.5 ± 7.2 s) compared to Fast rats (109.2 ±33.6 s). With repeated testing, however, the latency to leave the compartment in Slow rats lengthened dramatically, reaching 244.6 ± 66.9 s on the third test day, while latency in Fast rats became slightly shorter (80.3 ± 8.6 s). This finding is reminiscent of the profile seen

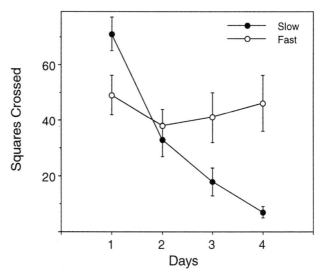

Figure 1. Mean (±SEM) squares crossed in an open-field test among Fast and Slow rats during a 5 min test on each of 4 consecutive days.

in an open-field exploratory test, where the Slow rats initially were more active than the Fast rats, but showed a pattern of rapid habituation over days that was not seen in the Fast rats, ultimately leading to much lower levels of activity in Slow rats. However, simply assessing open-field emergence itself may not be a good index of fear, since the behavior may be confounded by other factors. Thus, we re-addressed the experiment with new rats, which were now placed in the open arena, and their latency to enter the small, darkened chamber was recorded. During the initial trial, the latency to enter the darkened chamber in the two lines was similar (100.7 ± 73.8s and 97.0 ± 33.8s for Fast and Slow rats, respectively). However, over 3 test sessions the latency to enter the small chamber lengthened in the Slow rats (204.5 ± 82.5 s), while it decreased in the Fast rats (47.0 ± 26.6s). Thus, it seems likely again that there was an habituation of the initial behavior shown by the Slow rats, which was replaced by an 'opposite' behavioral profile, while the Fast rats changed comparatively little. Yet, as will be seen in ensuing sections, the behavioral repertoire of the two lines in response to a variety of experimental manipulations (including handling by the experimenter), precludes an explanation based simply on differences of habituation *per se*.

Response to Naturalistic Stressors

In an effort to identify more realistically the comorbid characteristics of the two lines, several experiments were undertaken to evaluate some of the behavioral and neuroendocrine responses that the rats displayed in response to different types of stressors. Rather than employ stressors such as footshock, we used more naturalistic stressors. In this regard, we chose (a) restraint, an experience that animals might undergo when captured, and (b) exposure to a ferret, a natural predator of the rat. The two lines displayed very different response profiles to these two stressors, but it appeared that the nature of the response depended on the specific stressor to which the animals were exposed. When placed in a triangular-shaped "baggie," which snuggly restrained the rat, the Slow rats immediately adopted a passive posture, rarely making any movements. In contrast, for almost half of the 15 min restraint period, the Fast rats struggled vigorously and gnawed at the restrainer (Anisman et al., 1997).

Unlike the behavioral profiles seen in response to restraint, when exposed to a ferret for a 15 min period, the Fast rats spent about 90% of their time in an immobile posture, while the Slow rats remained fairly active, moving away from the ferret as best they could (Anisman et al.,1997; McIntyre et al., 1999c). Furthermore, it was observed that pituitary ACTH release was associated with the defensive styles that rats adopted in response to the stressors. Among Slow rats, plasma ACTH was elevated to a similar degree in response to both stressors. However, in Fast rats, the ACTH increase was markedly greater in response to restraint than to the ferret (Anisman et al., 1997). In additional experiments, where blood was collected over time following stressor exposure (i.e., through an indwelling carotid cannula), plasma corticosterone levels in the Slow rats were greater in response to the ferret, while in the Fast rats the corticosterone levels were greater in response to restraint (Merali, Michaud, Kent, McIntyre, McIntosh, and Anisman, 1997).

Clearly, the defensive posture adopted by the two rat lines, as well as the hypothalamic-pituitary-adrenal (HPA) activation that occurred, was dependent upon the nature of the stressor to which they had been exposed. In his influential work, Bolles (1970) argued that in analyzing avoidance learning, it was essential to consider the species-specific defensive styles that animals displayed. Thereafter, Shettleworth (1972) advanced the theme that in addition to these defensive behaviors, it was important to consider the link between the warning signals and the stressor to which the animal was exposed (or the degree to which an animal was prepared to associate these stimuli). The findings in the Fast and Slow kindling rat lines makes it clear that defensive styles between lines may be exceedingly different, and that conclusions pertaining to these defensive styles need to consider, among other things, the specific stressor to which an animal is exposed. Thus, it may be premature to conclude that the Slow rats were more anxious in response to stressors in general, but rather it may be important to qualify such conclusions in terms of specific stressor events.

At this juncture, it seems judicious to raise an important caveat. Specifically, in some of the tests described above, the behavior of the animal was assessed under conditions of minimal stress (although some stress is obviously present even by placing an animal in an open-field), whereas in other situations, the response of an animal was assessed in response to clearly defined stressors (startle, restraint, ferret). It is certainly possible that basal levels of anxiety in the strains differ, and that anxiety levels differ yet again in response to specific stressors or in the presence of specific contextual cues that had been associated with stressors. Indeed, such an outcome was observed with respect to monoamine alterations elicited by various types of challenges in these rat lines. For instance, Merali, Michaud, McIntyre and Anisman (reported in Anisman and Merali, 1999) observed that under basal conditions, NA release in the amygdala, as determined *in vivo* in samples collected by microdialysis, was similar between the two rat lines. However, when exposed to a cytokine (in this instance interleukin-1β, as we were interested in evaluating immune-brain interactions), the release of NA was modest (~50%) and transient in the Fast line, whereas in the Slow line the increase was far more dramatic (~400%) and longer lasting (>2.5 hr). Likewise, analyses of postmortem tissues have indicated that while comparable monoamine levels and turnover were apparent in the lines under basal conditions, following stressor exposure, marked stressor- and amine-specific differences were observed between the strains (McIntyre et al., 1999c). Clearly, in considering the comorbid characteristics of pathological states (including epilepsy), it is important to distinguish between existent comorbidity versus vulnerability to such factors.

ASSOCIATIVE DISTURBANCES

It would appear that in many respects the Fast rats exhibit several aberrant behavioral styles beyond that simply of relatively lower levels of fear/anxiety. For example, rats placed in an open-field ordinarily display a progressive decrease of motor activity, reflecting habituation to environmental stimuli. Because the Fast rats did not show such habituation in the open-field task, the question arose as to whether they suffered attentional and/or associative deficits, which might be reflected in different situations. Accordingly, to test this possibility, we examined the two rat lines in several different learning tasks (beyond the active and inhibitory avoidance learning tasks described earlier) for performance differences associated with acquisition/retention of learning/memory. Most of these tests included opportunities for the rats to display differences in both reference memory and working memory. Reference memory, of course, refers to those aspects of the task that are consistent from trial to trial, like basic procedures, and are generally not vulnerable to interference effects; working memory holds information that is critical for successful performance of the immediate trial, but may not be relevant to subsequent trials, and generally is vulnerable to interference effects.

Delayed Alternation Performance

One sensitive test of working memory is found in the paired (information and choice) trials of the delayed alternation paradigm. In this paradigm, rats are trained to run down the alleyway of a T-maze, and are directed at the intersection of the T to either the left or right compartment in order to receive a reinforcement (information trial). On the ensuing trial (choice trial), which may occur at either short or long intervals after the information trial (thereby challenging working memory over varying intervals), the rats are required to respond by standard procedural or reference memory rules to select the same arm (matching) or the alternate arm (nonmatching) in order to obtain the reinforcement. In our *nonmatching* version of this task, the Fast rats were very inferior to Slow rats in reaching the performance criterion level for successful acquisition of the T-maze discrimination response (McLeod and McIntyre, 1995). Yet, over the first few days of acquisition, the speed of the Fast rats to run to the T-maze choice point was actually faster than that of the Slow rats (although eventually the latencies of both lines were equivalently short). Thus, it appeared that the Fast rats were always well motivated to reach the goal, and had acquired *part* of the basic concept, which involved running down the alleyway, at least as well as the Slow rats (reference memory); however, on the choice trials (working memory), the Fast rats seemed not to have benefited much from (or paid attention to?) the outcome of the previous information trials, as they usually chose inaccurately. In part, the poor choices among the Fast rats seemed to reflect the fact that when they arrived at the choice point, they would *rush* to whichever goal they were facing, rather than 'making a thoughtful' choice (as the Slow rats appeared to do) by looking back and forth at the goals (vacillating) before responding. It was not surprising then that increasing the delay between the information and choice trials (progressively from 1-5 min), which further challenges working memory, additionally degraded the performance of the Fast rats, while it had little or no effect on the Slow rats.

In this same experiment, after reaching the performance criterion of 80% correct choices, two parallel groups of pretrained Fast and Slow rats were then exposed to daily amygdala kindling – during the ongoing learning procedure. Each daily amygdala stimulation was followed 23 hr later by T-maze training. With the progressive development of convulsive stage-5 seizures, the T-maze performance of the Fast rats was significantly compromised, while similar stage-5 seizures had no measurable effect on the Slow rats. Even shortening the interval between the triggered kindled convulsion and the learning trials, from 23 hr to 1 hr to 10 min, did not change subsequent T-maze performance of the Slow rats, while it devastated the Fast rats, who now only performed at chance levels. Indeed, at the shortest interval (10 min), many of the Fast rats were unable to correctly perform even some of the basic reference memory requirements, but with no obvious effect on their motivation to perform in the task or their mobility.

Given the poor T-maze acquisition performance of the Fast rats, reflected largely by their working memory impairments, it seems possible that these rats suffer from a basic associative disturbance, which could be exacerbated by triggered seizures. Alternatively, or additionally, the Fast rats might experience impulsivity problems, which rendered them relatively inattentive to environmental cues during the information trials, and created the apparent working memory deficits.

Spatial and Cue Learning: Attentional Factors

To further assess the possibility of associative deficits, we evaluated performance in several variations of the Morris Water-maze (MWM). Even though the principle excitability differences seen in kindling between our two rat lines was in the amygdala and adjacent cortices (piriform and perirhinal), the hippocampus also showed intrinsic differences between lines (albeit to a lesser extent) (McIntyre et al., 1999a). We selected the MWM task to assess associative deficits because the integrity of hippocampus and parahippocampal cortices (including the perirhinal cortex) are believed to be critical for its acquisition. Although the cues by which a rat normally learns the MWM are based heavily on spatial or distal cues, one can train rats in this task with proximal cues; in the latter case, even hippocampal damaged rats usually appear normal (Aggleton, Hunt and Rawlins, 1986).

In the first form of the MWM task that we employed, the rats had to find the submerged platform to escape from the water with no previous training in the maze or assistance from proximal cues. The position of the platform remained *fixed* over the 4 days of testing, while the start position for each of the 4 successive daily trials varied; one min was allotted between trials. Although the position of the platform was quickly learned by both strains, the performance of the Slow rats was markedly superior to the Fast rats, during the first 2 days. A deficit in acquisition might reflect poorer working memory (i.e., remembering where the platform was on the preceding *trial* that day) or it might reflect poorer reference memory (i.e., the rat may not recall the platform position from the previous *day*, or even the *concept* that a submerged platform exists). In view of the latter possibility, we again examined

38

acquisition with the *fixed* position procedure, as above, but preceded this with pretraining using a raised, visible platform (4 trials on one day only). The Fast rats appeared to benefit substantially from this pretreatment session, as subsequent MWM performance was indistinguishable from that of the Slow rats. In effect, in this simple version of the MWM, the concept of what to do was needed by the Fast rats to allow them to perform at the level of the Slow rats.

This simple task can be made more difficult by moving the platform location between days, but holding it constant within a day. This manipulation gives information about working memory within a day versus reference memory between days that is not readily available using the fixed platform procedure (Whishaw, 1985). In this experiment, after minimal pretraining with the raised platform (1 trial on the first day only), the rats received 6 days of acquisition, with the submerged platform in a new location each day (8 trials/day). Thus, a between-days improvement of first trial latencies might be indicative of rats learning the concept of an escape platform, and improving performance following the first trial (trials 2-8) should be reflecting working memory (i.e., remembering that day's platform location). As seen in Figure 2, the performance of the Fast rats in this paradigm

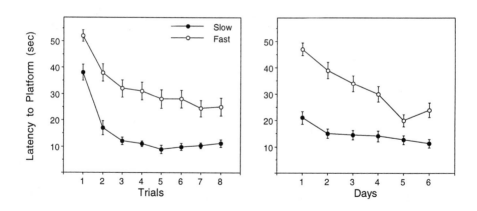

Figure 2. Mean (±SEM) latencies to reach the platform over trials (collapsed over 6 days; left-hand panel) and over days (right-hand panel). Fast and Slow rats were tested in a variable position Morris Water Maze task.

indicated very poor working memory relative to Slow rats. Having found the platform on the first trial each day, their response latencies on the ensuing 7 trials that day were much longer than the Slow rats. In effect, it appeared that Fast rats did not remember the position of the platform from the information trial it received 1 min earlier.

A second difference between the lines in that experiment concerned the first trial response each day. The Slow rats showed a steady 'first trial' improvement over days, such that the first trial latencies decline progressively by about 55% by the 6th day. The improvement over days in the Fast rats was far less evident. In their case, by the 6th day, their first trial latencies only declined by about 10% from that of the first day. In effect, these rats again were not acquiring/remembering the general concept (procedural strategy) or applying well it over days.

However, if the rats were given pretraining, consisting of 3 trials with the raised platform the day before beginning this experiment, the latency difference between the two lines was substantially reduced, and with 8 such pretraining trials, the latency differences were almost entirely eliminated. In effect, if the concept was well established that an escape platform existed, then subsequent deficits of both reference and working memory were markedly attenuated. Thus, again it appeared that the primary difficulty faced by the Fast rats was acquiring the basic concept (or effecting a strategy) of accessing the escape platform.

It is well established that spatial learning deficits, such as those associated with hippocampal disturbances, are not evident in tests where the position of the platform is cued by *proximal* stimuli (e.g., Aggleton, Hunt and Rawlins, 1986). Thus we considered the possibility that the performance deficits in Fast rats were additionally related to their poorer use of distal cues in the spatial learning task, deficits that might be ameliorated by appropriately placed proximal cues. In several experiments, with no pretraining, we evaluated the performance of the 2 lines in either the fixed or variable position MWM paradigms, but in each instance the position of the platform was cued (proximal) by a 12 cm long x 3 cm wide black object hanging 15 cm above the platform. Regardless of whether the platform position was fixed or varied over days, the performance of the Fast rats was inferior to the Slow rats. Thus, the proximal cue did not appear to facilitate acquisition in the Fast rats (beyond that seen in Slow rats), unlike the pretraining raised platform manipulation. The behavioral impairments, particularly evident on the first trial in both the fixed or variable position paradigms, again suggested that the Fast rats encountered difficulty in retaining the concept (established the previous day) of a *cued* escape platform.

In an effort to establish whether, the two rat lines were responding differentially to the proximal cue (possibly reflecting attentional differences), we trained the rats for 4 days in the *fixed* position paradigm with the cue hanging above the platform; but then, on the 5th day, either the platform or the cue was moved to a new location, diagonally opposite to the original training quadrant. Importantly, if the *cue was moved* (but the platform remained in the original position*)*, there was a substantial disruption across all 4 trials that day in the Fast rats, while only a slight disruption was evident in the Slow rats (Figure 3, right-hand panel). By contrast, when the cue remained over the original training quadrant on that 5th day, but the *platform was moved*, performance in both lines was dramatically disrupted (Figure 3, left-hand panel). However, in this case, the Slow rats reacquired their usual short latencies by the 3rd of 4 trials, while the Fast rats did not. These two different manipulations seem to suggest that Slow rats largely learn the MWM using spatial (distal) cues, given that altering the position of the proximal cue hardly disrupted their performance. In contrast, given the opportunity, the Fast rats will use both distal and proximal cues. Thus, moving the proximal cue negatively impacted mostly on the Fast rats. (Parenthetically, it is often thought that an animal does not use two cues when they are relevant but redundant. However, in fact, the proximal and distal cues were not totally redundant, as the distal cues signalled general location, while the proximal cue identified the precise location of the platform.) When the position of the platform was moved (which changed the distal cue information and dissociated it from the proximal cue information), both lines were affected, but more so in the Fast rats. Indeed, unlike the Slow rats, the Fast rats did not behaviorally recover from the cue movement during the 4 test trials.

To further understand the importance of distal versus proximal cues use in the MWM by the two lines, we trained them in the variable platform version of the task, where a new platform location was assigned each day but where that location was also signaled by the over-hanging proximal cue. Again, as in the fixed position task, the Fast rats remained slightly but significantly inferior to the Slow rats after 4 days of training. On the 5th day, the platform was again located in a new position (as on previous days), but this time the cue was moved to the diagonally opposite quadrant. Not surprisingly, this change impacted negatively on the Fast rats, but it also affected the Slow rats (albeit much less than in the Fast rats). Thus, it appears that in this task both strains increased their use of proximal cue information, perhaps

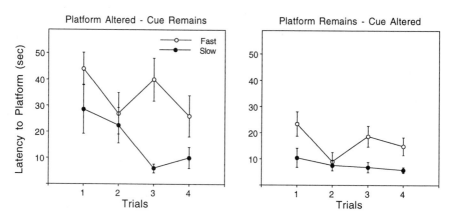

Figure 3. Mean (±SEM) latencies to reach the platform on 4 consecutive test day trials. Fast and Slow rats had been trained in a fixed-position Morris water-maze test where the position of the platform was proximally cued. On the test day, the platform position was altered and the cue remained in the original location (left-hand panel) or the platform remained in the original location and the cue position was altered (right-hand panel).

because on the first trial, the latter was a good predictor of the platform location for that day. Yet, even when that cue no longer predicted the platform location (at least not in the previous manner) on that 5th day, the Slow rats quickly reacquired short latency responses, while the Fast rats did not. Hence, the Slow rats either now ignored the cue or perhaps used it in a different way to predict the platform location (diagonally opposite to the cue, rather than beneath it). In future experiments, one could separate these two possibilities by moving the cue randomly on each of the 4 trials on this 5th day (i.e., so it had no predictive value).

Summarizing these various MWM results, we observed that the Fast rats can perform at levels similar to the Slow rats when given *pretraining*, where concepts pertinent to the problem solution might be acquired. Without this pretraining, the Fast rats showed significant acquisition deficits compared to the Slow rats, which included inferior performance on the *first* trial of each day (reflecting reference or long-term memory) and inferior improvement over the 4 daily trials (reflecting working memory). Further, when spatial or distal cues alone could predict the location of the platform, the Slow rats used them almost exclusively, while the Fast rats additionally relied on proximal cues when available. By contrast, Slow rats gave evidence of proximal cue use only if the latter predicted the platform location when distal cues did not (i.e., the first daily trial of the variable platform procedure). Clearly, the Fast rats show associative deficits in the MWM, but these deficits did not result from ubiquitous inattention to cues *per se*, but rather to particular cues. For example, the Fast rats appeared not to use the spatial or distal cues in the same manner as the Slow rats, so that without pretraining (raised platform) the Fast rats were more reliant on proximal cues, which would not ordinarily be used by the Slow rats. Further, if the proximal cues were no longer useful in a particular situation (e.g., first daily trial in the variable platform procedure or when the position of the cue and/or platform is altered), the Slow rats readily abandoned them for an alternative strategy, while the Fast rats did not. This observation, interestingly, is similar to many clinical examples of adult humans with learning disabilities, who have difficulty solving problems in the same facile manner as persons without learning disabilities, and where the therapist helps them discover alternative approaches and strategies to 'accommodate their special needs.'

IMPULSIVITY

Thus, all of the above data suggested two obvious possibilities. First, in some paradigms, the Fast rats may suffer associative deficits involving connections between stimuli or between stimuli and response outcomes. Second, the Fast rats may suffer from a problem related to impulsivity and/or an inability to attend to appropriate environmental stimuli, culminating in associative types of deficits. Of course, it is fairly well established that in humans, attention deficit hyperactivity disorder is frequently accompanied by a learning disability, and both these characteristics exhibit high comorbidity with numerous other disorders, including depression, anxiety disorder, conduct disorder, and substance abuse (e.g., Hooper and Olley, 1996). Indeed, a characteristic feature that we have observed in the Fast rats, in numerous situations, is their high level of disinhibition (or impulsive behavioral styles). In this regard, it will be recalled that the Fast rats did not habituate normally in open field environments, they could not easily withhold responses in an inhibitory avoidance paradigm and, in a T-maze appetitive task, they 'accidentally selected' the arm into which they over-ran from the stem approach.

However, the impulsive response style of the Fast rats is not limited to exploratory or appetitive tests. In our recent experiments (Michaud et al., 1999), the impulsivity of the Fast rats was dramatically apparent in their sexual response to conspecific females. Ordinarily, rats will attempt to mate with a female based on specific cues, which include visual, auditory, and olfactory stimuli. Thus, in rodents, as in other mammals, an estrous female will elicit sexual behaviors from the male that are not forthcoming to a non-estrous female. In our experiments, it was observed that Slow males *never* attempted to mount a non-estrous female. On the other hand, after introduction of a female, Fast males quickly attempted to mount her, independent of her state of estrous. Further, even when vigorously rebuffed, they persevered in this behavior. Thus, the sexually aggressive response of the Fast males to females was not diminished by the absence of estrous or estrous-associated behaviors (i.e., appropriate social signals) in the females. We suggest that the immediate and sustained inappropriate responses of the Fast rats to nonestrous females is a manifestation of their high impulsivity. Interestingly, this inappropriate Fast rat behavior was evident even in the face of significantly lower testosterone levels compared to Slow rats. We do not know whether the impulsivity comorbid with inappropriate sexually related responses in Fast rats suggests this as a model

42

for sexual predatory behavior, but it certainly and dramatically indicates very socially inappropriate behavior by the Fast rats.

CONCLUSION

At the present time, our data are consistent with the proposition that a *predisposition* for rapid amygdala kindling is associated with learning impairments, perhaps secondary to impulsivity and/or deficits of attention, whereas the *predisposition* to resist amygdala kindling is associated with relatively high levels of fear/anxiety and a very 'conservative personality'. Although the Fast and Slow rats also differ across numerous biological dimensions, including differences of HPA axis activation and $GABA_A$ subunit expression, it is still premature to make conclusions about the specific relations between the behavioral and neurochemical substrates in these two lines. While it is our contention that the Fast rats may be useful in modelling human attentional/impulse control disorders, this conclusion must await tests in the Fast rats evaluating the efficacy of pharmacological treatments known to attenuate such behaviors in humans (e.g., methylphenidate, amphetamine, etc.).

[1] Supported by Grants from the Medical Research Council of Canada and from the Natural Sciences and Engineering Research Council of Canada. H.A. is Senior Research Fellow of the Ontario Mental Health Foundation. We are indebted to Charlene Dodds, Tammy Legault, Nathalie Lukenbil, Owen Kelly, Matt D'Angelis for their work in the collection of some of the Morris Water-maze and anxiety data. As well, Zul Merali, Dave Michaud, Pam Kent, Shawn Haley, Jerzy Kulczycki, who were responsible for the *in vivo* neurochemical work, as well as the documentation of male sexual behaviors in response to estrous and nonestrous female rats.

REFERENCES

Aggleton, J.P., Hunt, P.R., Rawlins, J.N.P. (1986) The effects of hippocampal lesions upon spatial and non-spatial tests of working memory. Behav Brain Res. 19: 133-146.
Alemayehu, S., Bergey, G.K., Barry, E., Krumholz, A., Wolf, A., Fleming, C.P., Frear, E.J. (1995) Panic attacks as ictal manifestations of parietal lobe seizures. Epilepsia 36: 824-830.
Altshuler, L.L., Devinsky, O., Post, M.D., Theodore, W. (1990) Depression, anxiety, and temporal lobe epilepsy: Laterality of focus and symptoms. Arch Neurol. 47: 284-288.
Anisman, H., Zalcman, S., Shanks, N., Zacharko, R.M. (1991) Multisystem regulation of performance deficits induced by stressors: An animal model of depression. In: A.Boulton, G. Baker, M. Martin-Iverson M. eds. Neuromethods, vol. 19: Animal Models of Psychiatry, II. New Jersey: Humana Press, 1-59.
Anisman, H., Lu, Z.W., Song, C., Kent, P., McIntyre, D.C., Merali, Z. (1997) Influence of psychogenic and neurogenic stressors on endocrine and immune activity: differential effects in fast and slow seizing rat strains. Brain Behav Immun. 11: 63-74.
Anisman, H. and Merali, Z. (1999) Anhedonic and anxiogenic effects of cytokine exposure. Adv Exp Med Biol. 461: 199-233.
Binnie, C.D. and Marston, D. (1992) Cognitive deficits of interictal discharges. Epilepsia 33: S11-S17.
Bolles, R.C. (1970) Species-specific defense reactions and avoidance learning. Psychol. Rev. 77: 32-48.
Corcoran, M.E. and Mason, S.T. (1980) Role of forebrain catecholamines in amygdaloid kindling. Brain Res. 190: 473-484.
de Albuquerque, M. and de Campos, C.J. (1993) Epilepsy and anxiety. Arq Neuropsiquiatr. 51: 313-318.
DePaulis, A., Helfer, V., Deransart, C., Marescaux, C. (1997) Anxiogenic-like consequences in animal models of complex partial seizures. Neurosci Biobehav Rev. 21: 767-774.
Dodrill, C.B. (1992) Interictal cognitive aspects of epilepsy. Epilepsia 33: S7-S10.

Ettinger, A.B., Weisbrot, D.M., Nolan, E.E., Gadow, K.D., Vitale, S.A., Andiola, M.R., Lenn, N.J., Novak, G.P., and Hermann, B.P. (1998) Symptoms of depression and anxiety in pediatric epilepsy patients. Epilepsia 39: 595-599.

Freund, T., Buzsaki, G. (1996) Interneurons of the hippocampus. Hippocampus. 6: 345-474.

Genton, P., Bartolomei, F., Guerrini, R. (1995) Panic attacks mistaken for relapse of epilepsy. Epilepsia 36: 48-51.

Helfer, V., Deransart, C., Marescaux, C., DePaulis, A. (1996) Amygdala kindling in the rat: anxiogenic-like consequences. Neuroscience 73: 971-978.

Hermann, B.P. (1982) Neuropsychological functioning and psychopathology in children with epilepsy. Epilepsia 23: 545-554.

Hermann, B.P. and Whitman, S. (1984) Behavioral and personality correlates of epilepsy: A review, methodological critique, and conceptual model. Psychol Bull. 95: 451-497.

Hooper, S.R. and Olley, J.G. (1996) Psychological comorbidity in adults with learning disabilities. In N. Gregg, C. Hoy and A.F. Gay eds. Adults With Learning Disabilities. The Guilford Press, New York, pp. 162-183.

Kanner, A.M. and Nieto, J.C. (1999) Depressive disorders in epilepsy. Neurology 53: S26-S32.

McIntyre, D.C., Saari, M., and Pappas, B.A. (1979) Potentiation of amygdala kindling in adult or infant rats by injection of 6-hydroxydopamine. Exp. Neurol. 63: 527-544.

McIntyre, D.C., Kelly, M.E., Dufresne, C. (1999a) FAST and SLOW amygdala kindling rat strains: comparison of amygdala, hippocampal, piriform and perirhinal cortex kindling. Epilepsy Res., 35: 197-209.

McIntyre, D.C., Hutcheon, B., Poulter, M.O. (1999b) Altered $GABA_A$ receptor kinetics in the perirhinal cortex of seizure-prone and resistant rats. Soc Neurosci Abstr. 25: 539.

McIntyre, D.C., Kent, P., Hayley, S., Merali, Z., and Anisman, H. (1999c) Influence of psychogenic and neurogenic stressors on neuroendocrine and central monoamine activity in fast and slow kindling rats. Brain Res. 840: 65-74.

McIntyre, M., Pritchard, P.B., Lombroso, C.T. (1976) Left and right temporal lobe epileptics: a controlled investigation of some psychological differences. Epilepsia 17: 377-386.

McLeod, W.S. and McIntyre, D.C. (1995) The effects of amygdala kindling on T-maze performance in epileptogenetically Fast and Slow kindling rat strains. Soc Neurosci Abstr. 21: 2115.

Mendez, M.F., Cummings, J.L., and Benson, D.F. 1986. Depression in epilepsy. Arch Neurol. 43, 766-770.

Merali, Z., Michaud, D., Kent, P., McIntyre, D.C., McIntosh, J., Anisman, H. (1997) Effects of psychological (ferret exposure) and restraint stressors on amygdalar CRF release and endocrine responses in two differentially stress-sensitive rat strains. Soc Neurosci Abst 23: 1077.

Michaud, D., McIntyre, D.C., Anisman, H, and Merali, Z. (1999) Rat strains with high versus low sexual reactivity: Behavioral and lateralized amygdala CRH responses of males. Soc Neurosci Abst. 25: 346.

Mohapel, P. and McIntyre, D.C. (1998) Amygdala kindling-resistant (SLOW) or -prone (FAST) rat strains show differential fear responses. Behav Neurosci. 112: 1402-1413.

Poulter, M.O., Brown, L.A., Tynan, S., Willick, G., William, R., McIntyre, D.C. (1999) Differential expression of α_1, α_2, α_3, and α_5 $GABA_A$ receptor subunits in seizure-prone and seizure-resistant rat models of temporal lobe epilepsy. J Neurosci. 19: 4654-4661.

Racine, R.J. (1972) Modification of seizure activity by electrical stimulation: II. Motor seizure. Electroencephalogr Clin Neurophysiol. 32: 281-294.

Racine, R.J., Steingart, M., and McIntyre, D.C. (1999) Development of kindling-prone and kindling-resistant rats: selective breeding and electrophysiological studies. Epilepsy Res. 35:183-195.

Roberston, M.M., Trimble, M.R., Townsend, H.R.A. (1987) Phenomenology of depression in epilepsy. Epilepsia, 28: 364-368.

Shettleworth, S.J. (1972) Constraints on learning. In D.S. Lehrman, R.A. Hinde, E. Shaw, eds. Advances in the Study of Behavior. Academic Press, New York.

Traub, R.D., Whittington, M.A., Colling, S.B., Buzsaki, G., and Jefferys, J.G. (1996) Analysis of gamma rhythms in the rat hippocampus in vitro and in vivo. J Physiol. 493: 471-484.

Traub, R.D., Whittington, M.A., Stanford, I.M., and Jefferys, J.G. (1996) A mechanism for generation of long-range synchronous fast oscillations in the cortex. Nature 383: 621-624.

Traub, R.D., Spruston, N., Soltesz, I., Konnerth, A., Whittington, M.A., and Jefferys, J.R. (1998) Gamma-frequency oscillations: a neuronal popultation phenomenon, regulated by synaptic and intrinsic cellular process, and inducing synaptic plasticity. Prog Neurobiol. 55: 563-575.

Weilburg, J.B., Bear, D.M., Sachs, G. (1987) Three patients with concomitant panic attacks and seizure disorder: possible clues to the neurology of anxiety. Am J Psychiat. 144: 1053-1056.

Whishaw, I. Q. (1985) Formation of a place learning-set by the rat: a new paradigm for neurobehavioral studies. Physiol Behav. 35: 139-143.

4 BEHAVIORAL AND NEUROHORMONAL SEQUELAE OF PRENATAL STRESS: A SUGGESTED MODEL OF DEPRESSION

Marta Weinstock

INTRODUCTION

Although the etiology of depressive mood disorders is still unclear, it is strongly influenced by genetic (McGuffin, 1988; Kendler et al., 1992) and environmental factors which include the maternal milieu during gestation (Weinstock, 1997). Recurring inescapable or uncontrollable stress can lead to chronic anxiety, feelings of hopelessness and defeat, and depression. This is associated with overactivity of corticotropin releasing hormone (CRH) and dysregulation of the hypothalamic-pituitary adrenal (HPA) axis (Chrousos and Gold, 1992; Behan et al., 1997). Mood disorders have also been reported in the offspring of women that were exposed during pregnancy to physical and psychological stress, such as marital and family discord (Stott, 1973), the threat of impending war (Meier, 1985), or death of the spouse in World War II (Huttunen and Niskanen, 1978). Those children exhibited excessive crying and clinging to the mother and unsociable or inconsiderate behavior towards other children. In prenatally-stressed (PS) teenagers, there was a higher incidence of alcohol intake, antisocial and criminal behavior, depressive and neurotic episodes (Huttunen and Niskanen, 1978). Since of necessity, such analyses in humans are retrospective and cannot be controlled for genetic and postnatal environmental factors, most of our information about the behavioral and neurochemical sequelae of gestational stress is derived from studies in experimental animals. This chapter describes the experimental evidence obtained in such studies in support of the hypothesis that prenatal stress can induce permanent changes in the behavior, regulation of the HPA axis and corticotropin releasing hormone (CRH) that are consistent with those seen in depressive mood disorders.

BEHAVIORAL EFFECTS OF PRENATAL STRESS

Disturbed Social Interaction

It is well recognized that disturbed social behavior occurs in almost all mood disorders and may not only be a consequence of the disorder but an intrinsic component of the underlying pathological process. The disturbance in social behavior seen in PS children has also been described in experimental animals. The young offspring of Rhesus monkeys that had been removed from their home cages and repeatedly subjected to noise stress during mid-late gestation showed abnormal clinging behavior to other monkeys (Clarke and Schneider, 1993). Rats born to mothers that had been stressed during the last week of pregnancy by uncontrollable electric foot-shock or thrice daily restraint had a reduced propensity for juvenile play and for social interaction (Ward and Stehm, 1991; Takahashi et al., 1992). This showed that prenatal stress in animals causes long-lasting abnormalities in social behavior, reminiscent of those seen in humans.

Learned Helplessness or Behavioral Despair

The tendency to adopt a passive behavior when faced with inescapable unpleasant events is one characteristic of depressed subjects. Lack of control over aversive environmental events results in the expectancy that subsequent aversive stimuli will also be uncontrollable and leads to a behavior designated as "learned helplessness" (Seligman 1972). This forms the basis of a model of depression in experimental animals (Porsolt et al., 1978; Willner, 1986). Although the degree of learned helplessness displayed by rats appears to be genetically determined (Weiss et al., 1998), it can also be increased by prenatal stress. Secoli and Teixeira, (1998), found a greater degree of learned helplessness in PS rats than in controls 24 hours after subjection to inescapable footshock.

A type of passive behavior indicative of learned helplessness can be induced in mice and rats by forcing them to swim for 15 min in a narrow cylinder from which there is no escape and in which their movements are restricted. When re-exposed to the cylinder the following day for 5 minutes, many of them stop struggling after a short while and adopt an immobile posture. Pretreatment of the animals with electroconvulsive shock, or different classes of drugs that have antidepressant activity in human subjects, decreases the duration of immobility (Porsolt et al., 1978; Kitada et al., 1981). Although the exact mechanism of action of the drugs is not yet clear, the findings suggest that there may be some common features between depressive mood disorders in humans and this behavior in rats. Table 1 summarizes the data from three studies showing the effect of prenatal stress on this form of learned helplessness. The proportion of time spent by control male Sprague-Dawley rats in floating or immobile behavior after re-exposure to the swimming chamber was already high compared with that of females leaving little room to demonstrate a significant increase after prenatal stress (Alonso et al., 1991; Barros and Ferigolo, 1998). Two different types of prenatal stress, daily restraint and unpredictable loud noise and flashing light increased immobility in females, while daily immersion in cold water (5°C) also increased learned helplessness in Wistar male rats.

Table 1. Effect of prenatal stress on behavior in the forced swim test

Type of maternal stress	Rat strain and sex	% of time in immoblity	
		Controls	PS
Daily restraint, day 15-parturition[1]	Sprague-Dawley males	68 ± 3	70 ± 5
Daily restraint, day 15-parturition[1]	Sprague-Dawley females	50 ± 4	67 ± 3*
Unpredictable noise thrice weekly[2]	Sprague-Dawley males	55.5 ± 9.9	67.4 ± 4.0
Unpredictable noise thrice weekly[2]	Sprague-Dawley females	27.6 ± 5.0	45.2 ± 5.6*
Daily immersion in cold water from day 5 gestation	Wistar males	60.0 ± 5.7	81.1± 6.7*

Significantly different from control rats, P<0.05. [1] Alonso et al., 1991;
[2] Poltyrev and Weinstock (unpublished observations) [3] Drago et al., 1999.

It was possible to induce immobile behavior in normal rats similar to that seen in PS rats by the infusion of CRH into the locus coeruleus (Butler et al., 1990). Moreover, the duration of immobility was significantly decreased by adrenalectomy (Mitchell and Meaney, 1991) and metyrapone, which inhibits corticosterone synthesis (Baez and Volosin, 1994). This suggested that greater activity of CRH and release of corticosterone may mediate the development of learned helplessness.

Hedonic Deficit

Anhedonia, or an inability to feel joy or pleasure is a characteristic feature of depression. Such a condition can be induced in rats by chronic unpredictable or inescapable stress, and is indicated by a disruption of appetite and a decreased desire to consume sweet food or drink. The latter include saccharine that has no nutritive value but its ingestion is thought to be pleasurable in this species (Katz, 1982). The deficit induced by uncontrollable stress in the consumption of sweet substances can be corrected by chronic treatment with different types of antidepressant drugs (Willner et al., 1987; Moreau et al., 1994).

Sex differences are also found in the amount of consumption of sweet solutions by rats, with females generally consuming higher amounts than males. In a test of sweet preference in which the rats could choose freely between saccharine solution (3mM) or tap water, PS females, but not male littermates, showed a significantly reduced sweet preference compared to controls (Keshet and Weinstock, 1995). The findings that prenatal stress can also induce a hedonic deficit provided further support for its ability to cause long-term alterations in behavior that are reminiscent of depression.

Heightened Anxiety

A state of chronic anxiety often accompanies or precedes that of depression and both can result from persistent or uncontrollable stress (Chrousos and Gold, 1992). Several studies have shown that prenatal stress induces behavior that is compatible with greater timidity or anxiety. For example, PS rats markedly suppress their normal activities of food seeking and pup-retrieval under aversive conditions (Fride et al., 1985; 1986) and show a higher incidence of defecation accompanied by less exploration in an intimidating novel environment (Thompson, 1957; Wakshlak and Weinstock, 1990). The conflict that is induced in rodents by their desire to explore and their fear of open spaces and heights, which they find aversive, forms the basis of the plus-maze test of anxiety. The greater the fear or anxiety, the less time the rat spends in the open arms of the maze. This has been validated by its sensitivity to agents that are either anxiolytic or anxiogenic in human subjects, which increase or decrease the amount of time in the open arms, respectively (Pellow and File, 1986).

Several studies have shown that different types of prenatal stress in three different rat strains reduce by about 50% the proportion of time spent in the open arms of the maze (Table 2). This behavior is consistent with greater anxiety in a novel, intimidating situation and is associated with increased activation of the HPA axis (File et al., 1994).

Table 2. Effect of prenatal stress on open arm entries in plus maze

Type of maternal stress	Rat strain	Sex	% of time in open arms	
			Control rats	PS rats
Unpredictable noise and light[1]	Sabra	F	23.2 ± 3.4	10.2 ± 2.7*
Unpredictable noise and light[2]	Sprague-Dawley	M	15.5 ± 3.8	4.9 ± 2.9*
Daily restraint[3]	Sprague-Dawley	M	26.5 ± 2.4	18.0 ± 2.8*
Daily restraint[4]	Long-Evans	M	12.1 ± 1.8	6.3 ± 1.6*

[1]Wakshlak and Weinstock, 1990; [2]Poltyrev et al., 1996; [3]Vallee et al., 1997; [4]Zimmerberg and Blaskey, 1998.

A similar reduction in the amount of time spent in the open arms of the plus maze was seen in normal rats after the intracerebral injection of CRH. The effects of the peptide and of prolonged inescapable stress on anxiogenic behavior were prevented by pretreatment with a CRH antiserum or a specific antagonist (Dunn and Berridge, 1990). These findings support the role of CRH in the mediation of both anxiety and despair and suggest that its increased release and/or activity may be responsible for the behavioral abnormalities induced by prenatal stress. This suggestion could be substantiated by the demonstration that a specific CRH antagonist can abolish the difference in behavior between PS and control rats.

NEUROCHEMICAL EFFECTS OF PRENATAL STRESS

Dysregulation of the Hypothalamic-pituitary Adrenal Axis

Repeated exposure of an individual to situations that are uncontrollable, aversive or unrewarding result in a failure of the individual to adapt to them. This induces dysregulation of the HPA axis through a reduction in the negative feedback by glucocorticoids on CRF and ACTH release and on the adrenal itself (Delbende et al., 1992). Such dysregulation occurs in individuals with endogenous depression and is indicated by the finding of higher levels of circulating cortisol at rest and after stress, and a failure of the glucocorticoid, dexamethasone to suppress them, testifying to an impairment in the negative feedback control (Holsboer et al., 1994). Depressed individuals also have increased amounts of CRH in the CSF (Nemeroff, 1984). This peptide is not only instrumental in causing the release of ACTH from the pituitary, but also serves as a neurotransmitter. CRH-containing neurones are found in several brain areas including the amygdala, septum and brainstem nuclei controlling the activity of the sympathetic nervous system (Delbende et al., 1992).

In 1986, we showed that the HPA axis of PS rats, unlike that of controls, failed to adapt to repeated exposure to the same novel environment and responded with an increased release of corticosterone even after 8 exposures (Fride et al., 1986). Subsequently, we and others reported that PS rats showed a delayed return to normal in plasma B and had a lower number of hippocampal glucocorticoid receptors (Weinstock et al., 1992; Henry et al., 1994; Maccari et al., 1995). No differences were found in the amounts of CRH in the median eminence of PS rats and controls at rest, or after exposure to noise stress (Weinstock and Tilders, unpublished observations). However, PS rats had higher levels of the peptide in the amygdala and a greater amount was released in response to stimulation (Cratty et al., 1995). CRH cell bodies in the amygdala contains glucocorticoid receptors, suggesting that the steroid may act at this site as part of the negative feetback loop to control the release of the peptide (Gray, 1993). Long-lasting up-regulation may occur in CRH-ergic transmission in the amygdala, partly due to impaired feedback, which could be important in the generation of hyperemotional offspring by gestational stress.

In response to footshock stress PS rats showed significantly greater increases than controls in plasma noradrenaline in addition to corticosterone. This indicated that they had enhanced activation of the sympatho-adrenal and HPA systems that could have resulted from greater activity of CRH on brainstem noradrenergic neurones (Weinstock et al., 1998). Mild stress and intracerebroventricular (icv) injection of CRH in PS rats also caused the release of significantly larger amounts of acetylcholine in the hippocampus than in control rats (Day et al., 1998). This effect of CRH was independent of its ability to release corticosterone, further testifying to an influence of prenatal stress on the neurotransmitter role of CRH.

Depression, CRH and Immune Function

A significant correlation has been found between the severity of depressive symptoms and anxiety and suppression of immune competence (Irwin, 1995). The latter may result at least in part, from increased activity of CRH, since its injection (icv) in rats decreases some measures of immune function through activation of brainstem noradrenergic nuclei and the sympatho-adrenal system (Irwin, 1994). Prenatal stress also suppressed a number of indices of immune function in adult male and female rats. These included natural killer cell cytotoxicity in splenic and circulating lymphocytes and the proliferation of lymphocytes in response to a B-cell mitogen (Kay et al., 1998). Prenatal stress did not induce any alteration in the distribution of subsets of lymphocytes in either the spleen or blood indicating that the changes in proliferative and cytotoxic activity resulted from functional modifications of effector mechanisms in the cells rather than from alterations in their migration between immune compartments. These data showed that prenatal stress may compromise immune function and could explain the higher incidence of respiratory disease in infants born to mothers that had experienced uncontrollable psychological stress during pregnancy (Stott, 1973).

Disturbance in Circadian Rhythm in Depression and After Prenatal Stress

Alterations in circadian rhythms of body temperature and plasma cortisol are found in subjects with endogenous depression and have been suggested to play an aetiological role in this illness (Goodwin et al., 1982). Treatment with antidepressants can restore normal rhythm together with their ability to improve the depressive symptomatology. Prenatal stress induced a phase shift in the circadian rhythm for circulating corticosterone in rats in a similar direction to that seen in depression (Koehl et al., 1997). Although the mechanism by which this phase-shift is produced is not yet clear, the possibility should be considered that it is due to the action of an excess of maternal steroid released during stress on developing fetal glucocorticoid receptors in the suprachiasmatic nucleus (see below).

Maternal Stress Hormones Mediate Alterations in HPA Axis and Behavior in Offspring

In 1957, Thompson suggested that the development and maturation of the fetal HPA axis is sensitive to maternal hormones reaching it during a critical period in gestation and genetic differences in anxiety-related behavior may be mediated by the level of corticosterone in the maternal circulation. This was demonstrated recently by the finding that rats from the Wistar strain, bred for high levels of anxiety in the plus maze and forced swim test, had significantly greater plasma concentrations of corticosterone during pregnancy than those with low anxiety (Neumann et al., 1998). Corticosterone is lipid soluble and readily passes from the maternal into the fetal circulation (Zarrow et al., 1970). Restraint, intermittent loud noise or footshocks all increase corticosterone in the maternal blood and can affect fetal brain development during the last week of gestation (Weinstock et al., 1988). This was demonstrated recently in pregnant rats subjected to footshocks, which had higher plasma corticosterone even 48 hours after the shock. Moreover, on day 20 of gestation the plasma concentration in the fetuses of stressed mothers was higher than that in controls (Takahashi et al., 1998). This showed that fetal blood levels of corticosterone are increased by the stress at a time when the control of fetal HPA axis is independent of that of the mother (Milkovic et al., 1973).

Direct evidence in support of a role for maternal corticosterone in mediating the dysregulation of the HPA axis in the offspring was provided by Barbazanges et al., (1996). They showed that maternal adrenalectomy, with the addition of corticosterone to maintain normal levels, (but not those reached during stress) prevented the development of an abnormal response to stress in their adult offspring. These included the slower return to normal of stress-induced elevations in corticosterone and a lower number of hippocampal corticosteroid receptors. While these findings showed that the excess levels of maternal corticosterone could have been instrumental in impairing the feedback regulation in the HPA axis of the offspring, we do not know whether they are also responsible for the induction of the learned helplessness type of behavior seen in PS rats. Neither is it known if the action of excess corticosterone on the fetal brain during gestation can also increase the neurotransmitter actions of CRH, and whether they can be prevented by adrenalectomy and maintenance of normal levels of the steroid in the presence of maternal stress.

However, evidence from other studies suggested that excess amounts of opioid peptides are also released during maternal stress and produce alterations in the fetal opioid systems and subsequent behavior (Poltyrev and Weinstock, 1997). The opioid antagonist, naltrexone administered continuously to the pregnant rat during the last week of gestation, prevented the appearance in the adult PS offspring of heightened anxiety in the plus maze test (Keshet and Weinstock, 1995) and aberrant sexual behavior (Ward et al., 1986). It is not yet known whether the abnormalities in behavior in PS rats are related to an imbalance between the actions of CRH and opioid peptides. It also remains to be determined whether chronic opioid receptor blockade during gestation in stressed rats can also normalize the regulation of the HPA axis in the offspring.

CONCLUSIONS

The foregoing data show that prenatal stress can induce several of the behavioral symptoms associated with depressive illness. They include abnormalities in social behavior, a hedonic deficit, a greater intensity of leaned helplessness in the face of inescapable stress and increased anxiety in intimidating situations. PS animals also show a phase-shift in the circadian rhythm of plasma corticosterone and abnormalities in the feedback regulation of the HPA axis similar to that in depressed human subjects. There are indications that PS rats may have increased neuronal activity of CRH that could be responsible for their hyperanxiety and suppressed immune function. The alterations in the HPA axis appear to be due to the action of excess amounts of corticosterone, released into the maternal blood by the stress, on the developing fetal brain. It is not clear however, whether the steroid is also responsible for the behavioral abnormalities or whether other maternal hormones, like opioid peptides also play a role in their aetiology.

REFERENCES

Alonso, S.J., Arevalo, R., Afonso, D., Rodriguez, M. (1991) Effects of maternal stress during pregnancy on forced swimming test behavior of the offspring, Physiol. Behav. 50: 511-517.

Baez, M. and Volosin, M. (1994) Corticosterone influences forced swimming immobility. Pharmacol. Biochem. Behav. 49: 729-736.

Barbazanges, A. Piazza, P.V., Le Moal, M., Maccari, S. (1996) Maternal glucocorticoid secretion mediates long-term effects of prenatal stress. J. Neurosci. 16: 3963-3969.

Barros, H.M., Ferigolo, M. (1998) Ethopharmacology of imipramine in the forced swim test: gender differences. Neurosci. Biobehav. Revs. 23: 279-286.

52

Behan, D.P., Grigoriadis, D.E., Lovenberg, T., Chalmers, D., Heinrichs, S., Liaw, C., et al. (1994) Stress, antidepressant drugs, and the locus coeruleus. Brain Res. Bull. 35: 545-556.

Britton, D.R., Koob,; G.F., Rivier J., Wale, W. (1982) Intraventricular corticotrophin-releasing factor enhances behavioral effects of novelty. Life Sci. 31: 363-367.

Butler P.D., Weiss, J.M., Stout, J.C., Nemeroff, C.B. (1990) Corticotrophin-releasing factor produces fear-enhancing and behavioral activating effects following infusion into the locus coeruleus. J. Neurosci. 10: 176-183.

Chrousos, G.P., and Gold, P.W. (1992) The concepts of stress and stress system disorders,-overview of physical and behavioral homeostasis. JAMA 267: 1244-1253.

Clarke, A.S., Schneider, M.L. (1993) Prenatal stress has long-term effects on behavioral responses to stress in juvenile rhesus monkeys. Dev. Psychobiol. 26: 293-304.

Cratty, M.S., Ward, H.E., Johnson, E.A., Azzaro, A.J., Birkle, D.L. (1995) Prenatal stress increases corticotropin-releasing factor (CRF) content and release in rat amygdala minces. Brain Res. 675: 297-302.

Day, J.C., Koehl, M., Deroche, V. LeMoal, M., Maccari, S. (1998) Prenatal stress enhances stress- and corticotropin-releasing factor-induced stimulation of huppocampal acetylcholine release in adult rats. J. Neurosci. 18: 1886-1892.

Delbende, C., Delarue, C., Lefebvre, H., Tranchard Bunel, D., Szafarczyk, A., Mocaer, E. et al. (1992). Glucocorticoids, transmitters and stress. Brit. J. Psychriatr. 160 (suppl. 15): 24-34.

Drago, F., Di-Leo, F., Giardina L. (1999) Prenatal stress induces body weight deficit and behavioral alterations in rats: the effect of diazepam. Eur. Neuropsycopharmacol. 9: 239-245.

Dunn, A.J., Berridge, C.W. (1990) Physiological and behavioral responses to corticotrophin-releasing factor administration: is CRF a mediator of anxiety or stress responses? Brain Res. Revs. 15: 71-100.

File, S.E., Zangrossi H. Jr., Saunders, F., Mabbutt, P.S. (1994) Raised corticosterone in the rat after exposure to the elevated plus maze. Psychopharmacol. 113: 543-546.

Fride, E., Dan, Y., Feldon, J., Halevy, G., Weinstock, M. (1986) Effects of prenatal stress on vulnerability to stress in prepubertal and adult rats, Physiol. Behav. 37: 681-687.

Fride, E., Dan, Y., Gavish, M., Weinstock, M. (1985) Prenatal stress impairs maternal behavior in a conflict situation and reduces hippocampal benzodiazepine receptors. Life Sci. 36: 2103-2109.

Goodwin, F.K., Wirz-Justice, A., Wehr, T.A. (1982) Evidence that the pathophysiology of depression and the mechanism of action of antidepressant drugs both involve alterations in circadian rhythms. Adv. Biochem. Psychopharmacol. 32: 1-11.

Gray, T.S. Amygdaloid pathways. (1993) Role in autonomic, neuroendocrine, and behavioral responses to stress. Ann. N.Y. Acad. Sci. 697: 53-60.

Henry, C., Kabbaj, M., Simon, H., Le Moal, M., Maccari, S. (1994) Prenatal stress increases the hypothalamic-pituitary-adrenal axis response to stress in young and adult rats. J. Endocrinol. 6: 341-345.

Holsboer, F., Grasser, A., Friess, E., and Wiedemann, K. (1994) Steroid effects on central neurons and implications for psychiatric and neurological disorders. Ann. N.Y. Acad. Sci. 746: 345-359.

Huttenen, M.O. and Niskanen, P. (1978) Prenatal loss of father and psychiatric disorders. Arch. Gen. Psychiatry 35: 429-431.

Irwin, M. (1995) Stress Induced Immune Dysfunction. In: M.R. Brown, G.F. Koob, C., Rivier, eds. Stress: Neurobiology and Neuroendocrinology. New York, Marcel Dekker: 585-615.

Irwin, M. (1994) Stress-induced immune suppression: Role of brain corticotropin releasing hormone and autonomic nervous system mechanisms. Adv. Neuroimmunol. 4: 29-47.

Katz, R. (1982) Animal model of depression: pharmacological sensitivity of a hedonic deficit. Pharmacol. Biochem. Behav. 16: 965-968.

Kay, G., Tarcic, N., Poltyrev, T., Weinstock, M. (1998) Prenatal stress depresses immune function in rats. Physiol. Behav. 63: 397-402.

Kendler, K.S., Neale, M.C., Kessler, R.C., Heath, A.C., Eaves, L. (1992) Major depression and generalized anxiety disorder. Same genes (partly) different mechanisms? Arch. Gen. Psychiatry 49: 716-722.

Keshet, G.I., and Weinstock, M. (1995) Maternal naltrexone prevents morphological and behavioral alterations induced in rats by prenatal stress. Pharmacol. Biochem. Behav. 50: 413-419.

Kitada, Y., Miyauchi, T., Satoh, A., Satoh, S. (1981) Effect of antidepressants in the rat forced swim test. Eur. J. Pharmacol. 72: 145-152.

Koehl, M., Barbazanges, A., Le Moal, M., Maccari, S. (1997) Prenatal stress induces a phase advance of circadian corticosterone rhythm in adult rats which is prevented by postnatal stress. Brain Res. 759: 317-320.

Maccari, S., Piazza, P.V., kabbaj, M., barbazanges, A., Simon, H., LeMoal, M. (1995) Adoption reverses the long-term impairment in glucocorticoid feedback induced by prenatal stress. J. Neurosci. 15: 110-116.

McGuffin, P. (1988) Major genes for affective disorder? Br. J. Psychiatry 153: 591-596.

Meijer, A. (1985) Child psychiatric sequelae of maternal war stress. Acta Psychiatr. Scand. 72: 505-511.

Milkovic, S., Milkovic, K., Pannovic, J. (1973) The initiation of fetal adrenocorticotrophic activity in the rat. Endocrinology 92: 380-384.

Mitchell, J.B. and Meaney, M.J. (1991) Effects of corticosterone on response consolidation and retrieval in the forced swim test. Behav. Neurosci. 105: 798-803.

Moreau, J.-L., Jenck, F., Martine, J.R., Mortas, P. (1994) Curative effects of the atypical antidepressant mianserin in the chronic mild stress-induced anhedonia model of depression. J. Psychiatr. Neurosci. 19: 51-56.

Nemeroff, C.B., Widerlov, E., Bisette, G. et al. (1984) Elevated concentrations of CSF corticotropin-releasing factor-like immunoreactivity in depressed patients. Science 226: 1342-1344.

Neumann, I.D., Wigger, A., Liebsch, G., Holsboer, F., Landgraf, R. (1998) Increased basal activity of the hypothalamic-pituitary adrenal axis during pregnancy in rats bred for high anxiety-related behavior. Psychoneuroendocrinology 23: 449-463.

Pellow, S. and File, S.E. (1986) Anxiolytic and anxiogenic drug effects on exploratory activity in an elevated plus maze: A novel test of anxiety in the rat. Pharmacol. Biochem. Behav. 24: 525-529.

Poltyrev, T., Keshet, G.I., Kay, G., Weinstock, M. (1996) Role of experimental conditions in determining differences in exploratory behavior of prenatally-stressed rats. Dev. Psychobiol. 29: 453-462.

Poltyrev, T. and Weinstock, M. (1997) Effect of prenatal stress on opioid component of exploration in different experimental situations. Pharmacol. Biochem. Behav. 58: 387-393.

Porsolt, R.D., Anton, G., Blavet, N., Jalfre, M. (1978) Behavioral despair in rats: A new model sensitive to antidepressant treatments. Eur. J. Pharmacol. 47: 379-391.

Secoli, S.R. and Teixeira, N.A. (1998) Chronic prenatal stress affects development and behavioral depression in rats. Stress 2: 273-280.

Stott, D.H. (1973) Follow-up study from birth of the effects of prenatal stresses. Develop. Med. Child Neurol. 5: 770-787.

Takahashi, L.K., Haglin, N.H., Kalin, N.H. (1992) Prenatal stress potentiates stress-induced behavior and reduces propensity to play in juvenile rats. Physiol. Behav. 51: 319-323.

Takahashi, L.K., Turner, J.G., Kalin, N.H. (1998) Prolonged stress-induced elevation in plasma corticosterone during pregnancy in the rat: Implications for prenatal stress studies. Psychoneuroendocrinology 23: 571-581.

Thompson, W.R. (1957) Influence of prenatal maternal anxiety on emotionality in young rats. Science 15: 698-699.

Vallee, M., Mayo, W., Dellu, F., Le Moal, M., Simon, H., Maccari, S. (1997) Prenatal stress induces high anxiety and postnatal handling induces low anxiety in adult offspring: correlation with stress-induced corticosterone injection. J. Neurosci. 17: 2626-2636.

Wakshlak, A., and Weinstock, M. (1990) Neonatal handling reverses behavioral abnormalities induced in rats by prenatal stress. Physiol. Behav. 48: 289-292.

Ward, O.B., Monaghan, E.P., Ward, I.L (1986) Naltrexone blocks the effects of prenatal stress on sexual behavior differentiation in male rats Pharmacol. Biochem. Behav. 25: 573-576.

Ward, I.L., Stehm, (1991) Prenatal stress feminizes juvenile play patterns in male rats. .Physiol. Behav. 50: 601-605.

Weinstock, M. (1997) Does prenatal stress impair coping and regulation of the hypothalamic-pituitary-adrenal axis? Neurosci. Biobehav. Revs. 21: 1-10.

Weinstock, M., Fride, E., Hertzberg, R. (1988) Prenatal Stress Effects on Functional Development of the Offspring, In G.J. Boer, M.G.P. Feenstra, M. Mirmiran, D.F. Swaab, F. Van Haaren, eds. Biochemical Basis of Functional Neuroteratology, Progress in Brain Research, vol. 73. Amsterdam: Elsevier, 319-331.

Weinstock, M., Matlina, E., Maor, G.I., Rosen, H., McEwen, B.S. (1992) Prenatal stress selectively alters the reactivity of the hypothalamic-pituitary adrenal system in the female rat. Brain Res. 595: 195-200.

Weinstock, M., Poltyrev, T., Schorer-Apelbaum, D., Men, D., McCarty, R. (1998) Effect of prenatal stress on plasma corticosterone and catecholamines in response to footshock in rats. Physiol. Behav. 64: 439-444.

Weiss, J.M., Goodman, P.A., Losito, B.G., Corrigan, S., Charry, J.M., Bailey, W.H. (1981) Behavioral depression produced by an uncontrollable stressor: Relationship to norepinephrine, dopamine and serotonin levels in various regions of the rat brain. Brain Res. Rev. 3: 167-205.

Weiss, J.M., Cierpial M.A., West, C.H.K. (1998) Selective breeding of rats for high and low motor activity in a swim test: toward a new model of depression. Pharmacol. Biochem. Behav. 61: 49-66.

Willner, P. (1986) Validation criteria for animal models of human mental disorders. Learned helplessness as a paradigm case. Psychopharmacol. Biolog. Psychiat.10: 677-690.

Willner, P., Towell, A., Sampson, D., Muscat, R., Sopokleous, S. (1987) Reduction of sucrose preference by chronic mild stress and its restoration by a tricyclic antidepressant. Psychopharmacology, 93: 358-364.

Zarrow, M.O., Philpott, J., Denenberg, V. (1970) Passage of ^{14}C-corticosterone from the rat mother to the foetus and neonate. Nature 226: 1058-1059.

5 PROMISES AND LIMITATIONS OF TRANSGENIC AND KNOCKOUT MICE IN MODELING PSYCHIATRIC SYMPTOMS

Andrew Holmes and Jacqueline N. Crawley

INTRODUCTION

Targeted gene mutation provides a powerful tool for dissecting the biological substrates of neuropsychiatric diseases. *Transgenic* mice contain a new gene, such as the human gene for a disease, or an extra copy of a normal mouse gene. *Knockout* mice contain a DNA construct that effectively deletes a gene from the mouse genome. The targeted gene mutation approach is particularly useful for testing discrete hypotheses about genes linked to major psychiatric syndromes. Neurochemical, anatomical, neurophysiological, and behavioral sequelae of the mutation of a homologous gene in mice are compared to the symptoms characterizing the human disease state (Burright et al., 1997; Campbell and Gold, 1996; Crawley, 1999, 2000; Crawley and Paylor, 1997; Crawley et al., 1997; Jucker and Ingram, 1997; Kieffer, 1999; Nelson and Young, 1997; Picciotto, 1999).

In addition, targeted gene mutations can be used to test potential therapeutic interventions. Both gene therapies and standard pharmacological treatments can be evaluated in mice with mutations relevant to the predicted disease substrate. For example, a mutation in a neurotransmitter receptor subtype generates a mouse deficient selectively in that one subtype of interest. The mutant line is used to test the pharmacological specificity of drug candidates at that receptor subtype. Gene deletions for each of the receptor subtypes are also useful to determine which behavioral function is mediated by which receptor subtype. If administration of the naturally occurring receptor agonist fails to produce an expected behavioral action, then the mutated receptor subtype mediates that behavioral effect in some way.

This chapter will describe behavioral methods to analyze phenotypes of transgenic and knockout mice, with emphasis on mutations in genes relevant to anxiety and schizophrenia. The advantages and successes of the new technology will be contrasted with the limitations and pitfalls of targeted gene mutation models of anxiety and schizophrenia.

EXPERIMENTAL DESIGN

False positives arise when a mutation produces a variety of interacting biological actions. If only a small subset of behavioral tests are conducted, the deduced phenotype may be due to a sensory or motor defect rather than a mouse analog of a human psychiatric symptom. *False negatives* arise when a mutation produces subtle effects. If only one or two behavioral tasks within a domain are conducted, the phenotypic effects of the mutation may be missed. Our laboratory is refining a strategy to minimize both false positives and false negatives in the first analyses of a new transgenic or knockout mouse (Crawley, 1999, 2000; Crawley and Paylor, 1997).

Several factors must be considered when first designing the targeted gene mutation to model a neuropsychiatric syndrome. The first is *breeding strategy*. Most mutations are generated in embryonic stem cells originating from one of the 129 inbred substrains of mice. Several of the 129 substrains contain background genes that produce aberrant behavioral phenotypes. For example, 129/J mice fail to develop the corpus callosum fiber bundle that connects the right and left cerebral cortex hemispheres, and show severe deficits on learning and memory tasks (Livy and Wahlsten, 1997; Montkowski et al., 1997). In addition, blastula donation and breeding contributes a new set of background genes. Good breeding strains such as CD-1 are outbred, which dramatically increases the variability within the control group, thereby requiring a much bigger effect of the mutation to be detectable above the baseline variability of the controls.

The best approach for behavioral phenotyping is to backcross into an inbred strain with characteristics appropriate for the hypothesized functions of the gene of interest. Characteristics of several inbred strains of mice, on a wide variety of behavioral tests, are available from several good reviews of mouse strain distributions (Banbury Conference, 1997; Crawley et al., 1997; Wehner and Silva, 1996). Choosing the optimal background strain for breeding will avoid complications of background genes that mask the behavioral phenotype of the mutation. For example, a strain with low levels of anxiety-like behaviors is useful if the gene to be mutated is hypothesized to increase anxiety. A strain with high levels of prepulse inhibition is useful if the gene to be mutated is predicted to decrease sensorimotor gating. A strain such as C57BL/6J shows moderate scores on most behavioral tests, making it a reasonable choice in many cases. Once the breeding strain is chosen, backcrossing for at least seven generations is required to produce a relatively pure genetic background (Silver, 1995). Five generations may be sufficient using the speed congenic breeding strategy, wherein breeding males are selected by their scores on the relevant behavioral tests (Markel et al., 1997).

Genotypes and *group size* are determined by the power criteria of the appropriate statistical tests. The genotype comparison is between homozygous (null) mutant (-/-), heterozygous mutant (+/-) and homozygous wild type littermate controls (+/+). Environmental factors such as parental care, birth order, and dominance hierarchy in the home cage influence behavioral traits in mice. Use of littermates serves to control for these variables. Group size is a minimum of 10 mice per treatment group, to achieve sufficient power for the standard statistical tests used in behavioral neuroscience. The treatment groups are males and females of each of the three genotypes. Thus, at least 60 mice are tested in the first experiments. If no gender differences are detected, the data from males and females can be combined for each genotype, to increase the power of the statistical analysis.

Gender data can then be pooled in future replication experiments, thereby reducing the required Ns.

If it is impractical to obtain the full complement of mice all at once, a series of smaller group sizes can be tested. The critical design feature is inclusion of some individuals from all three genotypes and both genders within each day's experiments. Data from the groups tested at different times can subsequently be combined for statistical analysis of genotype effects, unless a statistically significant difference is detected between the time points.

Genotyping is first conducted on all mice. The molecular geneticist confirms that the mutation is expressed as expected, and that the gene product is overexpressed in the transgenics or missing in the knockouts, in the generation of mice to be used for behavioral phenotyping. Confirmations of expected anatomical and biochemical sequelae of the mutation are best performed before the start of the labor-intensive behavioral testing.

Identification of individual mice is critical for behavioral experiments, since each animal is used for multiple behavioral tests. Firmly attached ear tags and/or subcutaneous bar code chips work well. *Housing* in the vivarium is by genotype, or as mixed genotypes, with genders separately housed. For behavioral experiments, the animals live in a quiet, temperature-controlled, humidity-controlled environment, on a fixed daily lighting schedule, and are not simultaneously used for any other experiments.

PRELIMINARY TESTS TO AVOID ARTIFACTS

Our laboratory first conducts a series of *general observations* for the initial evaluation of a new set of mutant mice. The goal is to identify gross physiological abnormalities. A sick mouse will perform poorly on all behavioral tasks. A blind mouse cannot learn a visual task; a deaf mouse will fail on acoustic startle tests; motor dysfunctions will impair performance on every behavioral task that requires movement. Recognizing gross functional abnormalities is particularly important for *conventional mutations*. When the mutation is expressed in all tissues of the body, from the earliest stages of development, peripheral organs may be impaired in ways that dramatically affect behaviors. Technological advances in *conditional, inducible, and conditional/inducible mutations* will avoid some of these complications, by expressing the mutation only in the brain region of interest, and only during the experimental time period.

False positives are avoided by recognizing the limitations of the mouse and designing specific behavioral tasks around the limitations. For example, learning and memory tests that employ olfactory and auditory cues can be used to test mice with visual impairment. *True positives* are often revealed in the course of the general observations. For example, audiogenic seizures and elevated body weight were detected during general observations in mice with mutations in the serotonin 5-HT2C receptor subtype (Applegate and Tecott, 1998). Dopamine transporter knockouts demonstrate dramatic hyperlocomotion in the home cage, analogous to the hyperlocomotion induced by treatment with drugs that increase synaptic dopamine levels (Giros et al., 1996). High levels of aggressive behavior were first detected in the home cage in nitric oxide synthase knockout mice (Nelson et al., 1995). Unusual nesting patterns led to the discovery of social interaction abnormalities in dishevelled-1 knockout mice (Lijam et al., 1997).

Mice are first observed daily in their home cages. Overall health and condition of the fur and whiskers are noted. Home cage activity, grooming, nesting, and sleeping patterns are observed. Any unusual patterns of locomotion, hyperreactivity to handling, or fighting in the home cage are noted. Body weight is recorded by weighing each mouse in a standard triple beam or pan balance. Body temperature is measured by rectal thermister. Abnormal appearance, barbered whiskers, unusual body weight, and unusual home cage social behaviors are noted, for further investigation.

Batteries of reflexes have been described by Irwin (1968), Moser (1995), and the SHIRPA team (Rogers et al., 1997), and Richard Paylor in our laboratory (Crawley and Paylor, 1997; Paylor et al., 1998). The righting reflex test measures the time it takes for the mouse to right itself to an upright posture, after being turned on its back. The eye blink reflex is elicited by approaching the eye with a cotton-tip swab. The ear twitch reflex is elicited by touching the ear with a cotton-tip swab. The whisker-orienting reflex is measured by touching the vibrissae on one side; the whiskers will normally stop moving and the head will turn to the side on which the whiskers were touched. Visual cliff behavior is rapidly evaluated by observing whether the mouse walks off the edge of a high table. Acoustic startle is rapidly evaluated by observing the flinch response to a sudden loud sound. Most mice are normal on all of the tests for simple neurological reflexes. If a reflex is abnormal, then the mutation has produced a gross physiological or behavioral phenotype that can be fruitfully investigated with more sophisticated tests.

Motor skills are integral to the performance of most behavioral tasks. If the mutation induces severe deficits in the ability of the mouse to walk, grip, balance, climb, swim, etc., the mouse is likely to show performance deficits on the procedures necessary for more sophisticated behavioral tasks. Several good automated tests are routinely used to evaluate motor functions. Open field exploratory activity is quantitated in a photocell-equipped automated Digiscan apparatus that records several parameters of locomotion and rearings. The ability of the mouse to balance on a rotating cylinder is quantitated with an automated accelerating rotarod apparatus. These two tests are sensitive to major abnormalities in spinal motor neurons and cerebellum. Grip tests, such as hanging wire grip time, measure neuromuscular strength. Footprint pathway analysis detects abnormal gait.

Specific sensory abilities are required for the performance of many behavioral tasks. Sensitive sensory tests for mice involve neurophysiological recording during presentation of the sensory stimulus. The auditory brainstem response is a neurophysiological measurement of the auditory nerve activity in response to a series of tones. The electroretinogram measures optic nerve activity in response to grades flashes of light. Visual response to light is determined by measuring constriction and subsequent dilation of the pupil when a small flashlight beam is directed at the eye. Visual acuity is measured by responses to visual stimuli, after mice have been trained in a conditioned reward paradigm. Pain sensitivity is evaluated by a threshold determination, using jumps, vocalizations, and running in response to a graded series of footshocks, or with the graded diameters of Von Frey hairs touched to the base of a foot. Olfactory ability is evaluated in a choice test for a series of odors delivered through a specialized airflow system, in a conditioned reward paradigm. Olfactory acuity is measured by neurophysiological recording from the olfactory cortex during presentation of scents. Taste discriminations and taste preference is measured in a choice test with graded gustatory stimuli. All of these tests require specialized equipment and multiple training sessions. Simpler methods for evaluating sensory abilities in mice would be of great benefit to the behavioral phenotyping armamentarium.

MOUSE BEHAVIORAL TESTS RELEVANT TO SYMPTOMS OF PSYCHIATRIC DISEASES

Behavioral neuroscience has a rich literature encompassing many well-established and carefully validated tests for mouse behaviors over a wide variety of domains. Several excellent reviews (Campbell and Gold, 1996; Crawley, 1999, 2000; Crawley et al., 1997, 1999; Crawley and Paylor, 1997; Jucker and Ingram, 1997; Nelson and Young, 1997; Wehner and Silva, 1996) cite the primary literature on the best tests to evaluate learning and memory, feeding, sexual behaviors, parenting behaviors, social interactions, aggression, anxiety-like behaviors, depression-like behaviors, addictive behaviors, schizophrenia-like symptoms, as well as vision, hearing, smell, taste, pain threshold, locomotion, balance, muscle strength, ataxia, and seizures.

Successful behavioral phenotyping of mice with mutations in genes relevant to psychiatric diseases depends on the quantity and quality of the relevant behavoral tests. Our laboratory generally selects two or three tests from each behavioral domain relevant to the gene of interest. Each test measures a slightly different behavior, with different underlying mechanisms, and requiring different sensory and motor modalities. The likelihood of *true positives*, detecting a specific behavioral abnormality revealing the function of the gene, is increased by conducting multiple, complementary tests within a given domain, thus avoiding *false negatives* when only a single test is used. If the same behavioral abnormality is detected across two or three complementary tests, the interpretation of the behavioral phenotype is very strong. If the behavioral abnormality is detected in only one of the complementary tests, the specific type of abnormality can be further explored in additional tests that focus on that component. For example, if cued and contextual conditioning is impaired but the Morris water task and radial maze acquisition are normal, future research will focus on fear-related learning tasks.

Mouse Tasks Relevant to Anxiety Disorders

Behavioral Assays for Anxiety-like Behavior in Mice

There are currently over 30 models used to study anxiety-like behaviors in animals, with many specifically designed for use with rodents (Griebel, 1995; Lister, 1990). While many of the rodent paradigms were initially designed and developed to test anti-anxiety drugs in rats, a number have been modified and validated for mice, thus providing a laboratory with a choice of tests to evaluate an hypothesized anxiety-like phenotype in a transgenic or gene knockout mouse. However, mice are not "little rats." Some tests with proven utility as models of anxiety-like behavior in rats, such as social interaction between conspecifics (File and Hyde, 1978), or punishment of appetitive behaviors (e.g., Vogel et al., 1980), have proven to be less well suited for measuring anxiety-like behavior in mice. Mice are naturally a very exploratory species, and many of the current tests for anxiety-like behaviors are constructed around this natural tendency (Crawley, 1985).

Originating from the pioneering work of Hall (e.g., Hall, 1936), the *open field* is the simplest of the exploration-based models of anxiety and has provided the forerunner to the more sophisticated paradigms. The apparatus comprises a large, novel, well-illuminated square or circular arena into which mice are placed and allowed to freely explore for a given amount of time (often 5-15 minutes). Behavior is assessed primarily in terms of line crossings or photocell beam breaks, with a low level of exploratory activity indicating a high baseline level of "anxiety" (e.g., Flint et al., 1995; Gray, 1979). Any observed differences between genotypes in defecation levels in the open field could be explained by unexpected alterations in gastrointestinal function in a mutant mouse, rather than an anxiety-related response. For this reason, caution should be exercised when adopting the measurement of defecation as an additional index of anxiety-related behavior in this, or any other, test for anxiety-like behavior.

While exploratory activity in the open field can be reduced by anxiolytics such as benzodiazepine agonists in mice (e.g., Christmas and Maxwell, 1970; Ongini et al., 1982), psychomotor depressants can produce a similar profile (e.g., Xu et al., 1994b). Therefore, concluding that reduced open field activity is evidence of anxiety-like behavior in a mutant mouse is potentially erroneous (e.g., Accili et al., 1996; Steiner et al., 1997). Indeed, an indication of hyperactivity or hypoactivity in a mutant mouse represents an interpretative problem for any exploration-based model of anxiety-like behavior. Dissociating general activity and anxiety-like behavior in novel/aversive environments is highly problematic because the two are related at a functional level; e.g., movement arrest is integral to rodent defensive behavior (e.g., Blanchard et al., 1998). Monitoring activity in the home cage is the surest way to quantitate locomotor activity uncontaminated by any reactivity to novelty/stressors.

To enhance the sensitivity of the open field to anxiety-related behaviors, activity in the center of the apparatus can be measured, and expressed as a ratio of center/total time, or center/total activity (e.g., Paylor et al., 1998; Ramboz et al., 1998). This measure is based on two observations: 1) rodents have a natural tendency to stay close to peripheral walls in an open environment (Barnett, 1963), and 2) such thigmotactic activity can be reliably reduced by anxiolytics (e.g., Grossen and Kelley, 1972; Treit and Fundytus, 1998). With this modification, the open field represents a good test for providing preliminary information on exploratory activity in a novel environment, and thereby gives an initial insight into anxiety-like behavior in a mutant mouse.

In the *light ↔ dark exploration test*, Crawley and colleagues (e.g., Crawley and Goodwin, 1980; Crawley et al., 1981) described an experimental situation in which mice explore two inter-connecting chambers: one large, open and brightly-lit, the other smaller, covered, and dimly-lit. The aversive properties of the brightly-lit compartment produce a robust preference for the dark compartment, while the number of transitions made between the two chambers and/or time spent in the light area over a 5-10 min test period can be increased by compounds selective for their anti-anxiety effects (e.g., Costall et al., 1987; Griebel et al., 1998; Mathis et al., 1994). As with the open field, an interpretative problem with the light ↔ dark exploration test concerns potential false positive effects of motor stimulants such as amphetamine (e.g., Crawley, 1985), and again analysis of locomotor behavior across genotypes in the home-cage will help clarify results. A more general strategy is to consider the weight of evidence from multiple tests for anxiety-like behavior before making firm conclusions about an anxiety-related phenotype in any one given test.

The *elevated plus-maze* has rapidly increased in popularity over the past decade and is now one of the most widely used animal models in anxiety research. One report confirms its regular use in over 100 different research laboratories (Hogg, 1996). The paradigm is also currently the test of choice for assessing anxiety-like behavior in knockout and transgenic mice (see Table 1). Based on the observation that rats prefer (elevated) enclosed alleys over (elevated) open alleys (Montgomery, 1955), Handley and Mithani (1984) designed the plus-maze as two open arms perpendicular to two enclosed arms (i.e., walled), interconnected by a single central platform, and elevated approximately 0.5m above floor level. Pellow et al. (1985) demonstrated that exploration of the open arms was bi-directionally sensitive to pro- and anti-anxiety compounds in rats. Subsequently, the test was reduced in size for use with mice (Lister, 1987), without compromising its sensitivity to drugs impacting anxiety in man, particularly benzodiazepine agonists (for reviews see Dawson et al., 1995; Rodgers, 1997). Thus, untreated mice show a preference for the enclosed arms, which can be accentuated by anxiogenic drugs (e.g., caffeine, pentylenetetrazole; Cole et al., 1995; Pellow et al., 1985), and reversed by anxiolytic compounds (e.g., chlordiazepoxide; Holmes and Rodgers, 1999). General activity levels in the elevated plus-maze can be indexed by total number of arm entries. However, a number of authors have suggested that the frequency of closed arm entries is a purer index of locomotor activity than total entries, the latter being a composite measure of closed and open arm entries, and therefore likely to correlate highly with changes in open arm exploration (e.g., Crestani et al., 1999; File et al., 1993). Evidence from factor analysis studies supports the dissociation, with closed entries and open arm entries loading on separate factors, and total entries co-loading across factors (e.g., Holmes and Rodgers, 1998).

Tests for anxiety-like behaviors are sensitive to various organismic and procedural variables. In line with this, performance on the elevated plus-maze is known to be influenced by subjects' age, strain, housing, prior handling, and test-experience (e.g., File et al, 1999; Holmes and Rodgers, 1999; Rodgers and Cole, 1993), as well the specific dimensions of the test apparatus *per se* (e.g., Fernandes and File, 1996; Hogg, 1996). Even in cases where attempts have been made to normalize many aspects of subjects' maintenance and experimental procedure, marked differences in elevated plus-maze behavior across laboratories have remained (Crabbe et al., 1999). Any studies with tests for anxiety-like behavior should be conducted with an acute awareness of the possible influence of extraneous variables. When comparing the behavior of mutant and wild-type mice in these tests, good experimental design, such as counterbalancing of test order across genotypes, is of the utmost importance.

Attempts at refinement of the traditional elevated plus-maze have stemmed directly from a greater understanding of rodent defensive behavior (e.g., Blanchard et al., 1990). Thus, in ethological versions of the elevated plus-maze, behavioral observations are broadened to include measures of vigilance or "risk assessment" that are argued to increase the pharmacological sensitivity of the model (e.g., Griebel et al., 1997), and which correlate highly with corticosterone-measured stress responses to test exposure (Rodgers et al., 1999). To date, a small number of

Table 1: Anxiety-related behaviors in gene knockout and transgenic mice. All examples refer to gene targeting studies unless otherwise stated.
(↑ higher anxiety-like behavior vs. wild-types; ↓ lower anxiety-like behavior vs. wild-types; ↔ no difference in anxiety-like behavior vs. wild-types).

	ELEVATED PLUS-MAZE	OPEN FIELD CENTER TIME	LIGHT↔DARK EXPLORATION	ELEVATED ZERO-MAZE	EMERGENCE TEST	FREE-EXPLORATION	NOVEL OBJECT EXPLORATION	SEPARATION-INDUCED USV
GABA								
GAD65 (1)	↑							
GABA-A-R γ2 +/- (2)	↑	↑	↑					
GABA-A-R γ2L (3)	↑					↑		
GABA-A-R δ (4)	↔							
GABA-A-R α1 (5)	↔		↔					
5-HT-R								
5-HT1A-R (6)		↑					↑	
5-HT1A-R (7)	↑	↑		↑				
5-HT1A-R (8)		↑						
5-HT1A-R (9)		↓						
5-HT1B-R (10)			↔					
5-HT1B-R (11)	↔						↓	
5-HT1B-R (12)	↔						↓	
5-HT1B-R (13)	↔							↓
5-HT2C-R (14)	↔	↔						
Monoamine								
MAOA (15)		↑						
MAOB (16)	↔							
COMT (17)			↑					
Dopamine D3R (18)	↓							
Dopamine D3R (19)	↔							
Dopamine D4R (20)		↑			↑		↑	
CRF								
CRF transgenic (21)	↑	↑						
CRF transgenic (22)			↑					
CRF (23)		↔						
CRF1-R (24)	↓		↓		↓			
CRF1-R (25)	↓							
CRF1-R (26)			↓					

(1) Kash et al., 1999; (2) Crestani et al., 1999; (3) Homanics et al., 1999; (4) Mihalek et al., 1999; (5) Rudolph et al., 1999; (6) Heisler et al., 1998; (7) Ramboz et al., 1998; (8) Parks et al., 1999; (9) Zhuang et al., 1999; (10) Ramboz et al., 1996; (11) Malleret et al., 1999; (12) Brunner et al., 1999; (13) Graille et al., 1999; (14) Tecott et al., 1998; (15) Kim et al., 1997; (16) Grimsby et al., 1997; (17) Gogos et al., 1998; (18) Steiner et al., 1996; (19) Xu et al., 1997; (20) Dulawa et al., 1999; (26) Timpl et al., 1998;

research groups have examined risk assessment behaviors in mutant mice (e.g., Brunner et al., 1999; Steiner et al., 1997).

A more wide-ranging modification of the elevated plus-maze resulted in the *elevated zero-maze* (Shepherd et al., 1994). Instead of a plus-maze shape, the zero-maze consists of a single annular platform divided into two open and two closed quadrants (i.e., no central platform). While this test has not been fully assessed for its utility as a valid screen for anxiety-related drugs in mice, a number of studies have reported anxiety-like phenotypes in mutant mice using this test (e.g., Heisler et al., 1998; Kash et al., 1999).

Some authors have noted that tests such as the elevated plus-maze measure the response to being forced into the test environment, and have described situations where the animal is provided a "safe" home base from which to explore the novel, more aversive parts of an environment (e.g., Crestani et al., 1999). Thus, in the *free-exploratory paradigm*, mice are given a lengthy (i.e., 24h) familiarization with one area, and subsequently allowed to explore the whole environment from this home base (e.g., Griebel et al., 1993). Operating along similar lines, the (dark) *emergence test* involves placing mice inside an opaque object (often a cylinder) which has one possible exit into a larger, unfamiliar open field (e.g., Smith et al., 1998b). A number of measures can be derived from behavior in this test, including the latency to emerge, time spent and exploratory activity in the open field, and transitions in and out of the cylinder. While this test has not been thoroughly validated for its sensitivity to anxiolytics, longer emergence times, fewer transitions, and less exploration of the novel arena in mutant mice have paralleled indices of anxiety-like behavior in well-validated tests, such as the light ↔ dark exploration test (e.g., Dulawa et al., 1999; Smith et al., 1998b). With further pharmacological validation, the emergence test may represent a useful test for anxiety-like behavior.

There are a number of tests to measure anxiety-like behavior that are not based around environmental exploration. Some of these may be particularly useful when examining anxiety-like behavior in a mutant mouse that has a significant hyperactive phenotype, or conversely, a general deficit in motor coordination. Notable among these are measurement of separation-induced ultrasonic distress vocalizations in pre-weanling pups (e.g., Brunner et al., 1999; Miczek et al., 1995; Olivier et al., 1994), measurement of the acoustic startle response (e.g., Grailhe et al., 1999; Trullas and Skolnick, 1993), the light-enhanced startle paradigm (e.g., Falls et al., 1997; Walker and Davis, 1997), novel object exploration (e.g., Belzung and LePape, 1993; Dulawa et al., 1999; Heisler et al., 1998; Malleret et al., 1999), and the shock-probe burying paradigm (e.g., Grailhe et al., 1999; Sluyter et al., 1996; Treit et al., 1981).

Anxiety-like Behaviors in Mutant Mice

Reports of the effects of genetic mutations on anxiety-like behaviors are ever growing (Table 1). In part, this has resulted from the fact that many laboratories now systematically screen for anxiety-like phenotypes in any mutant mouse grossly capable of performing tests designed to assay anxiety-like behavior. Even in cases for which there is only a weak *a priori* hypothesis for a mutation resulting in an anxiety-related phenotype, there have been some interesting findings (e.g., Chen et al., 1994; Köster et al., 1999; Walther et al., 1999). An alternative strategy has been to utilize gene knockout and transgenic techniques in order to study certain gene products (e.g., transmitters, receptors) that have been implicated by numerous lesion, pharmacological, and clinical investigations in the mediation of "anxiety." In this context, genetic manipulations of neurotransmitters/ neuromodulators that include the GABAergic, serotonergic/monoaminergic, and corticotropin-releasing hormone systems, have resulted in mouse phenotypes that arguably model aspects of "anxiety" in man. The next section provides a brief summary of these findings.

Mutations of the GABAergic System

Facilitation of GABAergic transmission, particularly via action at the benzodiazepine receptor site of the GABA-A receptor complex, is associated with a reduction in anxiety in man and animals (e.g., Tallman et al., 1980; Haefely et al., 1990). In line with this relationship, reducing the GABA synthesis by deleting GAD65, an isoform of the synthetic enzyme, glutamate decarboxylase, has been found to increase anxiety-like behaviors in mutant mice tested in the elevated zero-maze, and in an open field (Kash et al., 1999). In addition, GAD65-deficient mice failed to demonstrate any locomotor response to diazepam. GABA-A receptors are composed of some 20 protein subunits (e.g., Banard et al., 1998), and while they are known to vary in their distribution in the brain, their respective functional roles are poorly understood. The γ2 subunit is abundant throughout the brain, and targeted deletion of the γ2 subunit gene leads to massive depletion of benzodiazepine sites and a high percentage of perinatal lethality (Günther et al., 1995).

However, studying viable, generally healthy mice that are heterozygous for the γ2 subunit has strongly indicated a role for this subunit in anxiety-like behavior (Crestani et al., 1999). Thus, heterozygous γ2 mice displayed a clear anxiety-like phenotype in the elevated plus-maze, light ↔ dark exploration test, and free-exploratory paradigm. Furthermore, these mice showed an enhanced sensitivity to diazepam, thus simulating the heightened sensitivity to benzodiazepine anxiolytics in anxious humans (e.g., Glue et al., 1995). Crestani et al. (1999) attribute this phenotype to an impairment in GABA-A transmission, which in turn probably results from an evident reduction in GABA-A receptor clustering. Deletion of the long variant of the γ2 subunit gene has a less global impact on GABA-A receptor function, but also produces a higher level of baseline anxiety-like behavior in mice homozygous for the deletion, as assayed by the elevated plus-maze (Homanics et al., 1999a). Together, these observations clearly implicate the γ2 subunit in anxiety, and gene targeting of other GABA-A receptor subunits is helping to clarify their contribution to the mediating of anxiety (e.g., Mihalek et al., 1999; Rudolph et al., 1999).

Deletion of 5-HT Receptor Subtypes

An association between anxiety and the 5-HT system has long been proposed (e.g., Iversen et al., 1984). Drugs acting preferentially on the serotonergic system are now prescribed as anxiolytics (for review see Liebowitz, 1999). However, pharmacological dissection of the behavioral function of some 14 5-HT receptor subtypes has been hampered by the paucity of agents that are subtype selective. Therefore, as with the study of GABA-A receptor subunits, the use of genetic manipulations represents a powerful tool to study the role of 5-HT receptor subtypes in anxiety (for review see Murphy et al., 1999). For example, Grailhe et al. (1999) generated mice lacking a functional copy of the 5-HT5A receptor, and found these animals to exhibit little evidence of an anxiety-like phenotype in the elevated plus-maze, open field, defensive burying test, or in acoustic startle responses. Tecott et al. (1998) report that 5-HT2C receptor-deficient mice show significantly shorter latencies to emerge into a novel, brightly-lit open field in an emergence test, an observation indicative either of a reduced level of anxiety or increased spontaneous activity.

However, in the context of the relationship between anxiety and individual 5-HT receptor subtypes, the 5-HT1A receptor has to-date attracted the most interest. 5-HT1A agonists appear to decrease serotonergic transmission, and exert (albeit inconsistent) anxiolytic effects in various behavioral assays for anxiety in animals (e.g., De Vry, 1995). Indeed, the 5-HT1A partial agonist, buspirone, is used in the treatment of generalized anxiety disorder. A number of groups have generated 5-HT1A receptor knockout mice, and examined these mice for anxiety-like behaviors. Parks et al. (1998) report that 5-HT1A receptor knockout mice, especially males, spent significantly less time in the center of an open field, a finding replicated by Heisler et al. (1998), Ramboz et al. (1998), and Zhuang et al. (1999). In confirmation of an anxiety-like phenotype in 5-HT1A receptor knockout mice, these animals have shown less open arm exploration in the elevated zero-maze (Heisler et al., 1998), and elevated plus-maze tests (Ramboz et al., 1998), as well as less exploration of a novel object (Heisler et al., 1998), than wild-type controls.

Despite the strong phenotype in 5-HT1A mice, neither Heisler et al. (1998), nor Ramboz et al. (1998) found alterations in 5-HT (or metabolite) tissue concentrations in various brain regions examined. This finding suggests that compensatory adaptations, perhaps at the level of other 5-HT receptor subtypes, resulted from deletion of the 5-HT1A receptor deletion. Indeed, a possible upregulation of 5-HT1B receptors was indicated by the finding that the 5-HT1B agonist, CP93129, had an heightened inhibitory effect on electrically-evoked 5-HT release in hippocampal slices in 5-HT1A receptor-deficient mice, as compared to wild-types (Ramboz et al., 1998). These observations provide a good illustration of how interpretations of gene function based on conventional gene knockout technology, where the gene product of interest is absent throughout ontogeny, should always be made in the context of potentially adaptable *in vivo* systems.

While 5-HT1B agonists have demonstrable anxiogenic properties in humans (e.g., Murphy et al., 1989), an anxiety-related phenotype in mice lacking the 5-HT1B receptor has not been consistently demonstrated. In an early report, Ramboz et al. (1996) found no differences between wild-type and 5-HT1B receptor-deficient mice on the light ↔ dark exploration test, or in open field behavior. Similarly, Brunner et al. (1999), and Malleret et al. (1999) found no evidence of anxiety-like behaviors in the elevated plus-maze, or in a standard open-field. However, 5-HT1B receptor knockout pups have shown less separation-induced ultrasonic vocalizations than wild-types (Brunner et al., 1999), while adults have shown heightened exploration in an open field containing novel objects (Malleret et al., 1999). Such patterns of behavior represent some evidence of reduced anxiety-like behavior in 5-HT1B receptor knockout mice. In support of such a phenotype, there is one report that 5-HT1B receptor-deficient mice demonstrate more exploratory activity in a novel (but not familiar) open field (Zhuang et al., 1999).

Overall, however, the consequences of deleting the 5-HT1B receptor gene for anxiety-like behavior awaits further study. Clarification of this issue will benefit from the greater availability of techniques that permit the conditional knockout of 5-HT1B (and 5-HT1A) receptors in particular areas of the brain. For example, deletion of 5-HT autoreceptors in the raphé nuclei, may contrast with ubiquitous deletion of 5-HT receptors encompassing projection areas such as the septum and hippocampus.

Mutations of Monoamine Function

The enzyme monoamine oxidase A (MAO-A) inactivates monoaminergic neurotransmitters (e.g., dopamine, norepinephrine, 5-HT), and MAOA inhibitors have a long history in the treatment of anxiety (for review see Liebowitz et al., 1990). Kim et al. (1997) report that mice lacking MAO-A have elevated levels of 5-HT and norepinephrine in the frontal cortex, hippocampus, and cerebellum. In terms of anxiety-related behaviors, MAO-A-deficient mice were found to spend more time in the center of an open field than wild-type controls. However, in view of gross neurological abnormalities in the somatosensory cortices of these mutants, Cases et al. (1995) suggest that this behavior may have resulted from cognitive deficiencies. This observation demonstrates how reliance on a single index of anxiety-like behavior can be misleading when a mutation has potentially wide-ranging effects on brain function. Inactivation of the MAO-B gene did not result in any significant alterations in brain monoamine concentrations, nor did it affect open field or elevated plus-maze behavior (Grimsby et al., 1997). In contrast, inactivation of another major enzyme involved in the degradation of catecholamines, catechol-O-methyltransferase (COMT), resulted in substantially elevated levels of dopamine (but not norepinephrine or 5-HT) in the frontal cortex in mutant mice as compared to wild-types (Gogos et al., 1998). In terms of behavior, Gogos et al. (1998) found that female COMT-deficient mice exhibited a higher level of anxiety-like behavior in a modified light $\leftrightarrow$ dark exploration test.

More specific targeting of the dopaminergic system has involved deletion of the dopamine D3 receptor (D3R), normally highly expressed in the limbic system (e.g., Sokoloff et al., 1990). In terms of spontaneous locomotor activity, independently generated lines of dopamine D3R-deficient mice have yielded inconsistent phenotypes (Accili et al., 1996; Boulay et al., 1999; Xu et al., 1997). Similarly, while Steiner et al. (1997) report a reduced level of anxiety-like behavior in the elevated plus-maze in dopamine D3R knockout mice, Xu et al. (1997) report that behavior in this test was no different between D3R mutant mice and wild-type controls. Using multiple tests, Dulawa et al. (1999), report that D4R-deficient mice exhibit less center exploration in an open field. This behavior was more pronounced on first exposure to the open field than on subsequent exposures. As D4R-deficient mice also exhibited less novel object exploration, and greater preference for the home base in the emergence test, Dulawa et al. (1999) reason that these mice show reduced response to novelty, rather than heightened anxiety-like behavior *per se*. Finally, Campbell et al. (1999) have reported that transgenic potentiation of a restricted subset of dopamine D1R neurons in the amygdala and cortex produced a striking phenotype of excessive, repetitive stereotypies, and biting behavior. Given that these mice displayed no parallel signs of increased aggressive behavior,

Campbell et al. (1999) propose the phenotype may model certain symptoms of obsessive compulsive disorder.

Corticotropin Releasing Factor (CRF) Overexpression and CRF-Receptor Knockouts

The hypothalamic-pituitary-adrenal axis mediates stress responses that have been closely linked to anxiety disorders and anxiety-like behavior in animals. Of particular note, pharmacological studies have shown that intracranial administration of corticotropin-releasing factor (CRF) can markedly increase anxiety-like behavior in rats (e.g., Britton et al., 1986; Sutton et al., 1982). In line with these findings, Stenzel-Poore et al. (1994) report that mice overexpressing CRF exhibit heightened anxiety-like behavior in both the elevated plus-maze and the open field. As adrenalectomy failed to abolish anxiety-like behavior observed in the light $\leftrightarrow$ dark exploration test (Heinrichs et al., 1997), the phenotype of CRF-transgenic mice is likely to be centrally mediated (i.e., extrahypophyseal). In contrast to the positive phenotype evident in CRF overexpressing mice, Weninger et al. (1999) have found that CRF-deficient mice failed to show any significant differences in the elevated plus-maze as compared to wild-type controls.

Gene knockout studies that have targeted CRF receptors have provided further evidence for an important role for CRF in anxiety-related behavior. Of the two CRF receptors isolated to-date (e.g., Chen et al., 1993), CRFR-1 is more abundantly found in the brain, and is linked to anxiety-like behavior by studies which targeted the receptor with an antisense oligodeoxynucleotide (e.g., Liebsch et al., 1995). Two groups have independently reported that deleting CRFR-1 results in a phenotype of reduced anxiety-like behavior in a variety of test situations. Thus, Smith et al. (1998b) and Contarino et al. (1999) have found significantly reduced anxiety-like behavior in the elevated plus-maze, emergence, and light $\leftrightarrow$ dark exploration tests, while Timpl et al. (1998) report evidence of an anxiolytic-like phenotype in these mice in the light $\leftrightarrow$ dark exploration test. Therefore, there is preliminary evidence that genetic mutations of CRF processes at both the peptide and receptor level may represent useful models to examine the etiology of anxiety disorders.

Methodological Issues

Using classical knockout technology to remove a gene product is not analogous to using a "perfect" pharmacological antagonist which is 100% specific for a neurochemical target. The absence of a gene throughout the course of development may result in a cascade of molecular and neurochemical events, potentially amplifying a given phenotype, and rendering the attribution of a causative relationship between gene and behavior complex. Alternatively, the *in vivo* function of a gene product may be altered or even masked by compensatory adaptations (as discussed in the context of 5-HT1A and 5-HT1B receptor knockout mice), which could in itself reveal important information about the plasticity of particular neural systems. A major advantage of lesion and pharmacological studies is that specific brain regions can be manipulated. Manipulation of a gene throughout the brain (and body) not only provides less resolution of gene function, but inactivation or overexpression of a gene product could conceivably produce differing effects on anxiety-like behavior in different brain regions (e.g., autoreceptor versus postsynaptic 5-HT1A/5-HT1B receptors). Where a researcher is interested in developing a genetic model of anxiety (e.g., heterozygous GABA-A γ2 subunit mice; Crestani et al., 1999), the chronic, global manipulation of a gene product is preferable. Otherwise, the increasing availability of inducible and conditional gene knockout techniques will help address the limitations of classical knockout technology (for reviews see Gingrich and Roder, 1998; Nelson and Young, 1998).

A potentially more intractable problem concerns the influence of genetic background, discussed in detail elsewhere (e.g., Crawley, 1996; Gerlai, 1996). In the context of anxiety-like behavior, is it well known that mouse strains exhibit widely different profiles in tests for anxiety-like behavior, including the elevated plus-maze (e.g., Cole et al., 1995; Rodgers and Cole, 1993; Trullas and Skolnick, 1993), light ↔ dark exploration test (e.g., Beuzen and Belzung, 1995; Crawley and Davis, 1982; Mathis et al., 1994; 1995), free-exploratory paradigm (e.g., Beuzen and Belzung, 1995), and open field (e.g., Trullas and Skolnick, 1993). Simply considering the two inbred strains most commonly used as parental strains in the generation of gene knockout and transgenic mice, i.e., C57BL/6 and 129 substrains, marked differences in baseline anxiety-like behavior in the elevated plus-maze, light ↔ dark exploration test, acoustic startle response, and open field tests have been observed in our laboratory (Holmes et al., unpublished observations) and by others (e.g., Homanics et al., 1999a; Paulus et al., 1999). In this context, cases in which anxiety-like behavior has been observed in independent lines bred onto different genetic backgrounds (e.g., 5-HT1A receptor knockout; heterozygous GABA-A γ2 knockout), provide the most compelling evidence that the phenotype is a direct result of the mutation, and not an artifact of background genes.

On a final note, pathological anxiety is no longer thought of as a unitary phenomenon, although not all agree on the extent of its heterogeneity (e.g., Tyrer, 1990). DSM-IV divides anxiety into 12 sub-disorders, including generalized anxiety disorder, social phobia, specific phobia, panic disorder, obsessive compulsive disorder, and post-traumatic stress disorder (American Psychiatric Association, 1994). In the laboratory, there are suggestions that differences in pharmacological sensitivity across animal models might reflect important qualitative divergence between tests (e.g., Belzung and LePape, 1994; File et al., 1993; Griebel et al., 1995; Holmes and Rodgers, 1998). With further development and careful validation of behavioral situations which more closely model one form of anxiety, for example panic disorder, more than another, such as generalized anxiety disorder, testing for anxiety-like behaviors may more accurately reflect the heterogeneity of human anxiety. From this perspective, and in parallel with evidence from human genetic studies which are increasingly identifying possible candidate genes for susceptibility to particular anxiety disorders (e.g., Lesch et al., 1996), gene targeting and transgenic technologies provide an unprecedented opportunity to understand the neural basis of anxiety.

Mouse Tasks Relevant to Schizophrenia

There is no rodent model that encompasses the full symptomotology of schizophrenia. Further, mouse tests relevant to individual symptoms of schizophrenia are much less well developed than mouse tests relevant to anxiety. Discussion of mouse tasks relevant to schizophrenia will therefore be comparatively limited.

Rodent models of some of the components of schizophrenia are focused around several concepts. 1) The dopamine hypothesis of schizophrenia is tested with drugs and lesions that act on dopamine receptors and transporters. Exploratory locomotion and rewarded behaviors are tested, including open field activity, self-stimulation, and self-administration of drugs of abuse (Ellenbroek and Cools, 1990; Ingraham and Myslobodsky, this volume). 2) The serotonergic component of atypical antipsychotics such as clozapine is tested with drugs that act on serotonergic receptors and transporters, using similar behavioral tasks. 3) Psychostimulants such as amphetamine and cocaine can produce aberrant thought processes analogous to some components of schizophrenia. Repeated administration of psychostimulants to rats produces sensitization in terms of dopamine release and dopaminergic drug-induced locomotion (Kalivas, 1995; Kuczenski and Segal, 1999; discussed by Robinson, this volume). 4) The prefrontal cortex is the critical site for cognitive dysfunction in schizophrenia. Neonatal hippocampal lesions induce deficits in social behaviors, prepulse inhibition, and hyperlocomotion in rats, presenting a model of several aspects of schizophrenia (Sams-Dodd et al., 1997). 5) Attentional deficits in schizophrenic patients are modeled with the latent inhibition task in rats (Weiner et al, 1996; Weiner, this volume; Feldon et al., this volume). 6) Sensorimotor gating reflex deficits in schizophrenic patients are modeled with the prepulse inhibition task (Swerdlow and Geyer, 1998; Geyer, this volume). 7) Genes linked to schizophrenia are identified with linkage analysis from pedigrees of families with high incidence of schizophrenia (O'Donovan and Owen, 1999). Targeted gene mutation has been applied to investigate a small number of these components in transgenic and knockout mice.

Schizophrenia-Related Phenotypes of Knockout Mice

At least five dopamine receptor subtypes and two dopamine transporters have been identified to date (Sokoloff and Schwartz, 1995). Targeted gene mutations of each have been generated, and are being evaluated for their behavioral phenotypes. Analyses with tests relevant to schizophrenia have included the behavioral domains of prepulse inhibition, exploratory locomotion, stereotypy, grooming, learning, and responses to psychostimulants. D1 deficient mice were not significantly different from wild type littermate controls on open field locomotion, but failed to show the standard hyperlocomotion and stereotypy response to treatment with cocaine or with a D1 agonist, SKF 81297 (Xu et al., 1994a,b). D1 knockout mice displayed reduced grooming in response to novelty and to intraventricularly administered oxytocin, prolactin, ACTH, and β-endorphin (Drago et al., 1999). In contrast, D2 knockout mice displayed normal grooming and normal responses to novelty and neuropeptide administration (Drago et al., 1999). D1A deficient mice were not significantly different from wild type littermates on an olfactory discrimination, on distance traversed and time spent in three zones of a circular open field, or on swim speed and pattern in the Morris water task; however a significant impairment in place learning performance was detected in both the visible and hidden platform components of the Morris water task (Smith et al., 1998a). D2 deficient mice displayed reduced locomotion in the open field and poor performance on the rotarod (Balk et al., 1995). Amphetamine-induced deficits in prepulse inhibition were absent in D2 knockout mice, but not in D3 or D4 mutants (Ralph et al., 1999). In addition, D2 knockout mice failed to show conditioned place preference to morphine (Maldonado et al., 1997), indicating loss of rewarding effects of opiates. D3 deficient mice showed higher levels of locomotion in an open field (Accili et al., 1996). D4 deficient mice displayed reduced baseline horizontal activity and locomotion in an open field (Rubenstein et al., 1997; Dulawa et al., 1999), but increased locomotor activation in response to ethanol, cocaine, and methamphetamine administration (Rubenstein et al., 1997). D5 deficient mice, currently being tested, show preliminary indications of hyperlocomotion in the Digiscan open field (Sibley et al., 1998). Dopamine transporter knockout mice display very high baseline locomotion, and do not respond to amphetamine and cocaine treatments (Giros et al., 1996).

Less has been completed in mice with mutations in serotonin receptor subtypes for behaviors relevant to schizophrenia. 5-HT1B knockout mice showed slightly higher baseline levels of prepulse inhibition, and failed to respond to a 5-HT1A/1B agonist, RU24969, on habituation to prepulse inhibition (Dulawa et al., 1997). 5-HT5A knockout mice displayed increased exploratory activity in a novel environment, but attenuated hyperactivity in response to treatment with the hallucinogenic drug LSD (Grailhe et al., 1999). Serotonin transporter knockout mice displayed normal exploratory activity, but failed to show the normal hyperlocomotion response to the psychostimulant MDMA (Bengel et al., 1998).

Reduced prepulse inhibition, analogous to that seen in schizophrenic patients, was detected in several other mutant lines. Adrenergic $\alpha 2C$ receptor knockout mice showed diminished prepulse inhibition, in conjunction with an enhanced startle response (Sallinen et al., 1998). NCAM-180 knockout mice, deficient in a gene regulating neural migration, showed reduced prepulse inhibition (Wood et al., 1998). In contrast, interleukin-2 null mutants showed significantly greater prepulse inhibition (Petitto et al., 1999). Mice deficient in disheveled-1, a developmental gene, showed deficits in prepulse inhibition as well as reduced social interactions in the home cage and in a social dominance task, modeling several components of the symptoms of schizophrenia (Lijam et al., 1997).

CONCLUSIONS

The new technology of targeted gene mutation is just beginning to be successfully applied to the modeling of psychopathology. Methods for behavioral phenotyping of a mutation have been elaborated in mice, although additional methods are needed in some behavioral domains. Caveats have been clearly identified, as described above. Temporally inducible mutations, and tissue-specific conditional mutations, will need to be developed to avoid many of these caveats, and increase the power of the mutant mouse technology. However, the greatest challenge lies in formulating discrete hypotheses about genetic mechanisms underlying components of anxiety and schizophrenia, that can then be directly tested in mice.

The examples described above demonstrate the promise of the targeted gene mutation technique for evaluating hypotheses about individual symptoms of anxiety and schizophrenia. In some cases, the mutant mouse approach is best used to confirm the selectivity of receptor ligands on the behavioral function. In some cases, the mutant mouse approach tests the role of a neurotransmitter, receptor, signal tranducer, neurotrophic factor, transcriptional factor, etc. in the behavioral function. In the most interesting cases, the behavioral phenotype detects new functions for a gene product. The most exciting application of the targeted gene mutation technology will come from the discovery of highly replicable linkages of genes to anxiety and to schizophrenia, across many human pedigrees. Mutation of the homologous gene in the mouse will thus provide an excellent model system to evaluate the role of the identified gene in behaviors relevant to the human psychiatric diseases.

REFERENCES

Accili, D., Fishburn, C.S., Drago, J., Steiner, H., Lachowicz, J., Park, R.H., Gauda, E.B., Lee, E.J., Cool, M.H., Sibley, D.R., Gerfen, C.R., Westphal, H., Fuchs, S. (1996) A targeted mutation of the D_3 dopamine receptor gene is associated with hyperactivity in mice. Proc Natl Acad Sci USA. 93: 1945-1949.

American Psychiatric Association (1994) DSM-IV: Diagnostic and statistical manual of mental disorders. Fourth edition, Washington, DC: American Psychiatric Association.

Applegate, C.D. and Tecott, L.H. (1998) Global increases in seizure susceptibility in mice lacking 5-HT2C receptors: a behavioral analysis. Exp Neurol. 154: 522-530.

Balk, J.H., Picetti, R., Salardi, A., Thirlet, G., Dierich, A., Depaulis, A., Le Meur, M., Borrelli, E. (1995) Parkinsonian-like locomotor impairment in mice lacking dopamine D2 receptors. Nature. 377: 424-428.

Banbury Conference on Genetic Background in Mice. (1997): Neuron. 19: 755-759.

Barnard, E.A., Skolnick, P., Olsen, R.W., Mohler, H., Sieghart, W., Biggio, G., Braestrup, C., Bateson, A.N., Langer, S.Z. (1998) International Union of Pharmacology. XV. Subtypes of gamma-aminobutyric acidA receptors: classification on the basis of subunit structure and receptor function. Pharmacol Rev. 50: 291-313.

Barnett, S.A. (1963) The Rat: A Study in Behavior. London: Methuen.

Belzung, C. and Le Pape, G. (1994) Comparison of different behavioral test situations used in psychopharmacology for measurement of anxiety. Physiol Behav. 56: 623-628.

Bengel, D., Murphy, D.L., Andrews, A.M., Wichems, C.H., Feltner, D., Heils, A., Mossner, R., Westphal, H., Lesch, K.P. (1998) Altered brain serotonin homeostasis and locomotor insensitivity to 3,4-methylenedioxymethamphetamine ("ecstasy") in serotonin transporter-deficient mice. Mol Pharm. 53: 649-655.

Beuzen, A. and Belzung, C. (1995) Link between emotional memory and anxiety states: a study by principal component analysis. Physiol Behav. 58: 111-118.

Blanchard, D.C., Blanchard, R.J., Tom, P., Rodgers, R.J. (1990) Diazepam changes risk assessment in an anxiety/defense test battery. Psychopharmacology. 101: 511-518.

Blanchard, R.J., Hebert, M.A., Ferrari, P., Palanza, P., Figueira, R., Blanchard, D.C., Parmigiani, S. (1998) Defensive behaviors in wild and laboratory (Swiss) mice: the mouse defense test battery. Physiol Behav. 65: 201-209.

Boulay, D., Depoortere, R., Rostene, W., Perrault, G., Sanger, D.J. (1999) Dopamine D3 receptor agonists produce similar decreases in body temperature and locomotor activity in D3 knock-out and wild-type mice. Neuropharmacology. 38: 555-565.

Britton, K.T., Lee, G., Dana, R., Risch, S.C., and Koob, G.F. (1986) Activating and 'anxiogenic' effects of corticotropin releasing factor are not inhibited by blockade of the pituitary-adrenal system with dexamethasone. Life Sci. 39: 1281-1286.

Brunner, D., Buhot, M.C., Hen, R., Hofer, M. (1999) Anxiety, motor activation, and maternal-infant interactions in 5HT1B knockout mice. Behav Neurosci. 113: 587-601.

Burright, E.N., Orr, H.T., andClark, H.B. (1997) Mouse models of human CAG repeat disorders. Brain Pathol. 7: 965-977.

Campbell, I.L. and Gold, L.H. (1996) Transgenic modeling of neuropsychiatric disorders. Mol. Psychiatry. 1: 105-120.

Campbell, K.M., de Lecea, L., Severynse, D.M., Caron, M.G., McGrath, M.J., Sparber, S.B., Sun, L.Y., and Burton, F.H. (1999) OCD-Like behaviors caused by a neuropotentiating transgene targeted to cortical and limbic D1+ neurons. J Neurosci. 19: 5044-5053.

Cases, O., Seif, I., Grimsby, J., Gaspar, P., Chen, K., Pournin, S., Muller, U., Aguet, M., Babinet, C., Shih, J.C., and De Maeyer, E. (1995) Aggressive behavior and altered amounts of brain serotonin and norepinephrine in mice lacking MAOA. Science. 268: 1763-1766.

Chen, R., Lewis, K.A., Perrin, M.H., Vale, W.W. (1993) Expression cloning of a human corticotropin-releasing-factor receptor. Proc Natl Acad Sci U S A. 90: 8967-8971.

Chen, C., Rainnie, D.G., Greene, R.W., and Tonegawa, S. (1994) Abnormal fear response and aggressive behavior in mutant mice deficient for alpha-calcium-calmodulin kinase II. Science. 266: 291-294.

Christmas, A.J. and Maxwell, D.R. (1970) A comparison of the effects of some benzodiazepines and other drugs on aggressive and exploratory behaviour in mice and rats. Neuropharmacology. 9: 17-29.

Cole, J.C., Burroughs, G.J., Laverty, C.R., Sheriff, N.C., Sparham, E.A., Rodgers, R.J. (1995) Anxiolytic-like effects of yohimbine in the murine plus-maze: strain independence and evidence against alpha 2-adrenoceptor mediation. Psychopharmacology. 118: 425-436.

Contarino, A., Dellu, F., Koob, G.F., Smith, G.W., Lee, K.F., Vale, W., Gold, L.H. (1999) Reduced anxiety-like and cognitive performance in mice lacking the corticotropin-releasing factor receptor 1. Brain Res. 835: 1-9.

Costall, B., Hendrie, C.A., Kelly, M.E., Naylor, R.J. (1987) Actions of sulpiride and tiapride in a simple model of anxiety in mice. Neuropharmacology. 26: 195-200.

Crabbe, J.C., Wahlsten, D., Dudek, B.C. (1999) Genetics of mouse behavior: interactions with laboratory environment. Science. 284: 1670-1672.

Crawley, J.N. (1981) Neuropharmacologic specificity of a simple animal model for the behavioral actions of benzodiazepines. Pharmacol Biochem Behav. 15: 695-699.

Crawley, J.N. (1985) Exploratory behavior models of anxiety in mice. Neurosci Biobehav Rev. 9: 37-44.

Crawley, J.N. (1996) Unusual behavioral phenotypes of inbred mouse strains. Trends Neurosci. 19: 181-182.

Crawley, J.N. (1999) Behavioral phenotyping of transgenic and knockout mice: experimental design and evaluation of general health, sensory functionss, motor abilities, and specific behavioral tests. Brain Res. 835: 18-26.

Crawley, J.N. (2000) *What's Wrong With My Mouse? Behavioral Phenotyping of Transgenic and Knockout Mice.* New York: John Wiley and Sons, Inc.

Crawley, J.N., Belknap, J.K., Collins, A., Crabbe, J.C., Frankel, W., Henderson, N., Hitzemann, R.J., Maxson, S.C., Miner, L.L., Silva, A.J., Wehner, J.M., Wynshaw-Boris, A., and Paylor, R. (1997) Behavioral phenotypes of inbred mouse strains: implications and recommendations for molecular studies. Psychopharmacology. 132: 107-124.

Crawley, J.N. and Davis, L.G. (1982) Baseline exploratory activity predicts anxiolytic responsiveness to diazepam in five mouse strains. Brain Res Bull. 8: 609-612.

Crawley, J.N., Gerfen, C., McKay, R., Rogawski, M.A., Sibley, D.R., and Skolnick, P. (1999) *Current Procotols in Neuroscience.* New York: John Wiley and Sons, Inc.

Crawley, J. and Goodwin, F.K. (1980) Preliminary report of a simple animal behavior model for the anxiolytic effects of benzodiazepines. Pharmacol Biochem Behav. 13: 167-170.

Crawley, J.N. and Paylor, R. (1997) A proposed test battery and constellations of specific behavioral paradigms to investigate the behavioral phenotypes of transgenic and knockout mice. Hormones Behav. 31: 197-211.

Crestani, F., Lorez, M., Baer, K., Essrich, C., Benke, D., Laurent, J.P., Belzung, C., Fritschy, J.M., Luscher, B., and Mohler, H. (1999) Decreased GABAA-receptor clustering results in enhanced anxiety and a bias for threat cues. Nat Neurosci. 2: 833-839.

Dawson, G.R. and Tricklebank, M.D. (1995) Use of the elevated plus maze in the search for novel anxiolytic agents. Trends Pharmacol Sci. 16: 33-36.

De Vry, J. (1995) 5-HT1A receptor agonists: recent developments and controversial issues. Psychopharmacology. 121: 1-26.

Drago, F., Contarino, A., Busa, L. (1999) The expression of neuropeptide-induced excessive grooming behavior in dopamine D_1 and D_2 receptor-deficient mice. Europ J Pharmacol. 365: 125-131.

Dulawa, S.C., Grandy, D.K., Low, M.J., Paulus, M.P., Geyer, M.A. (1999) Dopamine D4 receptor-knockout mice exhibit reduced exploration of novel stimuli. J Neurosci. 19: 9550-9556.

Dulawa, S.C., Hen, R., Scearce-Levie, K., Geyer, M.A. (1997) Serotonin 1B receptor modulation of startle reactivity, habituation, and prepulse inhibition in wild-type and serotonin 1B knockout mice. Psychopharmacology. 132: 125-134.

Ellinbroek, B.A. and Cools, A.R. (1990) Animal models with construct validity for schizophrenia. Behav Pharmacol. 1: 469-490.

Falls, W.A., Carlson, S., Turner, J.G., Willott, J.F. (1997) Fear-potentiated startle in two strains of inbred mice. Behav Neurosc. 111: 855-861.

Fernandes, C. and File, S.E. (1996) The influence of open arm ledges and maze experience in the elevated plus-maze. Pharmacol Biochem Behav. 54: 31-40.

File, S.E. (1993) The interplay of learning and anxiety in the elevated plus-maze. Behav Brain Res. 58: 199-202.

File, S.E., Gonzalez, L.E., Gallant, R. (1999) Role of the dorsomedial hypothalamus in mediating the response to benzodiazepines on trial 2 in the elevated plus-maze test of anxiety. Neuropsychopharmacology. 21: 312-320.

File, S.E. and Hyde, J.R. (1978) Can social interaction be used to measure anxiety? Br J Pharmacol. 62: 19-24.

File, S.E., Zangrossi, H., Viana, M., Graeff, F.G. (1993) Trial 2 in the elevated plus-maze: a different form of fear? Psychopharmacology. 11: 491-494.

Flint, J., Corley, R., DeFries, J.C., Fulker, D.W., Gray, J.A., Miller, S., Collins, A.C. (1995) A simple genetic basis for a complex psychological trait in laboratory mice. Science. 8: 1432-1435.

Gerlai, R. (1996) Gene-targeting studies of mammalian behavior: is it the mutation or the background genotype? Trends Neurosci. 19: 177-181.

Gingrich, J.R. and Roder, J. (1998) Inducible gene expression in the nervous system of transgenic mice. Ann Rev Neurosci. 21: 377-405.

Giros, B., Jaber, M., Jones, S.R., Wightman, R.M., Caron, M.G. (1996) Hyperlocomotion and indifference to cocaine and amphetamine in mice lacking the dopamine transporter. Nature. 379: 606-612.

Glue, P., Wilson, S., Coupland, N., Ball., D., Nutt, D.J. (1995) The relationship between benzodiazepine sensitivity and neuroticism. J Anxiety Disord. 9: 33-45.

Gogos, J.A., Morgan, M., Luine, V., Santha, M., Ogawa, S., Pfaff, D., Karayiorgou, M. (1998) Catechol-O-methyltransferase-deficient mice exhibit sexually dimorphic changes in catecholamine levels and behavior. Proc Natl Acad Sci U S A. 95: 9991-9996.

Grailhe, R., Waeber, C., Dulawa, S.C., Hornung, J.P., Zhuang, X., Brunner, D., Geyer, M.A. and Hen, R. (1999) Increased exploratory activity and altered response to LSD in mice lacking the 5-HT(5A) receptor. Neuron. 22: 581-591.

Gray, J.A. (1979) Emotionality in male and female rodents: reply to Archer. Br J Psychol. 70: 425-440.

Griebel, G. (1995) 5-Hydroxytryptamine-interacting drugs in animal models of anxiety disorders: more than 30 years of research. Pharmacol Ther. 65: 319-95.

Griebel, G., Blanchard, D.C., Jung, A., Lee, J.C., Masuda, C.K. and Blanchard, R.J. (1995) Further evidence that the mouse defense test battery is useful for screening anxiolytic and panicolytic drugs: effects of acute and chronic treatment with alprazolam. Neuropharmacology. 34: 1625-1633.

Griebel, G., Belzung, C., Misslin, R., Vogel, E. (1993) The free-exploratory paradigm: an effective method for measuring neophobic behaviour in mice and testing potential neophobia-reducing drugs. Behav Pharm. 4: 637-644.

Griebel, G., Perrault, G., Sanger, D.J. (1998) Limited anxiolytic-like effects of non-benzodiazepine hypnotics in rodents. J Psychopharmacol. 12: 356-365.

Griebel, G., Rodgers, R.J., Perrault, G., Sanger, D.J. (1997) Risk assessment behaviour: evaluation of utility in the study of 5-HT-related drugs in the rat elevated plus-maze test. Pharmacol Biochem Behav. 57: 817-827.

Grimsby, J., Toth, M., Chen, K., Kumazawa, T., Klaidman, L., Adams, J.D., Karoum, F., Gal, J., Shih, J.C. (1997) Increased stress response and beta-phenylethylamine in MAOB-deficient mice. Nat Genet. 17: 206-210.

Grossen, N.E. and Kelley, M.J. (1972) Species-specific behavior and acquisition of avoidance behavior in rats. J Comp Physiol Psychol. 81: 307-310.

Gunther, U., Benson, J., Benke, D., Fritschy, J.M., Reyes, G., Knoflach, F., Crestani, F., Aguzzi, A., Arigoni, M., Lang, Y., Bluethman, H., Mohler, H, Luscher, B. (1995). Benzodiazepine-insensitive mice generated by targeted disruption of the gamma 2 subunit gene of gamma-aminobutyric acid type A receptors. Proc Natl Acad Sci U S A. 92: 7749-7753.

Haefely, W., Martin, J.R., Schoch, P. (1990) Novel anxiolytics that act as partial agonists at benzodiazepine receptors. Trends Pharmacol Sci. 11: 452-456.

Hall, C.S. (1936) Emotional behavior in the rat. I Defecation and urination as measures of individual differences in emotionality. J. Comp Psychol. 18: 385-403.

Handley, S.L. and Mithani, S. (1984) Effects of alpha-adrenoceptor agonists and antagonists in a maze-exploration model of 'fear'-motivated behaviour. Naunyn Schmiedebergs Arch Pharmacol. 327: 1-5.

Heinrichs, S.C., Min, H., Tamraz, S., Carmouche, M., Boehme, S.A., Vale, W.W. (1997) Anti-sexual and anxiogenic behavioral consequences of corticotropin-releasing factor overexpression are centrally mediated. Psychoneuroendocrinology. 22: 215-224.

Heisler, L.K., Chu, H.M., Brennan, T.J., Danao, J.A., Bajwa, P., Parsons, L.H., Tecott, L.H. (1998) Elevated anxiety and antidepressant-like responses in serotonin 5-HT1A receptor mutant mice. Proc Natl Acad Sci U S A. 95: 15049-15054.

Hogg, S. (1996) A review of the validity and variability of the elevated plus-maze as an animal model of anxiety Pharmacol Biochem Behav. 54: 21-30.

Holmes, A. and Rodgers, R.J. (1998) Responses of Swiss-Webster mice to repeated plus-maze experience: further evidence for a qualitative shift in emotional state? Pharmacol Biochem Behav. 60: 473-488.

Holmes, A. and Rodgers, R.J. (1999) Influence of spatial and temporal manipulations on the anxiolytic efficacy of chlordiazepoxide in mice previously exposed to the elevated plus-maze. Neurosci Biobehav Rev. 23: 971-908.

Homanics, G.E., Harrison, N.L., Quinlan, J.J., Krasowski, M.D., Rick, C.E., de Blas, A.L., Mehta, A.K., Kist, F., Mihalek, R.M., Aul, J.J., Firestone, L.L. (1999a) Normal electrophysiological and behavioral responses to ethanol in mice lacking the long splice variant of the gamma2 subunit of the gamma-aminobutyrate type A receptor. Neuropharmacology. 38: 253-265.

Homanics, G.E., Quinlan, J.J., Firestone, L.L. (1999b) Pharmacologic and behavioral responses of inbred C57BL/6J and strain 129/SvJ mouse lines. Pharmacol Biochem Behav. 63: 21-26.

Irwin, S. (1968) Comprehensive observational assessment: 1a. A systematic, quantitative procedure for assessing the behavioural and physiologic state of the mouse. Psychopharmacologia. 13: 222-257.

Iversen, S.D. (1984) 5-HT and anxiety. Neuropharmacology. 23: 1553-1560.

Jucker, M. and Ingram, D.K. (1997) Murine models of brain aging and age-related neurodegenerative diseases. Behav Brain Res. 85: 1-25.

Kalivas, P.W. (1995) Interactions between dopamine and excitatory amino acids in behavioral sensitization to psychostimulants. Drug Alc Depend. 37: 95-100.

Kash, S.F., Tecott, L.H., Hodge, C. and Baekkeskov, S. (1999) Increased anxiety and altered responses to anxiolytics in mice deficient in the 65-kDa isoform of glutamic acid decarboxylase. Proc Natl Acad Sci U S A. 96: 1698-1703.

Kieffer, B.L. (1999) Opioids: first lessons from knockout mice. Trends Pharmacol Sci. 20: 19-26.

Kim, J.J., Shih, J.C., Chen, K., Chen, L., Bao, S., Maren, S., Anagnostaras, S.G., Fanselow, M.S., De Maeyer, E., Seif, I., Thompson, R.F. (1997) Selective enhancement of emotional, but not motor, learning in monoamine oxidase A-deficient mice. Proc Natl Acad Sci U S A. 94: 5929-5933.

Koster, A., Montkowski, A., Schulz, S., Stube, E.M., Knaudt, K., Jenck, F., Moreau, J.L., Nothacker, H.P., Civelli, O., Reinscheid, R.K. (1999) Targeted disruption of the orphanin FQ/nociceptin gene increases stress susceptibility and impairs stress adaptation in mice. Proc Natl Acad Sci U S A. 96: 10444-10449.

Kuczenski, R. and Segal, D.S. (1999) Dynamic changes in sensitivity occur during the acute response to cocaine and methylphenidate. Psychopharmacology. 147: 96-103.

Lesch, K.P., Bengel, D., Heils, A., Sabol, S.Z., Greenberg, B.D., Petri, S., Benjamin, J., Muller, C.R., Hamer, D.H., Murphy, D.L. (1996) Association of anxiety-related traits with a polymorphism in the serotonin transporter gene regulatory region. Science. 274: 1527-1531.

Liebowitz, M.R. (1999) Update on the diagnosis and treatment of social anxiety disorder. J Clin Psychiatry. 18: 22-26.

Liebowitz, M.R., Hollander, E., Schneier, F., Campeas, R., Welkowitz, L., Hatterer, J., Fallon, B. (1990) Reversible and irreversible monoamine oxidase inhibitors in other psychiatric disorders. Acta Psychiatr Scand. 360: 29-34.

Liebsch, G., Landgraf, R., Gerstberger, R., Probst, J.C., Wotjak, C.T., Engelmann, M., Holsboer, F., Montkowski, A. (1995) Chronic infusion of a CRH1 receptor antisense oligodeoxynucleotide into the central nucleus of the amygdala reduced anxiety-related behavior in socially defeated rats. Regul Pept. 59: 229-239.

Lijam, N., Paylor, R., McDonald, M.P., Crawley, J.N., Deng, C.X., Herrup, K., Stevens, K.E., Maccaferri, G., McBain, C.J., Sussman, D.J., Wynshaw-Boris, A. (1997) Social interaction and sensorimotor gating abnormalities in mice lacking Dvl1. Cell. 90: 895-905.

Lister, R.G. (1987) The use of a plus-maze to measure anxiety in the mouse. Psychopharmacology. 92: 180-185.

Lister, R.G. (1990) Ethologically-based animal models of anxiety disorders. Pharmacol Ther. 46: 321-40.

Livy, D.J. and Wahlsten, D. (1997) Retarded formation of the hippocampal commissure in embryos from mouse strains lacking a corpus callosum. Hippocampus. 7: 2-14.

Maldonado, R., Saiardi., A., Valverde, O., Samad, T. A., Roques, B. P., Borrelli, E. (1997) Absence of opiate rewarding effects in mice lacking dopamine D2 receptors. Nature 388: 586-589.

Malleret, G., Hen, R., Guillou, J.L., Segu, L. and Buhot, M.C. (1999) 5-HT1B receptor knock-out mice exhibit increased exploratory activity and enhanced spatial memory performance in the Morris water maze. J Neurosci. 19: 6157-6168.

Markel, P., Shu, P., Ebeling, C., Carlson, G.A., Nagle, D.L., Smutko, J.S. and Moore, K.J. (1997) Theoretical and empirical issues for marker-assisted breeding of congenic mouse strains. Nature Genetics. 17: 280-284.

Mathis, C., Neuman, P. E., Gershenfeld, H., Paul, S. M., Crawley, J. N. (1995) Genetic analysis of anxiety-related drugs in AXB and BXA recombinant inbred mouse strains. Behav. Genet. 25: 557-568.

Mathis, C., Paul, S.M., Crawley, J.N. (1994) Characterization of benzodiazepine-sensitive behaviors in the A/J and C57BL/6J inbred strains of mice. Behav Genet. 24:171-180.

Miczek, K.A., Weerts, E.M., Vivian, J.A., Barros, H.M. (1995) Aggression, anxiety and vocalizations in animals: GABAA and 5-HT anxiolytics. Psychopharmacology. 121: 38-56.

Mihalek, R.M., Banerjee, P.K., Korpi, E.R., Quinlan, J.J., Firestone, L.L., Mi, Z.P., Lagenaur, C., Tretter, V., Sieghart, W., Anagnostaras, S.G., Sage, J.R., Fanselow, M.S., Guidotti, A., Spigelman, I., Li, Z., DeLorey, T.M., Olsen, R.W., Homanics, G.E. (1999) Attenuated sensitivity to neuroactive steroids in gamma-aminobutyrate type A receptor delta subunit knockout mice. Proc Natl Acad Sci U S A. 96: 12905-12910.

Montgomery, K.C. (1955). The relation between fear induced by novel stimulation and exploratory behaviour. J Comp Physiol Psychol. 48: 254-260.

Montkowski, A., Poettig, M., Mederer, A., Holsboer, F. (1997) Behavioural performance in three substrains of mouse strain 129. Brain Res. 762: 12-18.

Moser, V.C., Cheek, B.M., MacPhail, R.C. (1995) A multidisciplinary approach to toxicological screening: III. Neurobehavioral toxicity. J Toxicol Environ Health. 45: 173-210.

Murphy, D.L., Mueller, E.A., Hill, J.L., Tolliver, T.J., Jacobsen, F.M. (1989) Comparative anxiogenic, neuroendocrine, and other physiologic effects of m-chlorophenylpiperazine given intravenously or orally to healthy volunteers. Psychopharmacology. 98: 275-282.

Murphy, D.L., Wichems, C., Li, Q., Heils, A. (1999) Molecular manipulations as tools for enhancing our understanding of 5-HT neurotransmission. Trends Pharmacol Sci. 20: 246-252.

Nelson, R.J., Demas, G.E., Huang, P.L., Fishman, M.C., Dawson, V.L., Dawson, T.M., Synder, S.H. (1995) Behavioural abnormalities in male mice lacking neuronal nitric oxide synthase. Nature. 378: 383-386.

Nelson, R.J. and Young, K.A. (1998) Behavior in mice with targeted disruption of single genes. Neurosci Biobehav Rev. 22: 453-462.

O'Donovan, M.C. and Owen, M.H. (1999) Candidate-gene association studies of schizophrenia. Am J Human Genetics. 65: 587-592.

Olivier, B., Molewijk, E., van Oorschot, R., van der Poel, G., Zethof, T., van der Heyden, J., Mos, J. (1994) New animal models of anxiety. Eur Neuropsychopharmacol. 4: 93-102.

Ongini, E., Iuliano, E., Racagni, G. (1982) Cerebellar cyclic GMP and behavioral effects after acute and repeated administration of benzodiazepines in mice. Eur J Pharmacol. 80: 185-90.

Parks, C.L., Robinson, P.S., Sibille, E., Shenk, T., Toth, M. (1998) Increased anxiety of mice lacking the serotonin1A receptor. Proc Natl Acad Sci USA. 95: 10734-10739.

Paulus, M.P., Dulawa, S.C., Ralph, R.J., Geyer, M.A. (1999) Behavioral organization is independent of locomotor activity in 129 and C57 mouse strains. Brain Res. 835: 27-36.

Paylor, R., Nguyen, M., Crawley, J.N., Patrick, J., Beaudet, A., Orr-Urtreger, A. (1998) α7 nicotinic receptor subunits are not necessary for hippocampal-dependent learning or sensorimotor gating: A behavioral characterization of Acra7-deficient mice. Learning and Memory. 5: 302-316.

Pellow, S., Chopin, P., File, S.E., Briley, M. (1985) Validation of open:closed arm entries in an elevated plus-maze as a measure of anxiety in the rat. J Neurosci Methods. 14:149-167.

Petitto, J.M., McNamara, R.K., Gendreau, P.L., Huang, Z., Jackson, A.J. (1999) Impaired learning and memory and altered hippocampal neurodevelopment resulting from interleukin-2 gene deletion. J Neurosci Res. 56: 441-446.

Picciotto, M.R. (1999) Knock-out mouse models used to study neurobiological systems. Critical Reviews Neurobiol. 13: 103-149.

Ralph, R.J., Varty, G.B., Kelly, M.A., Wang, Y.M., Caron, M.G., Rubinstein, M., Grandy, D.K., Low, M.J., Geyer, M.A. (1999) The dopamine D2, but not D3 or D4, receptor subtype is essential for the disruption of prepulse inhibition produced by amphetamine in mice. J Neurosci. 19: 4627-4633.

Ramboz, S., Oosting, R., Amara, D.A., Kung, H.F., Blier, P., Mendelsohn, M., Mann, J.J., Brunner, D., Hen, R. (1998) Serotonin receptor 1A knockout: an animal model of anxiety-related disorder. Proc Natl Acad Sci U S A. 95: 14476-14481.

Ramboz, S., Saudou, F., Amara, D.A., Belzung, C., Segu, L., Misslin, R., Buhot, M.C., Hen, R. (1996) 5-HT1B receptor knock out - behavioral consequences. Behav Brain Res. 73: 305-312.

Rodgers, R.J. (1997) Animal models of 'anxiety': where next? Behav Pharmacol. 8: 477-496.

Rodgers, R.J., Cole, J.C. (1993) Influence of social isolation, gender, strain, and prior novelty on plus-maze behaviour in mice. Physiol Behav. 54: 729-736.

Rodgers, R.J. Haller, J., Holmes, A., Halasz, J., Walton, T.J., Brain, P.F. (1999) Corticosterone response to the plus-maze: high correlation with risk assessment in rats and mice. Physiol Behav. in press.

Rogers, D.C., Fisher, E.M.C., Brown, S.D.M., Peters, J., Hunter, A.J., Martin, J.E. (1997) Behavioral and functional analysis of mouse phenotype: SHIRPA, a proposed protocol for comprehensive phenotype assessment. Mammalian Genome. 8: 711-713.

Rubenstein, M., Phillips, T.J., Bunzow, J.R., Falzone, T.L., Dziewczapolski, G., Zhang, G., Fang, Y., Larson, J.L., McDougall, J.A., Chester, J.A., Saez, C., Pugsley, T.A., Gershanik, O., Low, M.J., Grandy, D.K. (1997) Mice lacking dopamine D4 receptors are supersensitive to ethanol, cocaine, and methamphetamine. Cell. 90: 991-1001.

Rudolph, U., Crestani, F., Benke, D., Brunig, I., Benson, J.A., Fritschy, J.M., Martin, J.R., Bluethmann, H., Mohler, H. (1999) Benzodiazepine actions mediated by specific gamma-aminobutyric acid(A) receptor subtypes. Nature. 401: 796-800.

Sallinen, J., Haapalinna, A., Viitamaa, T., Kobilka, B.K., Scheinin, M. (1998) Adrenergic alpha2C-receptors modulate the acoustic startle reflex, prepulse inhibition, and aggression in mice. J Neurosci. 18: 3035-3042.

Sams-Dodd, F., Lipska, B.K., Weinberger, D. (1997) Neonatal lesions of the rat ventral hippocampus result in hyperlocomotion and deficits in social behaviour in adulthood. Psychopharmacology. 132: 303-310.

Shepherd, J.K., Grewal, S.S., Fletcher, A., Bill, D.J., Dourish, C.T. (1994) Behavioural and pharmacological characterisation of the elevated "zero-maze" as an animal model of anxiety. Psychopharmacology. 116: 56-64.

Sibley, D.R., Hollon, T.R., Gleason, T.C., Lachowicz, J.E., Ariano, M.A., Huang, S.P., Westphal, H., Surmeier, D.J., Crawley, J.N. (1998) Generation and characterization of D5 dopamine receptor knock-out mice. American College of Neuropsychopharmacology 37th Annual Meeting. Abstract 56: page 287.

Silver, L. (1995) Mouse Genetics: Concepts and Applications. New York: Oxford University Press.

Sluyter, F., Korte, S.M., Bohus, B., Van Oortmerssen, G.A. (1996) Behavioral stress response of genetically selected aggressive and nonaggressive wild house mice in the shock-probe/defensive burying test. Pharmacol Biochem Behav. 54: 113-116.

Smith, D.R., Striplin, C.D., Geller, A.M., Mailman, R.B., Drago, J., Lawler, C.P., Gallagher, M. (1998a) Behavioural assessment of mice lacking D_{1A} dopamine receptors. Neuroscience. 86: 135-146.

Smith, G.W., Aubry, J.M., Dellu, F., Contarino, A., Bilezikjian, L.M., Gold, L.H., Chen, R., Marchuk, Y., Hauser, C., Bentley, C.A., Sawchenko, P.E., Koob, G.F., Vale, W., Lee, K.F. (1998b) Corticotropin releasing factor receptor 1-deficient mice display decreased anxiety, impaired stress response, and aberrant neuroendocrine development. Neuron. 20: 1093-1102.

Sokoloff, P., Giros, B., Martres, M.P., Bouthenet, M.L., Schwartz, J.C. (1990) Molecular cloning and characterization of a novel dopamine receptor (D3) as a target for neuroleptics. Nature. 347: 146-151.

Sokoloff, P. and Schwartz, J.C. (1995) Novel dopamine receptors half a decade later. Trends Pharmacol Sci. 16: 270-275.

Steiner, H., Fuchs, S., Accili, D. (1997) D3 dopamine receptor-deficient mouse: evidence for reduced anxiety. Physiol Behav. 63: 137-141.

Stenzel-Poore, M.P., Heinrichs, S.C., Rivest, S., Koob, G.F., Vale, W.W. (1994) Overproduction of corticotropin-releasing factor in transgenic mice: a genetic model of anxiogenic behavior. J Neurosci. 14: 2579-2584.

Sutton, R.E., Koob, G.F., Le Moal, M., Rivier, J., Vale, W. (1982) Corticotropin releasing factor produces behavioural activation in rats. Nature. 297: 331-333.

Swerdlow, N.R., and Geyer, M.A. (1998) Using an animal model of deficient sensorimotor gating to study the pathophysiology and new treatments of schizophrenia. Schizophrenia Bull. 24: 285-301.

Tallman, J. F., Paul, S. M., Skolnick, P., Gallager, D. W. (1980) Receptors for the age of anxiety: Pharmacology of the benzodiazepines. Science 207: 274-281.

Tecott, L.H., Logue, S.F., Wehner, J.M., Kauer, J.A. (1998) Perturbed dentate gyrus function in serotonin 5-HT2C receptor mutant mice. Proc Natl Acad Sci U S A. 95: 15026-15031.

Timpl, P., Spanagel, R., Sillaber, I., Kresse, A., Reul, J.M., Stalla, G.K., Blanquet, V., Steckler, T., Holsboer, F., Wurst, W. (1998) Impaired stress response and reduced anxiety in mice lacking a functional corticotropin-releasing hormone receptor. Nat Genet. 19: 162-166.

Treit, D. and Fundytus, M. (1988) Thigmotaxis as a test for anxiolytic activity in rats. Pharmacol Biochem Behav. 31: 959-962.

Treit, D., Pinel, J.P., Fibiger, H.C. (1981) Conditioned defensive burying: a new paradigm for the study of anxiolytic agents. Pharmacol Biochem Behav. 15: 619-626.

Trullas, R. and Skolnick, P. (1993). Differences in fear motivated behaviors among inbred mouse strains. Psychopharmacology. 111: 323-331.

Tyrer, P.J. (1990) The division of neurosis: a failed classification. J R Soc Med. 83: 614-616.

Vogel, R.A., Frye, G.D., Wilson, J.H., Kuhn, C.M., Koepke, K.M., Mailman, R.B., Mueller, R.A., Breese, G.R. (1980) Attenuation of the effects of punishment by ethanol: comparisons with chlordiazepoxide. Psychopharmacology. 71: 123-129.

Walker, D.L. and Davis, M. (1997) Double dissociation between the involvement of the bed nucleus of the stria terminalis and the central nucleus of the amygdala in startle increases produced by conditioned versus unconditioned fear. J Neurosci. 17: 9375-9383.

Walther, T., Voigt, J.P., Fukamizu, A., Fink, H., Bader, M. (1999) Learning and anxiety in angiotensin-deficient mice. Behav Brain Res. 100: 1-4.

Weninger, S.C., Dunn, A.J., Muglia, L.J., Dikkes, P., Miczek, K.A., Swiergiel, A.H., Berridge, C.W., Majzoub, J.A. (1999) Stress-induced behaviors require the corticotropin-releasing hormone (CRH) receptor, but not CRH. Proc Natl Acad Sci U S A. 96: 8283-8288.

Wehner J.M. and Silva, A. (1996) Importance of strain differences in evaluations of learning and memory processes in null mutants. Ment Retard Devel Disabilities Res Rev. 2: 243-248.

Weiner, I., Shadach, E., Tarrasch, R., Kidron, R., Feldon, J. (1996) The latent inhibition model of schizophrenia: Further validation using the atypical neuroleptic, clozapine. Biol Psychiat. 40: 834-843.

Wood, G.K., Tomasiewicz, H., Rutishauser, U., Magnuson, T., Quirion, R., Rochford, J., Srivastava, L.K. (1998) NCAM-180 knockout mice display increased lateral ventricle size and reduced prepulse inhibition of startle. NeuroReport. 16: 461-466.

Xu, M., Hu, X.T., Cooper, D.C., Moratalia, R., Graybiel, A.M., White, F.J., Tonegawa, S. (1994a) Elmination of cocaine-induced hyperactivity and dopamine-mediated neurophysiological effects in D1 receptor mutant mice. Cell. 79: 945-955.

Xu, M., Koeltzow, T.E., Santiago, G.T., Moratalla, R., Cooper, D.C., Hu, X.T., White, N.M., Graybiel, A.M., White, F.J., Tonegawa, S. (1997) Dopamine D3 receptor mutant mice exhibit increased behavioral sensitivity to concurrent stimulation of D1 and D2 receptors. Neuron. 19: 837-848.

Xu, M., Moratalia, R., Gold, L.H., Hiroi, N., Koob, G.F., Graybiel, A.M., Tonegawa, S. (1994b): Dopamine D1 receptor mutant mice are deficient in striatal expression of dynorphin and in dopamine-mediated behavioral responses. Cell. 79: 729-742.

Zhuang, X., Gross, C., Santarelli, L., Compan, V., Trillat, A.C., Hen, R. (1999) Altered emotional states in knockout mice lacking 5-HT1A or 5-HT1B receptors. Neuropsychopharmacology. 21: 52-60.

6 VIRAL MECHANISMS OF SCHIZOPHRENIA

Bradley D. Pearce

INTRODUCTION

The purpose of this review is to highlight the potential of a rodent model in providing clues to possible viral mechanisms in neuropsychiatric disorders. As evident from the various essays in this volume, the term "model" can be defined differently depending on its intended purpose. In my opinion, animal models aimed at elucidating the fundamental pathophysiology of psychiatric disorders are most informative when experimental results are used in a manner analogous to a mathematical result in a computer iteration. That is, the data from the animal model are used to construct a preliminary explanatory mechanism that is likely to be imprecise, but points nonetheless to a new set of experiments involving the actual human disease. The results from the human experiments in turn yield data which direct refinement of the model. As this process is repeated, successively better approximations of the human disease entity are attained. In contrast to models used expressly for the screening or evaluation of therapeutic drugs, all models directed at uncovering fundamental mechanisms of a given human disease will become obsolete as that disease becomes better understood. For many models "obsolescence" occurs relatively early in the process as the model no longer serves to suggest experiments related to the human disease.

This does not imply that the continued exploration of the hitherto model becomes less important, or that the basic science investigations of the experimental disease should be discontinued. Indeed constraining an experimental system to a particular disease can be counterproductive. For most neuropsychiatric diseases, multiple models will likely be needed to uncover various facets of the underling pathophysiology.

This review emphasizes an animal model of schizophrenia that examines the impact of a perinatal viral infection on the structure and function of the hippocampus. Given how little is known of the mechanisms by which viruses could give rise to schizophrenia, the model I describe is necessarily in its early stages of the "iterative" process, and the fundamental concepts revealed by these studies could prove applicable to other neurological or neurodegenerative diseases.

VIRAL INFECTIONS AND NEURODEVELOPMENT

Several decades of research have established viruses as important pathogens of the CNS (Johnson, 1996; Kristensson, 1992; Mohammed et al., 1993). Viral infections can be particularly devastating to the developing brain as exemplified by congenital rubella or cytomegalovirus (Griffith and Booss, 1994). Prenatal or early postnatal viral infections have been linked to mental retardation, seizure disorders, hydrocephalus, microencephaly, and sensorimotor abnormalities (Griffith and Booss, 1994; Volpe, 1995; Whitley and Stagno, 1997). In addition, humans are constantly confronted with emerging and undefined viral pathogens, and infections by known viruses are rarely recorded epidemiologically (Johnson, 1996). Indeed, many viral infections do not come to clinical attention even when they occur during pregnancy, and only in rare cases involving severe symptoms or clear diagnostic signs is the responsible virus isolated or identified. Moreover, because of the complex interrelationships between a virus and its host, the identification of a particular virus as being associated with a given neurological disease is only the first step in defining relevant pathophysiological mechanisms. This is particularly relevant for infections occurring in the context of the dynamic cellular and molecular events of neurodevelopment. Thus, while the capability of viruses to act as teratogens is well established (Griffith and Booss, 1994; Oberst, 1993; Volpe, 1995; Whitley and Stagno, 1997), uncloaking specific causal links between viral pathogens and neurological diseases in humans is confronted by numerous obstacles.

A multitude of viruses are capable of crossing the placenta (Kaplan, 1993; Nahmias and Kourtis, 1997), and the undeveloped fetal blood brain barrier may not offer adequate defense against viral invasion into the CNS (Lustig et al., 1992; Rodier, 1994). Viral infections during brain development entail pathogenic mechanisms that differ from those in the adult and hence may fail to produce the classical neuropathological hallmarks of a viral infection at autopsy (Volpe, 1995). Furthermore, modern virology has identified occult viral infections that are undetectable by conventional neuropathological techniques. For example, non-cytolytic viruses can infect neurons without diminishing cell vitality or causing signs of damage (Bilzer and Stitz, 1996; de la Torre and Oldstone, 1996; Kristensson and Norrby, 1986). Despite the lack of readily identifiable pathology, the differentiated or "luxury" function of these neurons can be disrupted by the infection leading to long term sequela (Bilzer and Stitz, 1996; de la Torre and Oldstone, 1996; Kristensson and Norrby, 1986). Thus, autopsy studies are constrained in their ability to ascribe an incompletely-defined disease to a given virus, and several lines of evidence support the concept that viral infections lacking overt or immediate clinical manifestations may nevertheless cause subtle or latent perturbation of brain structure and function. This evidence, along with the ubiquity of viruses in our environment, has fueled speculation that viral infections are involved in neurodegenerative and psychiatric disorders of unknown etiology (Crnic and Pizer, 1988; Kirch, 1993; Kristensson, 1992; Martyn, 1997; Yolken and Torrey, 1995).

VIRAL INFECTIONS IN NEUROPSYCHIATRIC DISORDERS

Recent epidemiological and neuropathological studies have focused on the potential role of viruses in causing neuropsychiatric disorders (Deykin and MacMahon, 1979; Kirch, 1993; Yolken and Torrey, 1995). Many such disorders, including autism, temporal lobe epilepsy, and schizophrenia, also have a neurodevelopmental component suggesting a prenatal or perinatal insult (O'Connor et al., 1996; Rapin and Katzman, 1998; Weinberger, 1995). Although the pathological characterization of most neuropsychiatric diseases is incomplete, and there is considerable heterogeneity even within a given diagnostic category, abnormalities of the hippocampal formation have been described in each of the disorders mentioned above (Bauman, 1991; Bogerts, 1993; Sagar and Oxbury, 1987). Perhaps this should not be surprising considering the proposed neurodevelopmental origin and clinical phenotypes of these disorders; and that the hippocampus develops late in neurohistogenesis (allowing for a subtle defect) and is pivotal to memory and sensory representations (Altman and Bayer, 1990; Humphrey, 1967; Swanson, 1983). In humans and experimental animals the developing hippocampus is vulnerable to diverse types of insults including several different families of viruses (Bilzer and Stitz, 1996; Mohammed et al., 1993). The importance of environmental factors such as viruses in causing hippocampal abnormalities in humans is underscored by a recent study of 15 sets of monozygotic twins who were discordant for schizophrenia; hippocampal volumes were consistently reduced only in the afflicted twins (Suddath et al., 1990). Nonetheless, many neuropsychiatric disorders including schizophrenia are believed to involve the interplay between genes and the environment, and a genetic diathesis for these disorders remains consistent with a viral etiology because host genes play an established role in determining individual responses and susceptibilities to viral infections (Abel and Dessein, 1997).

The epidemiological evidence for the involvement of a viral infection in schizophrenia is presented in Table 1. Most of this evidence is indirect. Furthermore, while the table presents positive findings, many of the findings have not been replicated and there are abundant unresolved discrepancies in the literature (Yolken and Torrey, 1995). Likewise, various reports of isolating viruses or viral nucleic acids from the brains of patients with schizophrenia have typically not withstood scientific scrutiny or are not confirmed in subsequent studies.

Epidemiological analysis of the viral hypothesis is an area of ongoing research, and as these studies are refined, and their findings are replicated (or fail to be replicated), the obscure concepts relating a viral infection to the etiopathology of schizophrenia should begin to be elucidated. In this regard, specific theories integrating the available data are beginning to emerge.

For example, Torrey and Yolken have hypothesized that schizophrenia could be caused by a virus transmitted from house cats (Torrey and Yolken, 1995). This hypothesis is consistent with some aspects of the geographical distribution of schizophrenia, and could explain the increase of pre-schizophrenia births during the winter and spring months when owners bring their cats into the house to protect them from the cold and rain. Cats are known to harbor a number of viruses, including retroviruses, and transmission of a human neuroteratogenic protozoan (toxoplasmosis) from house cats to their pregnant owners is well established (Torrey and Yolken, 1995). The proposed connection between cats and schizophrenia is being further investigated using patient questionnaires as well as

82

Table 1. Summary of epidemiological and serological studies of schizophrenia with specific relevance to the viral hypothesis.

Variable or Risk Factor Found in Schizophrenia Patients	Putative Implications for a Viral Etiopathology of Schizophrenia
↑ Exposure to influenza epidemics during 2nd trimester in utero	Maternal influenza (or ensuing immune response) causing disrupted fetal brain development
↑ Prenatal or postnatal exposure to enteroviruses (e.g., Poliovirus)	Subsets of neurons destroyed by neuro-invasive viral strains in susceptible hosts
↑ Incidence of urban versus rural birth, ↑ household crowding	Higher exposure to communicable viruses
↑ Number of siblings or ↑ probability of having older siblings	Transmission of (community acquired) virus to pregnant mother or younger (affected) sibling
↑ Probability of being born in late winter or early spring	Exposure to viral epidemics with seasonal cyclicality, indoors crowding
↑ Schizophrenia incidence among immigrant populations (including 2nd generation)	Immigrants contracting primary infections by novel viruses (e.g., fetus not protected by maternal antibodies)
↑ Exposure in utero to famine	Nutritional deprivation enhancing host vulnerability; heightened viral contact from atypical food sources
↑ Probability of dermatoglyphic or minor physical abnormalities	Altered morphogenesis by prenatal viral infection
↑ Probability of having been born with perinatal or obstetrical complications (OCs)	Virus-induced fetopathy causing OCs; heightened exposure of neonate to nosocomial viral infections
↑ Viral antibodies (in serum or CSF) to herpes viruses, influenza A, vaccinia, *and others*	Evidence of infection, virus reactivation, or virus-induced autoimmunity.

↑ Increased versus Controls
For references see: (DeLisi and Crow, 1986; Kirch, 1993; Squires, 1997; Watson et al., 1999; Yolken and Torrey, 1995).

virological studies that could point to a specific feline zoonosis (Torrey and Yolken, 1999).

The neurodevelopmental hypothesis of schizophrenia, which suggests a latency between the initial insult and the manifestation of symptoms, remains the prevailing paradigm for understanding schizophrenia pathogenesis (Weinberger, 1995). Discovering the nature of this "initial insult" has become a prominent goal of biological psychiatry, and viruses and bacteria remain prime candidates amongst environmental agents (Gilmore and Jarskog, 1997; Kirch, 1993:Yolken and Torrey, 1995). Unfortunately, investigations of viral pathogenesis are confounded when there is a long latency between infection and the development of neurological disease as illustrated by the human immunodeficiency virus (HIV), which enters the CNS early yet does not usually cause HIV encephalitis is until years later (Gray et al., 1992). The challenge in defining the role of viral infections in schizophrenia and other neurodevelopmental disorders hinges on understanding the cellular and molecular mechanisms by which viral insults during ontogenesis can cause latent pathology or dysfunction in the CNS.

CRITICISMS OF THE VIRAL HYPOTHESIS: A CALL TO REFINE THE PARADIGMS

Although there are an increasing number theories linking viral infections to schizophrenia, there are also valid and incisive criticisms of the "viral hypothesis." Clearly, the viral hypothesis is compelling but as yet unproven, and there is a need to refine the paradigms that are used to interpret available data and guide future studies. Some of the criticisms of the viral hypothesis are adumbrated below; suggested improvements of the hypothesis (put forth by various authors) are included to address these criticisms. For recent reviews see: Kirch, 1993; Squires, 1997; Torrey and Yolken, 1999; Yolken and Torrey, 1995.

1) *Schizophrenia is inarguably associated with genetic and familial variables.* The terms "familial" and "genetic" are by no means synonymous. Individuals within a family tend to be co-exposed to similar environments and thus similar sets of viral pathogens (Torrey and Yolken, 1999). Furthermore, viral and genetic etiologies for schizophrenia are conceptually complementary because host genes determine individual susceptibilities to viral infections. Hence, a genetic association with schizophrenia could be expressed as a polymorphism of a virus entry-receptor (allowing infection of a normally resistant cell type), or a failed immune response at the level of the mother, placenta, fetus or newborn. Furthermore, the ability of some viruses to integrate their DNA into the host genome blurs the distinction between genetic and infectious antecedents of disease (Yolken et al., 1999). For example, it is estimated that about 1% of the human genome consists of endogenous retroviral sequences (Sverdlov, 1998). These are thought to be mostly relics of infectious retroviruses which became integrated into the germ line and can therefore be transmitted vertically. Thus schizophrenia could be caused by maternal or fetal infection with a retrovirus, or result from the reactivation of a preexisting endogenous retrovirus by a new viral infection or the immune molecules it engenders.

2) *Most attempts to transmit a "schizogenic virus" from patients to experimental animals have failed.* Viruses are often species-specific and difficult to transmit to a species other than their natural host. Furthermore, a virus could initiate neuropathological and functional changes in the developing brain, and then be cleared by the immune system prior to the manifestation of symptoms. In such a case, autopsy tissue from patients with schizophrenia would not contain infectious virus. This issue is addressed specifically in the animal model described below.

3) *Various studies of antiviral antibodies point to the involvement of different viruses, and these serological data do not necessarily agree with the epidemiological findings.* Antibody findings may not be identifying the responsible virus per se, but rather could be risk indicators of increased susceptibility to a variety of viruses, one of which is the responsible agent. Likewise, epidemiological associations may be identifying a co-infection (e.g., influenza) which predisposes

the affected person to infection by another agent which ultimately causes schizophrenia. Conversely, the antibody increases in patients with schizophrenia may be indicators of a more vigorous B-cell response leading to autoantibodies. Indeed, the autoimmune hypothesis for schizophrenia is the subject of a rich and controversial literature (Ganguli et al., 1993), and there is accumulating evidence that viral infections can trigger autoimmune diseases in humans (Whitton and Fujinami, 1999). Thus schizophrenia could be triggered by a relatively common virus that only rarely generates an anti-CNS immune response; this is simply an extension of the generally-accepted idea that individual variations in the immune response can determine the degree and character of virus-induced CNS pathology. For example, only a small portion of people infected with HTLV-I develop tropical spastic paraparesis (HTLV-I associated myelopathy) but the risk of this complication is correlated with specific host HLA haplotypes (Jeffery et al., 1999; Usuku et al., 1988).

4) *Schizophrenia has been epidemiologically-correlated with a variety of nonviral environmental factors such as obstetrical complications and famine.* Although environmental variables are often difficult to disentangle, much of the epidemiology remains consistent with a viral etiology. For example, fetal or maternal infection are known causes of difficulties in labor and delivery, and conversely, obstetrical complications can increase neonatal exposure to nosocomial infections (Nahmias and Kourtis, 1997; Volpe, 1995). Furthermore, the critical factor in schizophrenia may be vulnerability of the pre-schizophrenia brain to variety of insults rather than exposure to a specific insult. In such a case, a viral infection would be one of many insults during pregnancy which, if occurring during a critical neurodevelopmental window in a genetically-susceptible individual, would cause brain alterations eventually leading to schizophrenia.

NEUROPATHOLOGY OF SCHIZOPHRENIA: THE LACK OF HALLMARKS

Schizophrenia is a complex disease involving abnormalities in numerous brain regions and several neurochemical systems (Arnold, 1997; Bachus and Kleinman, 1996; Benes, 1995; Bogerts, 1993; Harrison, 1999; Katsetos et al., 1997; Reynolds, 1995; Weinberger, 1995). An understanding of schizophrenia pathology has been hampered by methodological discrepancies, disease heterogeneity, and confounds caused by the common usage of antipsychotic medications. Owing to these factors, and the subtlety of the anatomical defects in schizophrenia, the consistency and reproducibility of relevant neuropathological findings has been disappointing. There are no neuropathological hallmarks of schizophrenia (Harrison, 1999). Nevertheless, recent advances in neurochemistry, cytoarchitectural analysis, and neuroradiology could provide clues to the origin of this devastating illness. Brain imaging studies and neuropathological observations have reported abnormalities in frontal cortex and temporal lobe structures, particularly the hippocampal formation (Arnold, 1997; Benes, 1995). Although lateral (temporal horn) ventricular dilation is the most consistent finding, a reduction of hippocampal volume and evidence for neuronal cell loss and decreased cell size in the hippocampus have also been reported (Arnold, 1997; Bogerts, 1993; Harrison, 1999). In addition, recent neurochemical studies have discovered that schizophrenia is associated with a preferential deficit in cortical and hippocampal inhibitory interneurons, including those expressing neuropeptides such as somatostatin (SS), neuropeptide-Y (NPY) and cholecystokinin (CCK) (Bachus et al., 1997; Benes, 1995; Benes et al., 1991; Gabriel et al., 1996; Powchik et al., 1998; Reynolds et al., 1990; Roberts et al., 1983).

One of the tenants of the neurodevelopmental hypothesis for schizophrenia is that once the developmental insult is complete and psychotic symptoms arise, the abnormalities in the brain are non-progressive (Weinberger, 1995). However, this statement deserves qualification because "developmental" changes can span two decades (Stevens, 1992; Woods, 1998). Therefore, it is important to consider when the well-described brain abnormalities (e.g., ventricular enlargement) arise in schizophrenia and determine if they progress during the latency period. Numerous investigators have suggested that regardless of when brain abnormalities are initially triggered, schizophrenia involves a series of subtle neural alterations occurring late in childhood or early adolescence. In some cases, alterations are more conspicuous like the progressive ventricular enlargement measured during childhood schizophrenia (Rapoport et al., 1997). Furthermore, a case can be made for a subtype of schizophrenia that has a progressive neurodegenerative course during adulthood (Knoll et al., 1998; Woods, 1998). Amongst the controversy concerning neuropathological progression in schizophrenia, the role of perinatal viral infections has received little attention. Therefore, our group is currently using an animal model to examine potential mechanisms by which some individuals may succumb to progressive degeneration following a neonatal viral infection (see below).

Regardless of whether the cytoarchitectural abnormalities in schizophrenia are static or progressive, the pertinent pathogenic mechanisms have not been determined. Excitotoxic damage to neurons by excitatory amino acids (EAA) is a well established phenomena and its relevance to neurodevelopmental disorders and viral infections is now becoming appreciated (Lipton, 1994; Lynn and Wong, 1995; Olney, 1990; Wasterlain and Shirasaka, 1994). Although a role for excitotoxicity in schizophrenia remains controversial, the relevance of alterations in EAA neurotransmission extends beyond the classical concept of excitotoxicity. Within brain regions relevant to schizophrenia (e.g., hippocampus), EAAs and inhibitory neurotransmitters such as GABA help regulate the birth, survival, and differentiation of neurons during ontogenesis (Gould et al., 1994; Marty et al., 1996), and consequently help determine the neuronal circuitry of the adult. Furthermore, the susceptibility of neuronal populations to excitotoxic damage induced by ischemia or hypoxia is dependent on the developmental stage of the brain (Olney, 1990). While the variables determining the susceptibility of neurons to excitotoxicity during ontogenesis have not been defined, recent data suggests that the extreme differences in susceptibility of individual cell types to EAA-mediated toxicity in the adult hippocampus are influenced by the anatomical and functional position of these neurons within the circuitry (Wasterlain and Shirasaka, 1994). Thus the balance between excitatory and inhibitory neurotransmission may exert a dual role in determining neuronal susceptibilities to excitotoxicity–first by influencing the original configuration of neuronal circuitry during development, and second by mediating the pathological consequences of abnormally-developed circuitry in the adult.

This concept has lead us to suggest that schizophrenia may be associated with a virus-induced imbalance between excitatory and inhibitory neurotransmission during neurodevelopment (Pearce et al., 1996; Pearce et al., 1997). Autopsy studies in schizophrenia broadly support such a mechanism.

Examination of brain regions implicated in schizophrenia has revealed a reduction of GABAergic axon terminals in the hippocampus as well as the temporal and prefrontal cortex (Reynolds, 1995; Reynolds et al., 1990; Simpson et al., 1989; Woo et al., 1998). Neurochemical and in situ hybridization studies in the frontal and temporal cortex indicate that the enzyme responsible for synthesizing GABA, GAD, is also reduced in schizophrenia (Akbarian et al., 1995; Sherman et al., 1991). Synaptosomal release of GABA is likewise thought to be impaired, and GABA itself may be reduced in some brain regions of patients with schizophrenia (Reynolds, 1995). The decrement of GABA is apparently accompanied by a compensatory upregulation of GABA-A receptors (Benes et al., 1992; Kiuchi et al., 1989).

These deficits in inhibitory neurons must be considered within the context of conflicting evidence for either a decrement or an increase in excitatory neurotransmission in schizophrenia (Benes, 1995; Kim et al., 1980; Moghaddam, 1994; Reynolds, 1995; Tsai et al., 1995). A thorough understanding of the pathophysiological implications of these findings will require hypothesis-driven investigations of the interaction between excitatory and inhibitory neurotransmitter systems over the course of the disease. One appealing mechanism proposes that a subset of GABAergic interneurons may be lost early in the disease during fetal or neonatal development, and that the resulting disinhibition of corticolimbic circuitry may lie dormant until triggered by the maturation of these circuits during adolescence (Benes, 1995). Nevertheless, the description of a pathogenic instigator which could bring about the early elimination of inhibitory neurons has been lacking. As described later, our data from an animal model presents the possibility of a viral-immune process causing the loss of select inhibitory interneurons as well as leading eventually to abnormalities in EAA neurotransmission.

Undoubtedly, schizophrenia is not a disease involving the wholesale loss of inhibitory neurons or a gross perturbation of EAA neurotransmission. As mentioned above, schizophrenia is associated with a deficit of (predominately inhibitory) interneurons expressing SS, CCK and NPY. Interestingly, each of these subclasses of peptidergic neurons has been shown to be dependent on brain derived neurotrophic factor (BDNF) for acquisition their of mature phenotypes (Jones et al., 1994; Marty et al., 1996; Nawa et al., 1993; Nawa et al., 1994). Because the activity and function of neurotrophic growth factors such as BDNF are determined by both genetic and environmental variables, these molecules are well poised as mediators of the putative neurodevelopmental insults in schizophrenia, and thus their involvement is consistent with a heterogeneous etiopathologly of the disease (Lauterborn et al., 1996; Proschel et al., 1992; Smith et al., 1995). Furthermore, there is emerging data to indicate abnormalities in the BDNF gene (or gene expression) in schizophrenia (Muglia et al., 1999). This raises the possibility that schizophrenia could have purely genetic subtypes as well as "sporadic" forms which arise due to environmental agents such as viruses acting on genetically susceptible individuals. Amongst endogenous substances commonly induced by environmental factors (especially infections), cytokines are immune molecules which deserve prominent consideration as intermediates in neurotrophic factor disruption.

THE CYTOKINE NEXUS BETWEEN INFECTION AND NEURODEVELOPMENT

There is increasing awareness that cytokines and neurotrophic factors constitute critical links in the cross-talk between the immune and nervous systems (Burns et al., 1993; Mehler and Kessler, 1995; Otten et al., 1994). Several cytokines which are elaborated during viral infection also appear to be involved in neurodevelopment, including IL-1, IL-2, IL-6, TNF-α, IFN-α/β and IFNγ (Burns et al., 1993; Mehler and Kessler, 1995; Otten et al., 1994; Patterson and Nawa, 1993; Plioplys, 1988; Pousset, 1994). Some of these cytokines have been shown to interact with neurotrophic factors (Lapchak et al., 1993; Montero-Menei et al., 1994). Thus a viral infection during neuromorphogenesis could induce high levels of cytokines that disrupt the developmental program, either by acting directly on developing neurons or by impairing the production of neurotrophic factors. In addition, neurotrophic factors regulate the development of inhibitory neurotransmitter systems, and there is growing evidence that the maturation of key limbic circuits is activity-dependent, which implies that programmed fluctuations of inhibitory and excitatory neurotransmission during neurodevelopment play a role in determining of the ultimate configuration of theses circuits in the adult (Gould et al., 1994; Marty et al., 1996). Thus cytokines can perturb neural circuitry formation at several levels, and in the context of the neurodevelopmental hypothesis for schizophrenia, investigating interactions between cytokines, neurotrophic factors, and inhibitory/excitatory neurotransmitters is a promising avenue of research.

Unfortunately, humans studies aimed at deciphering the role of these interactions in the genesis of schizophrenia are hampered by the long latency between the neurodevelopmental insult and the clinical diagnosis or neuropathological findings. For instance, neurochemical studies showing abnormalities in excitatory and inhibitory neurotransmission in schizophrenia are difficult to extrapolate to events occurring during development since autopsy studies characterize predominately end-stage disease, usually after a lengthy period of antipsychotic drug administration. Thus, animal models are needed to uncover the mechanisms by which an insult during neuro-ontogeny alters cytokine production, neurotrophic factors, and specific subsets of neurons--especially those expressing the major excitatory and inhibitory neurotransmitters.

To circumvent the conundrum of studying schizophrenia latency, it is desirable to have an animal model which displays the characteristic lag between the initial insult and the manifestation of disease. Our recent studies have focused on an animal model in which rats are infected soon after birth with lymphocytic choriomeningitis virus (LCMV). This perinatal viral infection causes the disruption of inhibitory and excitatory neurocircuitry, and a delayed loss of neurons in the hippocampus (Pearce et al., 1996, 1997). During the interval between the infection and stage at which the abnormalities become fully evident, many key neurodevelopmental events are taking place. For example, BDNF undergoes a developmentally-regulated increase in expression during the postnatal period which coincides with the period of active LCMV infection in our rats (Maisonpierre et al., 1990). Interestingly, our preliminary data suggest that the virus induces IL-1β in the developing hippocampus during this period (Pearce et al., 1997), and other laboratories have reported that systemic or intracranial injection of IL-1β (or LPS which elevates IL-1β) in adult rats causes a substantial decrease in hippocampal

BDNF mRNA (Lapchak et al., 1993; Montero-Menei et al., 1994). Considering that BDNF-dependent inhibitory circuits are developing during this period, the implications of this could be far reaching, and will be discussed later.

THE LCMV NEONATAL RAT MODEL

As described above, the ability of a viral infection to influence the development of specific neurotransmitter systems has potential implications for schizophrenia pathogenesis yet the mechanisms underlying the selective loss of subsets of neurons as a consequence of perinatal viral infections are enigmatic and poorly understood. To elucidate the relevant cellular and molecular interactions between viral infections and host neuronal circuitry we have undertaken a series of longitudinal studies examining the pathophysiological consequences of LCMV infection in neonatal rats (Baldridge et al., 1993; Pearce et al., 1996, 1997).

LCMV is an arenavirus which has a host range encompassing humans and many rodent species (Jahrling and Peters, 1992; Monjan et al., 1975; Wright et al., 1997). In many respects, LCMV is a quintessential non-cytolytic virus (Bilzer and Stitz, 1996; de la Torre et al., 1993; Oldstone and Dixon, 1974; Oldstone and Rall, 1993; Rodriguez et al., 1983). In vitro, LCMV causes a persistent non-cytopathic infection of cells including those with neuron-like phenotypes (de la Torre et al., 1993). In vivo, infection of neonatal or immune-suppressed mice further exemplifies the non-cytopathic nature of this virus. Specifically, a substantial portion of neurons are persistently infected in the hippocampus and other brain regions for the lifespan of the mouse yet there are no signs of neuronal loss or destruction (de la Torre and Oldstone, 1996; Rodriguez et al., 1983).

LCMV infection of rats has been less completely characterized and clearly involves distinct neuropathological processes which do not occur in the mouse. In neonatal rats, LCMV is reported to show a predilection to infect immature or undifferentiated neurons, particularly in the cerebellum, hippocampal dentate gyrus, taenia tectum and olfactory bulb (Baldridge et al., 1993; Monjan et al., 1973b). Once a neuron becomes infected, its fate is apparently determined by its neuroanatomical location or neuronal phenotype. Specifically, there is an acute degeneration of infected neurons in the cerebellum whereas infected neurons in some other brain regions are spared (Monjan et al., 1973a). In the hippocampus, there is a delayed loss of dentate granule cells which becomes apparent just prior to sexual maturity, and continues for months after infectious virus has been cleared (Monjan et al., 1975). The time course of hippocampal and cerebellar pathology (produced by infection of rats at 4 days old) is depicted in Figure 1.

Although the data are incomplete, current evidence indicates that the cerebellar and hippocampal pathology can be distinguished depending on the developmental stage of the rat at the time of infection. For instance, rats infected within a day of birth display little cerebellar pathology yet they eventually manifest the latent hippocampal disease (Monjan et al., 1975). This is pertinent to neurodevelopmental diseases such as schizophrenia because it demonstrates that pathology can be produced in different brain areas, and to different degrees of severity, as a function of the ontogenic stage during which the infection occurs. The cerebellum, like the hippocampus, develop relatively late in neuromorphogenesis (Humphrey, 1967; Jacobson, 1991).

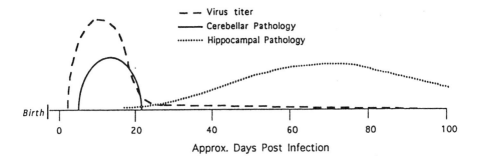

Figure 1. Diagram of pathological phases occurring in the cerebellum and hippocampus after infection with LCMV

Our studies have focused primarily on the hippocampus because of the importance of this structure in schizophrenia and temporal lobe epilepsy. However, several recent reports have suggested that the cerebellum is also involved in schizophrenia (Katsetos et al., 1997). As shown in Figure 2, our studies indicate that

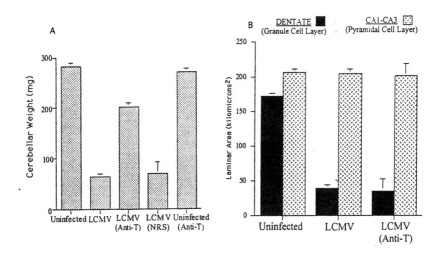

Figure 2. T-lymphocytes mediate cerebellar but not hippocampal pathology in LCMV infected rats. A) Immunosuppression with anti-thymocyte serum prevented LCMV induced cerebellar hypoplasia. Rats (3-5/group) were infected intracranially with LCMV, or received sham injections ("uninfected"), at 4 days old, and the mean cerebellar weight in each group was determined 90-93 days later. Rats which were LCMV-infected and received no treatment ("LCMV") had a significant loss of cerebellar mass compared to uninfected controls. Rats which were identically infected but received anti-thymocyte antibody (anti-T) treatment administered over the entire course of the experiment had cerebellar weights which were significantly greater than the untreated LCMV-infected group indicating protection by the immunosuppressive treatment. Equivalent treatment of LCMV-infected rats with non-immune serum immunoglobulin (NRS) had no protective effect. Treatment of sham-infected rats with anti-T did not significantly alter cerebellar weights as compared to the untreated controls. B) Quantitative analysis of cell loss in Nissl stained sections taken through the forebrain (at −3.90 mm relative to bregma) from the same rats used to determine cerebellar weights. The area of the dentate granule layer (solid bars) was

reduced in rats infected at 4 days old and assessed 90-93 days later. There was no protective effect of Anti-T treatment which was administered over the three month course of the experiment. The area corresponding to the pyramidal cell layer of Ammon's horn (stippled bars) was not significantly reduced by the infection. Error bars represent the standard error of the mean. One way ANOVA and Student-Newman-Keuls tests set at p<.05 significance were used for group comparisons. Figure reproduced from Pearce et. al., 1999.

while the cerebellar damage in LCMV-infected rats is mediated by T- lymphocytes, hippocampal abnormalities are not dependent on T-cell immunity (Pearce et al., 1999). Direct destruction of the neurons by LCMV also seems unlikely since most infectious virus has been cleared by the time the hippocampal pathology becomes evident (Monjan et al., 1975). As discussed in the next section, we suggest that the latent hippocampal pathology occurs by a previously undescribed mechanism.

We chose to infect rats at 4 days old because the developmental stage of the hippocampal dentate gyrus at this time corresponds to the stage attained in the human dentate gyrus during the second trimester in utero (Altman and Bayer, 1990; Humphrey, 1967), and neurodevelopmental theories of schizophrenia frequently point to this trimester as being critical for an insult to produce the type of abnormalities found in the disease (Yolken and Torrey, 1995). One of the cornerstones of the neurodevelopmental theory of schizophrenia is the lack of corticohippocampal gliosis, even in late stage schizophrenia and in cases where there is hippocampal cell loss (Jonsson et al., 1997). Therefore, (in unpublished studies) we examined whether a viral insult during neurodevelopment could cause hippocampal atrophy and neuronal loss without producing astrogliosis. Rats infected with the virus at 4 days old and examined as adults displayed varying degrees of lateral ventricular dilation along with an overt loss of dentate granule cells. However, using immunostaining for glial fibrillary acidic protein (GFAP) we found little evidence of gliosis accompanying these abnormalities in the hippocampus. Thus perinatal LCMV infection initiates latent cell loss in the hippocampus but fails to produce evident gliosis. Considering that signs of infectious virus would likewise not be detected in a perfunctory neuropathological examination of these adult rats, this pathology might be classified as a non-viral, non-degenerative disease, although the former is obviously not the case.

In a series of studies my collaborators and I have examined alterations in excitatory and inhibitory neurotransmitters in this model. To determine the long-term sequela of the LCMV infection, in vivo electrophysiological measures of hippocampal function were assessed in rats at 84-102 days following neonatal LCMV infection (Pearce et al., 1996). Figure 3 shows the results from paired-pulse experiments in which hippocampal evoked potentials were elicited by stimulation of perforant path afferents to the dentate gyrus.

The tracings in the top panel of Figure 3 demonstrate a decrease in EPSPs and a suppression of GABA-mediated recurrent inhibition in the dentate gyrus of LCMV-infected rats. While the decrease in EPSPs could result from dentate granule cell loss, the marked suppression of GABA-mediated recurrent inhibition indicates that the remaining dentate granule cells are hyperexcitable. As indicated in the graph derived from the paired pulse experiments (Figure 3, bottom panel), sham-infected rats showed absolute suppression of dentate granule cell population spike upon the second stimulus when interstimulus intervals were less than 20 ms. In contrast, a second population spike could be elicited in the LCMV infected animals even at the shortest interstimulus interval measured. In addition, when dentate

Figure 3. Neonatal infection with LCMV causes decreased recurrent inhibition in the adult hippocampus. The top panel shows representative in vivo recordings of evoked potentials in the dentate gyrus produced by paired equipotent stimuli (to the perforant path) measured in rats 84-102 days old. Comparisons are made between rats infected with LCMV at 4 days old, and sham-infected controls. Population spikes (immediately to the right of arrow heads) are thought to be produced by the synchronous firing of the dentate granule cells in response to the excitatory stimulus. The second stimulus of the pair does not normally illicit a second population spike as shown in the tracing from the sham-infected animal. This inhibition, observed at short interstimulus intervals, is mediated at least in part by GABA. The tracing from the LCMV infected rats suggests the infection has disabled inhibitory circuitry because the second stimulus is capable of eliciting another population spike representing the synchronous firing of the principle cells. The severity of the LCMV-induced abnormality is demonstrated in the bottom panel in which the population spike amplitude in response to the second stimulus (P2) is divided by the response to the first stimulus (P1) and this ratio is plotted against the time between the stimuli. Paired pulse inhibition is clearly and consistently suppressed in the dentate gyrus ($p < .001$) of infected rats indicating a profound disinhibition of dentate granule cells. Reproduced from Pearce et. al., 1996.

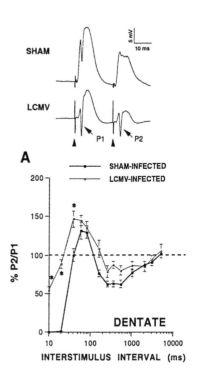

population spike amplitude was plotted against EPSP-slopes the resulting curve was steepened in the LCMV group thus further substantiating dentate granule cell hyperexcitability in response to perforant pathway stimulation. These electrophysiological findings cannot be explained by conventional models of viral pathogenesis. The data suggest that the dentate granule cells in these adult animals (who were originally infected as neonates) are hyperexcitable, most likely due to a decrement in the function of inhibitory interneurons (Pearce et al., 1997).

Recent studies are providing clues to the mechanism by which LCMV could be disrupting inhibitory interneurons. These studies have shown that while many of the cells infected in the hippocampus during the early acute phase of the disease are neurons that divide postnatally (e.g., the dentate granule cells), GABAergic interneurons are the exception, in that these cells are thought to be born prenatally yet they become infected (Pearce et al., 1997). Because GABAergic cells are undergoing the final stages of migration and differentiation during the acute infectious stage of the disease (Dupuy-Davies and Houser, 1999; Nitsch et al., 1990), the ability of these neurons to establish the appropriate connections within the hippocampal circuitry may be impaired by the infection.

Although LCMV is a non-cytopathic virus which is unlikely to kill GABAergic neurons directly, this virus has the well-established capacity to disrupt "luxury" functions of cells including neurotransmitter production (de la Torre and Oldstone, 1996; Lipkin et al., 1988). We have also observed LCMV infection in a subset of GABAergic neurons expressing parvalbumin (unpublished observations). These parvalbumin neurons are likewise differentiating during the acute infection –

which transpires prior observed loss of dentate granule cells (de Lecea et al., 1995; Monjan et al., 1975; Nitsch et al., 1990). Of note, rodent studies suggest that PVA neurons are dependant on BDNF, and thus share this characteristic with the peptidergic neurons discussed above (Jones et al., 1994). Our previous immunohistochemical studies in adult rats found a reduction in the number of these PVA inhibitory neurons (Pearce et al., 1996).

Thus the loss of inhibitory tone that was indicated by our electrophysiological experiments could be a consequence of an early disruption of infected GABAergic neurons, or a failure of parvalbumin neurons to thrive, perhaps because of a lack of neurotrophin support from BDNF or a virus-induced decrement in their production of their neuroprotective parvalbumin calcium binding protein (Celio, 1990). Alternatively, the impairment could be at the level of the dentate granule cells themselves; e.g., their improper differentiation under the strain of the infection could reconfigure the dentate circuitry. However, this alternative mechanism is not consistent with the latency of dentate granule cell loss, and furthermore fails to provide a parsimonious explanation for why a primary abnormality in the dentate granule cells would ultimately masquerade electrophysiologically as a loss of GABAergic function.

VIRUS INDUCED DISINHIBITION AND EXCITOTOXICITY (VIDE)

As described in the previous section, rats infected neonatally with LCMV develop hippocampal pathology which shows some parallels with the neurotransmitter and structural changes observed in schizophrenia. Studies of hippocampi from adult rats which have cleared infectious virus indicate a decrease in the number and function GABAergic interneurons, enlargement of lateral ventricles, and a gradual loss of dentate granule cells (Pearce et al., 1996). Because the infection evidently disables inhibitory circuits, glutamatergic input on dentate granule cells is apparently unleashed from its inhibitory control, and we suggest that the gradual death of the dentate granule cells is due to synaptically-mediated excitotoxicity. Although at present the data are not sufficient to prove every step in this mechanism– which I have termed Virus Induced Disinhibition and Excitotoxicity (VIDE)– the tenants I have described provide a conceptual framework linking perinatal viral infections with latently-expressed corticohippocampal abnormalities.

Before discussing the implications of VIDE for schizophrenia, I will elaborate on the VIDE mechanism as it is currently conceptualized. A central feature of the VIDE mechanism is that a prenatal or neonatal viral infection causes an impairment of inhibitory circuits that precedes the excitotoxic death of principle cells. Based on our data from the LCMV model, we have hypothesized two possible means by which this could occur (Figure 4). The first posits a direct viral infection of a vulnerable subset of inhibitory neurons. In our animal model this is exemplified by infection of the PVA subclass of GABAergic cells with LCMV; the infection occurs during a critical neurodevelopmental window. The second mechanism postulates virus-induced cytokines leading to a deficit in a neurotrophic factor (e.g., BDNF) and thus disrupted development of neurotrophin-dependent inhibitory circuits. This mechanism is consistent with our finding that LCMV induces IL-1β in the rat brain during the period when BDNF-dependent neurons are differentiating, These mechanisms are not mutually exclusive, and experiments are ongoing using the LCMV model to determine the relative contribution of direct neuronal infection versus an indirect effect mediated thorough neurotrophic factors in the disruption of inhibitory circuits.

In spite of the caveat that the LCMV model (and the VIDE mechanism) is in the first round of the iterative process that judges its validity as a model for schizophrenia, a critical inspection of its predictive and heuristic value is warranted in regard to schizophrenia pathogenesis. That is, our experimental infections with LCMV suggest a novel disease mechanism (VIDE) which could provide clues to a pathological process linking a viral infection with schizophrenia. If a VIDE mechanism is operating in schizophrenia what findings are expected in brains of patients, and what future experiments can be performed to support or refute this hypothesis?

The VIDE mechanism predicts that indices of GABAergic neurons would be consistently reduced in the affected brain regions of adult patients. Does this prediction hold true? As described in the previous sections, several studies have found evidence for a loss of GABAergic function in cerebral cortex and hippocampus of schizophrenia patients. However, these findings have not been uniformly replicated (Reynolds, 1995). Besides the usual explanations for these discrepancies (methodological or microneuroanatomical differences, patient heterogeneity, etiologic diversity) one possibility is that disease-related decreases in indices of GABA are masked by neuroleptic drug therapy. Indeed, some reports have indicated that dopamine antagonists can increase GABA release or upregulate GAD mRNA (Qin et al., 1994; Sherman et al., 1991). If this were the case, then one would expect to find evidence of impoverished GABAergic neurotransmission in patients who are not taking neuroleptics, but would measure normal or elevated levels in patients on high doses (or long-term therapy). In support of this idea, a recent study of GAD immunoreactivity in the hippocampus found lowest levels in patients not taking neuroleptic drugs, and revealed a positive correlation between GAD immunoreactivity and neuroleptic dose among all patients in the study (Todtenkopf and Benes, 1998). While the interpretation of this finding is open to speculation, it is compatible with the VIDE mechanism.

The indirect VIDE mechanism proposes a cytokine mediated decrease in BDNF retarding the maturation of neurons expressing SS, NPY and CCK (Jones et al., 1994; Marty et al., 1996; Nawa et al., 1993; Nawa et al., 1994). Deficits in each of these neuropeptides are found in limbic regions of schizophrenia patients, although (like virtually all post mortem studies in this disease) some of these findings have not been replicated (Bachus et al., 1997; Gabriel et al., 1996; Powchik et al., 1998; Reynolds et al., 1990; Roberts et al., 1983). Each of these neuropeptides has been shown to co-localize with GABA (Powchik et al., 1998). Therefore, the variable loss of these peptidergic neurons might be a reflection of the above mentioned decrement in GABAergic neurons. Postmortem analysis of peptidergic and GABAergic neurons in the same patients (e.g., taken from the same brain bank) would help determine what portion of patients have defects in either or both of these overlapping inhibitory systems.

The VIDE mechanism predicts that inhibitory neurotransmitter systems are compromised prior to schizophrenia diagnosis–which presumably occurs decades after the initial infection. Given the well know role of GABA systems in motor function, the subtle motor abnormalities observed in children prior to the development of schizophrenia could be in part a manifestation of disturbed

94

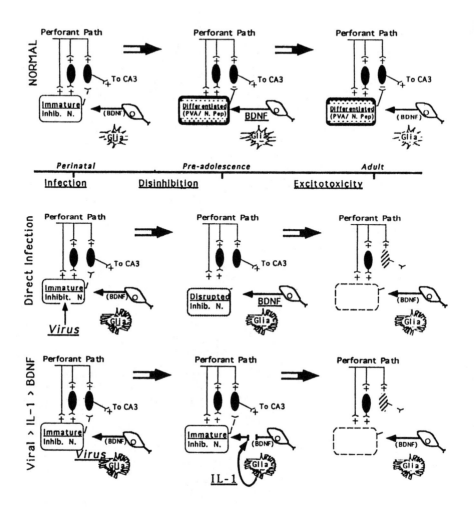

Figure 4. Proposed mechanism of Virus Induced Disinhibition and Excitotoxicity. Simplified diagram of the (rat) hippocampus showing consequences of viral infection on the development and interactions between dentate granule cells (black ovals) and inhibitory interneurons (shown as opaque squares) that express parvalbumin (PVA) or neuropeptides (N.Pep.) such as somatostatin. Excitatory and inhibitory synapses are shown as + or -, respectively. The top sequence depicts the normal differentiation and maturation of BDNF-dependent inhibitory (PVA/ N.Pep) neurons. At maturity, these neurons mediate feed forward and feed back inhibition that balances the excitatory influences coming from the perforant path and dentate granule cells. The consequences of direct viral infection of these inhibitory interneurons during neurodevelopment is shown in the middle panel. The virus is proposed to transiently interrupt the inhibitory function of these neurons without being directly cytocidal. The PVA/ N.pep neurons may nonetheless die because of impinging excitotoxic synapses from the perforant path of dentate granule cells. The bottom panel proposes an indirect VIDE mechanism in which infection of adjacent cells causes the release of IL-1 that in turn blocks the production of BDNF. The developmental program for the BDNF-dependent PVA/ N.Pep neurons is interrupted, and inhibition of the circuit is disabled. In both VIDE mechanisms, dentate granule cells receive unchecked excitatory input and consequently die later in the disease from excitotoxicity. At end stage disease, and overall loss of both GABA and EAA (normally supplied by the dentate granule cells) is expected.

GABAergic circuits (Walker et al., 1994). Furthermore, schizotypal symptoms (which can precede schizophrenia by years) might be a result of the decreased inhibitory modulation of excitatory principle cells leading to overactive output from the hippocampus or other limbic structures involved in schizophrenia (Benes, 1995; Benes et al., 1994; Walker et al., 1999). The VIDE mechanism also suggests a way by which schizotypal features could transition into frank psychotic symptoms sufficient to meet diagnostic criteria for schizophrenia. Within the hippocampus GABAergic neurons such as those expressing parvalbumin receive both excitatory and inhibitory inputs from other cells (Figure 4). During the quiescent or schizotypal prodrome of schizophrenia, a pathological cascade could be occurring in which the initial impairment of inhibitory modulation leads to increased excitatory input on GABAergic neurons, which in turn die as a consequence of excitotoxicity, leading to further disinhibition and corticolimbic over-stimulation that crosses the threshold needed to produce psychosis. Alternatively, first episode psychosis could be triggered by the maturation of excitatory lamina leading to the hippocampus (Benes et al., 1994), although the contribution of excitatory perforant path fibers to these late-maturing tracts remains questionable.

Ostensibly, VIDE predicts that older patients would manifest the latent excitotoxic component of Virus-Induced Disinhibition and Excitotoxicity. Such a mechanism could be predictive of the apparent progressive neurodegeneration (particularly in the hippocampal region) that is seen in at least some patients (Knoll et al., 1998; Woods, 1998). More importantly, VIDE is predictive of heterogeneity in both psychiatric symptom severity and neurodegeneration. Specifically, this concept is based on the likelihood of individual differences in the reserve capacity of inhibitory neuronal networks that can be brought to bear in a homeostatic effort to override the virus-induced disinhibition, and the subsequent excitotoxicity. Thus, individuals with inherently more robust inhibitory circuits, or resistance to the disruption of those circuits by the infection, would have more mild psychiatric symptoms, and presumably less degeneration. However, psychiatric and degenerative components of the disease could diverge because other compensatory mechanism would obviously come into play during the excitotoxicity stage.

In this regard, one can envisage a spectrum of outcomes as a consequence of the infection. At the worst end of the spectrum, perinatal infection of individuals with minimal inhibitory reserve could trigger a pathological concatenation of events. In such a scenario, the initial virus-induced death or dysfunction of a relatively select population of inhibitory cells (e.g., peptidergic) would result in excessive excitatory input onto other inhibitory populations which themselves would rapidly succumb to excitotoxicity leading to an accelerated VIDE cascade. Speculatively, the result could be a degenerative childhood schizophrenia, or temporal lobe epilepsy. Although seizure disorders are mechanistically diverse and the relationship between epilepsy and schizophrenia is dubious, the VIDE mechanism deserves mention in regard to an experimental epilepsy model which entails electrical stimulation of excitatory inputs to the hippocampus (Sloviter, 1987). This electrical model reveals a disinhibition similar to that seen in our infected rats, and thus implies that accentuated excitatory input can lead to disinhibition in the dentate gyrus. Furthermore, in the electrical stimulation model there is excitotoxic damage to select hippocampal neurons (Sloviter, 1987). Thus this model provides a parallel system that further supports the idea of a pathological cascade in VIDE. Interestingly, humans with temporal lobe epilepsy who have a history of CNS infection during hippocampal development, also have a loss of dentate granule cells and hippocampal hilar interneurons (O'Connor et al., 1996).

CONCLUSIONS AND CAVEATS

The hypothesis that VIDE is involved in schizophrenia or other neuropsychiatric diseases is clearly speculative. Since the LCMV model is in its first iteration, the VIDE mechanism has not been subjected to the refinement of the iterative process, and thus there are a multitude theoretical gaps that need to be filled, and criticisms to address. The VIDE mechanism represents only one of a series of more or less simpatico mechanisms which have been developed over the last several years to relate changes in inhibitory and excitatory neurotransmitters to schizophrenia pathogenesis (Benes, 1995; Benes et al., 1991; Lipska and Weinberger, 1993; Olney and Farber, 1995; Pearce et al., 1996; Reynolds et al., 1990; Tsai et al., 1995). Therefore, some of the most salient criticism have been addressed by others. For example, Reynolds and Benes have considered the role of dopamine (and the efficacy of neuroleptic drugs) in circuits with impaired GABAergic transmission (Benes, 1995; Reynolds et al., 1990). Although our emphasis has been on the hippocampus, schizophrenia clearly involves multiple interconnected brain areas. It is premature to consider VIDE in the broader context of associative neural networks or clinical subtypes. Nonetheless, Benes has described inhibitory and excitatory circuits in the cingulate cortex in which a mechanism analogous to VIDE could be operating (Benes, 1995). Olney and colleagues have indirectly addressed other potential criticisms of the VIDE mechanism in studies using an animal model that reveals how the apparent decrement in glutamatergic systems is actually compatible with a loss of limbic GABAergic function in the schizophrenia (Farber et al., 1998; Olney and Farber, 1995). Along similar lines, although the increase in excitatory influences on dentate granule cells in the LCMV model is ostensibly divergent from the proposed decrement in glutamatergic neurotransmission in schizophrenia, on closer inspection the parallels are maintained. In adult rats which have cleared the virus, dentate granule cells comprise the majority of neurons lost. Because these cells are themselves excitatory, their loss could recapitulate the decrease in hippocampal glutamate measured in schizophrenia at autopsy (Kim et al., 1980; Tsai et al., 1998). Thus it is important to determine how much of the brain atrophy in schizophrenia can be attributed to loss of excitatory neurons or axons, and further to define the quantitative relationship between such loss and CSF glutamate levels.

The VIDE mechanism would predict that patients with longer duration of disease would have more synaptically-mediated excitotoxicity, and in line with the aforementioned logic that most of the cells lost are excitatory, would also have fewer principle cells and thus lower CSF glutamate. Patients with recent onset disease would be expected to have higher CSF glutamate commensurate with ongoing excitotoxicity. This does not appear to be the case in the study by Tsai et al. which found no correlation between CSF glutamate levels and disease duration (Tsai et al., 1998). However, indices of glutamate neurons were found to be lower in patients evincing the greatest atrophy, which would support the VIDE mechanism.

The most straight-forward criticism of the VIDE mechanism (and the LCMV model) is that schizophrenia is not typically found to have the magnitude or character of degeneration seen in our adult LCMV-infected rats. This point deserves clarification. In spite of its ability to infect humans, I do not claim that LCMV is the cause of schizophrenia. And while it is conceivable that a similar virus could be involved in some cases of schizophrenia, it seems unlikely that a VIDE mechanism would be confined to the hippocampal dentate gyrus. Indeed, analogous circuits exist elsewhere in the hippocampus and cingulate cortex (Benes, 1995; Pearce et al., 1996), and different circuits could be affected depending on the timing of the neurodevelopmental insult. Even so, the dentate gyrus could be affected in some cases as reported by McLardy who measured a thinning of the dentate granule layer in the hippocampus of patients with early-onset schizophrenia (McLardy, 1973).

In summary, huge challenges lie ahead in defining the pathogenesis of schizophrenia and the relative contribution of viral infections. Perhaps it could be argued that designing an animal model to investigate viral mechanisms of schizophrenia is premature. However, considering the prevailing neurodevelopmental theory of schizophrenia and lack of pathological hallmarks, it could equally be argued that attempts to find vestiges of a viral infection in patients decades after viral exposure is tantamount to an unguided fishing tour.

I suggest the greatest strides can be made when both approaches are undertaken, and the human and animal studies are guided mutually in an iterative process.

ACKNOWLEDGEMENTS

The author wishes to acknowledge Dr. Andrew H. Miller, Cecilia Po, and Nojan Valadi for their support and assistance. Projects supported by NIH Grants #5-R29-NS37068, MH51761-01A1, and the Theodore and Vada Stanley Foundation.

REFERENCES

Abel, L. and Dessein, A. J. (1997). The impact of host genetics on susceptibility to human infectious diseases. Curr. Opinion Immun. 9, 509-16.

Akbarian, S., Kim, J. J., Potkin, S. G., Hagman, J. O., Tafazzoli, A., Bunney, W. E., Jr., Jones, E. G. (1995). Gene expression for glutamic acid decarboxylase is reduced without loss of neurons in prefrontal cortex of schizophrenics. Arch. of Gen. Psych. 52, 258-66; discussion 267-78.

Altman, A. and Bayer, S. A. (1990). Migration and distribution of two populations of hippocampal granule cell precursors during the perinatal and postnatal periods. J. of Comp Neurol. 301, 365-381.

Arnold, S. E. (1997). The medial temporal lobe in schizophrenia. J. of Neuropsych. & Clin. Neurosci. 9, 460-70.

Bachus, S. E., Hyde, T. M., Herman, M. M., Egan, M. F., Kleinman, J. E. (1997). Abnormal cholecystokinin mRNA levels in entorhinal cortex of schizophrenics. J. of Psychiat. Res. 31, 233-56.

Bachus, S. E. and Kleinman, J. E. (1996). The neuropathology of schizophrenia. J. Clin. Psych.57, 72-83.

Baldridge, J. R., Pearce, B. D., Parekh, B. S., Buchmeier, M. J. (1993). Teratogenic effects of neonatal arenavirus infection on the developing rat cerebellum are abrogated by passive immunotherapy. Virology 197, 669-677.

Bauman, M. (1991). Microscopic neuroanatomic abnormalities in autism. Pediatrics suppl., 791-796.

Benes, F. M. (1995). Is there a neuroanatomic basis for schizophrenia? an old question revisited. The Neuroscientist 1(2), 104-115.

Benes, F. M., McSparren, J., Bird, E. D., SanGiovanni, J. P., Vincent, S. L. (1991). Deficits in small interneurons in prefrontal and cingulate cortices of schizophrenic and schizoaffective patients. Arch. Gen. Psychiatry 48, 996-1001.

Benes, F. M., Turtle, M., Khan, Y., Farol, P. (1994). Myelination of a key relay zone in the hippocampal formation occurs in the human brain during childhood, adolescence, and adulthood. Arch.Gen. Psychiatry 51, 477-484.

98

Benes, F. M., Vincent, S. L., Alsterberg, G., Bird, E. D., SanGiovanni, J. P. (1992). Increased GABA receptor binding in superficial layers of cingulate cortex in schizophrenics. J. of Neuroscience *12*, 924-929.

Bilzer, T. and Stitz, L. (1996). Immunopathogenesis of virus diseases affecting the central nervous system. Critical Rev. Immunol. *16*, 145-222.

Bogerts, B. (1993). Recent advances in the neuropathology of schizophrenia. Schizophrenia Bull. *19*, 431-445.

Burns, T. M., Clough, J. A., Klein, R. M., Wood, G. W., Berman, N. E. J. (1993). Developmental regulation of cytokine expression in the mouse brain. Growth Factors *9*, 253-258.

Celio, M. R. (1990). Calbindin D-28 and parvalbumin in the rat nervous system. Neuroscience *35*, 375-474.

Crnic, L. S. and Pizer, L. I. (1988). Behavioral effects of neonatal herpes simplex type 1 infection of mice. Neurotoxicology & Teratology *10*, 381-6.

DeLisi, L. E. and Crow, T. J. (1986). Is schizophrenia a viral or immunologic disorder? Psych. Clin. N. America *9*, 115-32.

de la Torre, J. C. and Oldstone, M. B. A. (1996). Anatomy of viral persistence: mechanisms of persistence and associated disease. Adv. Virus Res. *46*, 311-471.

de la Torre, J. C., Rall, G., Oldstone, C., Sanna, P. P., Borrow, P., Oldstone, M. B. A. (1993). Replication of lymphocytic choriomeningitis virus is restricted in terminally differentiated neurons. J. of Virology *67*, 7350-7359.

de Lecea, L., del Rio, J. A., Soriano, E. (1995). Developmental expression of parvalbumin mRNA in the cerebral cortex and hippocampus of the rat. Mol. Brain Res. *32*, 1-13.

Deykin, E. Y. and MacMahon, B. (1979). Viral exposure and autism. Amer. J. Epidem. *109*, 628-638.

Dupuy-Davies, S. and Houser, C. R. (1999). Evidence for changing positions of GABA neurons in the developing rat dentate gyrus. Hippocampus *9*, 186-99.

Farber, N. B., Newcomer, J. W., Olney, J. W. (1998). The glutamate synapse in neuropsychiatric disorders. Focus on schizophrenia and Alzheimer's disease. Prog. Brain Res. *116*, 421-37.

Gabriel, S. M., Davidson, M., Haroutunian, V., Powchik, P., Bierer, L. M., Purohit, D. P., Perl, D. P., Davis, K. L. (1996). Neuropeptide deficits in schizophrenia vs. Alzheimer's disease cerebral cortex. Biol. Psychiatry *39*, 82-91.

Ganguli, R., Brar, J. S., Chengappa, K. N. R., Yang, Z. W., Nimgaonkar, V. L., Rabin, B. S. (1993). Autoimmunity in schizophrenia: a review of recent findings. Ann. Med. *25*, 489-496.

Gilmore, J. H. and Jarskog, L. F. (1997). Exposure to infection and brain development: cytokines in the pathogenesis of schizophrenia. Schizophr. Res. *24*, 365-7.

Gould, E., Cameron, H. A., McEwen, B. S. (1994). Blockade of NMDA receptors increases cell death and birth in the developing rat dentate gyrus. J. Comp. Neurol *340*, 551-565.

Gray, F., Lescs, M., Keohane, C., Paraire, F., Marc, B., Durigon, M., Gherardi, R. (1992). Early brain changes in HIV infection: neuropathological study of 11 HIV seropositive, non-AIDS cases. J. of Neuropath. and Exp. Neurol. *51*, 177-185.

Griffith, B. P. and Booss, J. (1994). Neurologic infections of the fetus and newborn. Neurologic Clinics *12*, 541-564.

Harrison, P. J. (1999). The neuropathology of schizophrenia. A critical review of the data and their interpretation. Brain *122*, 593-624.

Humphrey, T. (1967). The development of the human hippocampal fissure. J. of Anatomy *101*, 655-676.

Jacobson, M. (1991). Histogenesis and morphogenesis of cortical structures. In Developmental Neurobiology, N.Y.: Plenum, pp. 401-451.

Jahrling, P. B. and Peters, C. J. (1992). Lymphocytic choriomeningitis virus, a neglected pathogen of man. Arch. Pathol. Lab. Med. *116*, 486-488.

Jeffery, K. J., Usuku, K., Hall, S. E., Matsumoto, W., Taylor, G. P., Procter, J., Bunce, M., Ogg, G. S., Welsh, K. I., Weber, J. N., Lloyd, A. L., Nowak, M. A., Nagai, M., Kodama, D., Izumo, S., Osame, M., Bangham, C. R. (1999). HLA alleles determine human T-lymphotropic virus-I (HTLV-I) proviral load and the risk of HTLV-I-associated myelopathy. PNAS (USA) *96*, 3848-53.

Johnson, R. T. (1996). Emerging Viral Infections. Arch. Neurol. *53*, 18-22.

Jones, K. R., Farinas, I., Backus, C., Reichardt, L. F. (1994). Targeted disruption of the BDNF gene perturbs brain and sensory neuron development but not motor neuron development. Cell *76*, 989-999.

Jonsson, S. A., Luts, A., Guldberg-Kjaer, N., Brun, A. (1997). Hippocampal pyramidal cell disarray correlates negatively to cell number: implications for the pathogenesis of schizophrenia. Eur. Arch. of Psych. & Clin. Neurosci. *247*, 120-7.

Kaplan, C. (1993). The placenta and viral infections. Sem. Diag. Path. *10*, 232-50.

Katsetos, C. D., Hyde, T. M., Herman, M. M. (1997). Neuropathology of the cerebellum in schizophrenia--an update: 1996 and future directions. Biol. Psychiatry *42*, 213-24.

Kim, J. S., Kornhuber, H. H., Schmid-Burgk, W., Holzmuller, B. (1980). Low cerebrospinal fluid glutamate in schizophrenic patients and a new hypothesis on schizophrenia. Neurosci. Lett. *20*, 379-82.

Kirch, D. G. (1993). Infection and autoimmunity as etiologic factors in schizophrenia: a review and reappraisal. Schizophrenia Bull. *19*, 355-370.

Kiuchi, Y., Kobayashi, T., Takeuchi, J., Shimizu, H., Ogata, H., Toru, M. (1989). Benzodiazepine receptors increase in post-mortem brain of chronic schizophrenics. European Arch. Psych. Neurol. Sci. *239*, 71-8.

Knoll, J. L. t., Garver, D. L., Ramberg, J. E., Kingsbury, S. J., Croissant, D., McDermott, B. (1998). Heterogeneity of the psychoses: is there a neurodegenerative psychosis? Schizophrenia Bull. *24*, 365-79.

Kristensson, K. (1992). Potential role of viruses in neurodegeneration. Mol. Chem. Neuropathol. *16*, 45-58.

Kristensson, K. and Norrby, E. (1986). Persistence of RNA viruses in the central nervous system. Ann. Rev. Microbiol. *40*, 159-184.

Lapchak, P., Araujo, D. M., Hefti, F. (1993). Systemic interleukin-1 beta decreases brain-derived neurotrophic factor messenger RNA expression in the rat hippocampal formation. Neuroscience *53*, 297-301.

Lauterborn, J. C., Rivera, S., Stinis, C. T., Hayes, V. Y., Isackson, P. J., Gall, C. M. (1996). Differential effects of protein synthesis inhibition on the activity-dependent expression of BDNF transcripts: evidence for immediate-early gene responses from specific promoters. J. Neurosci. *16*, 7428-7436.

Lipkin, W. I., Battenberg, E. L. F., Bloom, F. E., Oldstone, M. B. A. (1988). Viral infection of neurons can depress neurotransmitter mRNA levels without histologic injury. Brain Res. *451*, 333-339.

Lipska, B. K. and Weinberger, D. R. (1993). Delayed effects of neonatal hippocampal damage on haloperidol-induced catalepsy and apomorphine-induced stereotypic behaviors in the rat. Brain Res. Dev. Brain Res. *75*, 213-22.

Lipton, S. A. (1994). HIV-related neuronal injury: potential therapeutic intervention with calcium channel antagonists and NMDA antagonists. Mol. Neurobiol. *8*, 181-196.

Lustig, S., Danenberg, H. D., Kafri, Y., Kobiler, D., Ben-Nathan, D. (1992). Viral neuroinvasion and encephalitis induced by lipopolysaccharide and its mediators. J. Exp. Med. *176*, 707-12.

Lynn, W. S. and Wong, P. K. Y. (1995). Neuroimmunodegeneration: do neurons and T cells use common pathways for cell death? FASEB J. *9*, 1147-1156.

Maisonpierre, P. C., Belluscio, L., Friedman, B., Alderson, R. F., Wiegand, S. J., Furth, M. E., Lindsay, R. M., Yancopoulos, G. D. (1990). NT-3, BDNF, and NGF in the developing rat nervous system: parallel as well as reciprocal patterns of expression. Neuron *5*, 501-509

Marty, S., Berninger, B., Carroll, P., Thoenen, H. (1996). GABAergic stimulation regulates the phenotype of hippocampal interneurons through the regulation of brain-derived neurotrophic factor. Neuron *16*, 565-570.

Martyn, C. N. (1997). Infection in childhood and neurological diseases in adult life. Brit. Med. Bull. *53*, 24-39.

McLardy, T. (1973). Deficit and paucity of dentate granule cells in some schizophrenic brains. International Res. Communications System *March* (73-3) 16, 1-1

Mehler, M. F. and Kessler, J. A. (1995). Cytokines and neuronal differentiation. Crit. Rev. Neurobiol. *9*, 419-446.

Moghaddam, B. (1994). Recent basic findings in support of excitatory amino acid hypothesis of schizophrenia. Prog. Neuro-Psychopharmacol. & Biol. Psychiat. *18*, 859-870.

Mohammed, A. H., Norrby, E., Kristensson, K. (1993). Viruses and behavioural changes: a review of clinical and experimental findings. Rev. Neurosciences *4*, 267-86.

Monjan, A. A., Bohl, L. S., Hudgens, G. A. (1975). Neurobiology of LCM virus infection in rodents. Bull.World Health Organiz. *52*, 487-491.

Monjan, A. A., Cole, G. A., Gilden, D. H., Nathanson, N. (1973a). Pathogenesis of cerebellar hypoplasia produced by lymphocytic choriomeningitis virus infection of neonatal rats 1. Evolution of disease following infection at 4 days of age. J. Neuropath. Exp. Neurol. *32*, 110-124.

Monjan, A. A., Cole, G. A., Nathanson, N. (1973b). Pathogenesis of LCMV disease in the rat. In: F. Lehmann-Grube ed. Lymphocytic choriomeningitis virus and other arenaviruses. Berlin, Heidelberg, & New York: Springer, pp. 195-206.

Montero-Menei, C. N., Sindji, L., Pouplard-Barthelaix, A., Jehan, F., Denechaud, L., Darcy, F. (1994). Lipopolysaccharide intracerebral administration induces minimal inflammatory reaction in rat brain. Brain Res. *653*, 101-111.

Muglia, P., Macciardi, F., Kennedy, J. L. (1999). The neurodevelopmnetal hypotheisis of schizophrenia: Genetic investgations. CNS Spectrums *4*, 78-90.

100

Nahmias, A. J. and Kourtis, A. P. (1997). The great balancing acts. The pregnant woman, placenta, fetus, and infectious agents. Clinics Perinat. 24, 497-521.

Nawa, H., Bessho, Y., Carnahan, J., Nakanishi, S., Mizuno, K. (1993). Regulation of neuropeptide expression in cultured cerebral cortical neurons by brain-derived neurotrophic factor. J. Neurochem. 60, 772-775.

Nawa, H., Pelleymounter, M. A., Carnahan, J. (1994). Intraventricular administration of BDNF increases neuropeptide expression in newborn rat brain. J. of Neurosci. 14, 3751-3765.

Nitsch, R., Bergman, I., Kuppers, K., Mueller, G., Frotscher, M. (1990). Late appearance of parvalbumin-immunoreactivity in the development of GABAergic neurons in the rat hippocampus. Neurosci. Lett. 118, 147-150.

O'Connor, W. M., Masukawa, L., Freese, A., Sperling, M. R., French, J. A., O'Conner, M. J. (1996). Hippocampal cell distributions in temporal lobe epilepsy: a comparison between patients with and without an early risk factor. Epilepsia 37, 440-449.

Oberst, R. D. (1993). Viruses as teratogens. Vet. Clinics of N. Amer.: Food Anim. Prac. 9, 23-31.

Oldstone, M. B. A. and Dixon, F. J. (1974). Aging and chronic virus infection: is there a relationship? Federation Proc. 33, 2057-2059.

Oldstone, M. B. A. and Rall, G. F. (1993). Mechanism and consequence of viral persistence in cells of the immune system and neurons. Intervirology 35, 116-121.

Olney, J. W. (1990). Excitotoxin-mediated neuron death in youth and old age. Prog. Brain Res. 86, 37-51.

Olney, J. W. and Farber, N. B. (1995). Glutamate receptor dysfunction and schizophrenia. Arch. Gen. Psych. 52, 998-1007.

Otten, U., Scully, J. L., Ehrhard, P. B., Gadient, R. A. (1994). Neurotrophins: signals between the nervous and immune systems. Prog. Brain Res. 103, 293-305.

Patterson, P. H.,and Nawa, H. (1993). Neuronal differentiation factors/cytokines and synaptic plasticity. Neuron 10, 123-137.

Pearce, B. D., Po, C., Jones, S., Pisell, T. L., Miller, A. H. (1997). The role of the immune response and inhibitory circuits in latent virus-induced hippocampal degeneration. Neuroscience Abstract : Society of Neuroscience.

Pearce, B. D., Po, C. L., Pisell, T. L., Miller, A. H. (1999). Lymphocytic responses and the gradual hippocampal neuron loss following infection with lymphocytic choriomeningitis virus (LCMV). J. of Neuroimmunol. 101, 137-147.

Pearce, B. D., Steffensen, S. C., Paoletti, A. D., Henriksen, S. J., Buchmeier, M. J. (1996). Persistent dentate granule cell hyperexcitability after neonatal infection with lymphocytic choriomeningitis virus. J. Neurosci. 16, 220-228.

Plioplys, A. V. (1988). Expression of the 210 kDa neurofilament subunit in cultured central nervous system from normal and trisomy 16 mice: regulation by interferon. J. Neurosci. 85, 209-222.

Pousset, F. (1994). Development expression of cytokine genes in the cortex and hippocampus of the rat central nervous system. Dev. Brain Res. 81, 143-146.

Powchik, P., Davidson, M., Haroutunian, V., Gabriel, S. M., Purohit, D. P., Perl, D. P., Harvey, P. D., Davis, K. L. (1998). Postmortem studies in schizophrenia. Schizophrenia Bull. 24, 325-41.

Proschel, M., Saunders, A., Roses, A. D., Muller, C. R. (1992). Dinucleotide repeat polymorphism at the human gene for the brain-derived neurotrophic factor (BDNF). Human Molec. Genetics 1, 353.

Qin, Z. H., Zhang, S. P., Weiss, B. (1994). Dopaminergic and glutamatergic blocking drugs differentially regulate glutamic acid decarboxylase mRNA in mouse brain. Brain Res. Mol. Brain Res. 21, 293-302.

Rapin, I. and Katzman, R. (1998). Neurobiology of autism. Ann. Neurol. 43, 7-14.

Rapoport, J. L., Giedd, J., Kumra, S., Jacobsen, L., Smith, A., Lee, P., Nelson, J., Hamburger, S. (1997). Childhood-onset schizophrenia. Progressive ventricular change during adolescence. Arch. of Gen. Psych. 54, 897-903.

Reynolds, G. P. (1995). Neurotransmitter systems in schizophrenia. Int. Rev. Neurobiol. 38, 305-39.

Reynolds, G. P., Czudek, C., Andrews, H. B. (1990). Deficit and hemispheric asymmetry of GABA uptake sites in the hippocampus in schizophrenia. Biol. Psychiatry 27, 1038-1044.

Roberts, G. W., Ferrier, I. N., Lee, Y., Crow, T. J., Johnstone, E. C., Owens, D. G., Bacarese-Hamilton, A. J., McGregor, G., O'Shaughnessey, D., Polak, J. M. (1983). Peptides, the limbic lobe and schizophrenia. Brain Res. 288, 199-211.

Rodier, P. M. (1994). Vulnerable periods and processes during central nervous system development. Environmental Health Perspectives 102 Suppl 2, 121-4.

Rodriguez, M., Buchmeier, M. J., Oldstone, M. B. A., Lampert, P. W. (1983). Ultrastructural localization of viral antigens in the CNS of mice persistently infected with lymphocytic choriomeningitis virus (LCMV). American J. Path. 110, 95-100.

Sagar, H. J. and Oxbury, J. M. (1987). Hippocampal neuron loss in temporal lobe epilepsy: correlation with early childhood convulsions. Ann. Neurol. 22, 334-340.

Sherman, A. D., Davidson, A. T., Baruah, S., Hegwood, T. S., Waziri, R. (1991). Evidence of glutamatergic deficiency in schizophrenia. Neurosci. Lett. 121, 77-80.

Simpson, M. D., Slater, P., Deakin, J. F., Royston, M. C., Skan, W. J. (1989). Reduced GABA uptake sites in the temporal lobe in schizophrenia. Neurosci. Lett. 107, 211-5.

Sloviter, R. S. (1987). Decreased hippocampal inhibition and a selective loss of interneurons in experimental epilepsy. Science 235, 73-76.

Smith, M. A., Makino, S., Kvetnansky, R., Post, R. M. (1995). Stress and glucocorticoids affect the expression of brain-derived neurotrophic factor and neurotrophin-3 mRNAs in the hippocampus. J. Neurosci. 15, 1768-1777.

Squires, R. F. (1997). How a poliovirus might cause schizophrenia: a commentary on Eagles' hypothesis. Neurochem. Res. 22, 647-56.

Stevens, J. R. (1992). Abnormal reinnervation as a basis for schizophrenia: a hypothesis. Arch. Gen. Psychiatry 49, 238-243.

Suddath, R. L., Christison, G. W., Torrey, F. E., Casanova, M. F., Weinberger, D. R. (1990). Anatomical abnormalities in the brains of monozygotic twins discordant for schizophrenia. The NEJM 322, 789-794.

Sverdlov, E. D. (1998). Perpetually mobile footprints of ancient infections in human genome. FEBS Lett. 428, 1-6.

Swanson, L. W. (1983). The hippocampus and the concept of the limbic system. In: W. Seifert, ed. Neurobiology of the Hippocampus. New York: Academic Press, pp. 3-19.

Todtenkopf, M. S. and Benes, F. M. (1998). Distribution of glutamate decarboxylase65 immunoreactive puncta on pyramidal and nonpyramidal neurons in hippocampus of schizophrenic brain. Synapse 29, 323-32.

Torrey, E. F., Yolken, R. H. (1995). Could schizophrenia be a viral zoonosis transmitted from house cats? Schizophrenia Bull. 21, 167-171.

Torrey, E. F. and Yolken, R. H. (1999). Familial and genetic mechanisms in schizophrenia. Brain Res. In press.

Tsai, G., Passani, L. A., Slusher, B. S., Carter, R., Baer, L., Kleinman, J. E., Coyle, J. T. (1995). Abnormal excitatory neurotransmitter metabolism in schizophrenic brains. Arch. Gen. Psychiatry 52, 829-836.

Tsai, G., van Kammen, D. P., Chen, S., Kelley, M. E., Grier, A., Coyle, J. T. (1998). Glutamatergic neurotransmission involves structural and clinical deficits of schizophrenia. Biol. Psychiatry 44, 667-74.

Usuku, K., Sonoda, S., Osame, M., Yashiki, S., Takahashi, K., Matsumoto, M., Sawada, T., Tsuji, K., Tara, M., Igata, A. (1988). HLA haplotype-linked high immune responsiveness against HTLV-I in HTLV-I-associated myelopathy: comparison with adult T-cell leukemia/lymphoma. Ann. Neurol. 23 Suppl, S143-50.

Volpe, J. J. (1995). Neurology of the Newborn. Philadelphia: W.B. Sanders Company, pp. 675-729.

Walker, E. F., Diforio, D., Baum, K. (1999). Developmental neuropathology and the precursors of schizophrenia. Acta Psychiatrica Scandinavica, Suppl. 395, 12-9.

Walker, E. F., Savoie, T., Davis, D. (1994). Neuromotor precursors of schizophrenia. Schizophrenia Bull. 20, 441-51.

Wasterlain, C. G. and Shirasaka, Y. (1994). Seizures, brain damage and brain development. Brain and Devel. 16, 279-295.

Watson, J. B., Mednick, S. A., Huttunen, M., Wang, X. (1999). Prenatal teratogens and the development of adult mental illness. Devel. Psychopath. 11, 457-466.

Weinberger, D. R. (1995). From neuropathology to neurodevelopment. Lancet 346, 552-7.

Whitley, R. J. and Stagno, S. (1997). Perinatal viral infections. In W. M. Scheld, R. J. Whitley and D. T. Durack, eds. Infections of the Central Nervous System. Philadelphia: Lippencott-Raven, pp. 223-242.

Whitton, J. L. and Fujinami, R. S. (1999). Viruses as triggers of autoimmunity: facts and fantasies. Curr. Opinion Microbiol. 2, 392-7.

Woo, T. U., Whitehead, R. E., Melchitzky, D. S., Lewis, D. A. (1998). A subclass of prefrontal gamma-aminobutyric acid axon terminals are selectively altered in schizophrenia. PNAS (USA) 95, 5341-6.

Woods, B. T. (1998). Is schizophrenia a progressive neurodevelopmental disorder? Toward a unitary pathogenetic mechanism. Am. J. of Psych. 155, 1661-70.

Wright, R., Johnson, D., Neumann, M., Ksiazek, T. G., Rollin, P., Keech, R. V., Bonthius, D. J., Hitchon, P., Grose, C. F., Bell, W. E., Bale, J. F., Jr. (1997). Congenital lymphocytic choriomeningitis virus syndrome: a disease that mimics congenital toxoplasmosis or Cytomegalovirus infection. Pediatrics 100, 1-6.

Yolken, R. H., Karlsson, H., Yee, F., Wilson, N. L., Torrey, E. F. (1999). Retroviruses and Schizophrenia. Brain Res. *In press*

Yolken, R. H. and Torrey, E. F. (1995). Viruses, schizophrenia, and bipolar disorder. Clin. Microbiol. Rev. *8*, 131-145.

7 PREPULSE INHIBITION AS A CROSS-SPECIES MODEL OF SENSORIMOTOR GATING DEFICITS IN SCHIZOPHRENIA

Mark A. Geyer

SENSORIMOTOR GATING IN SCHIZOPHRENIA

Theories addressing the processes involved in schizophrenia have emphasized abnormalities in the processing of information, and specifically difficulties in the filtering or gating of both external sensory stimuli and internal cognitions. Most theories describing the group of disorders included within the broad term "schizophrenia" have conceptualized the common aspect of these disorders as involving deficits in one or more of the multiple mechanisms that enable normal individuals to filter or inhibit responding to most of the sensory stimuli they receive (Braff and Geyer, 1990; Geyer and Braff, 1987; McGhie and Chapman, 1961). As a group, such mechanisms are referred to as sensorimotor gating. In theory, impairments in gating lead to sensory overload and subsequently to cognitive fragmentation. The hypothetical construct of sensorimotor gating has been operationalized and studied in both human and animal paradigms. One important operational measure of sensorimotor gating is provided by prepulse inhibition of the startle response (PPI), which can be measured in humans or animals using virtually identical approaches. Prepulse inhibition refers to the reduction in the startle response produced by a weak non-startling stimulus (the prepulse) presented between 30 and 500 msec before the startle stimulus (Hoffman and Ison, 1980).

The first report of deficits in PPI of acoustic startle in schizophrenia appeared in 1978 (Braff et al., 1978). Subsequently, the deficit in PPI has been confirmed in studies of medicated, but still-ill patients with schizophrenia in different countries and by investigators using a variety of methods (Bolino et al., 1994; Braff et al., 1992; Grillon et al., 1992; Hamm et al., 1995). Deficits in PPI in schizophrenia patients do not simply result from medications or psychotic behavior *per se*, because schizotypal patients who exhibit behavioral abnormalities but are not receiving antipsychotic medications and are not grossly psychotic also exhibit PPI deficits (Cadenhead et al., 1993). The deficits in sensorimotor gating seen in schizophrenia have now been linked experimentally as well as theoretically with measures of increased distractibility, cognitive fragmentation, and thought disorder (Karper et al., 1996; Perry et al., 1999).

ANIMAL MODELS OF SENSORIMOTOR GATING

In view of the evidence of a deficit in PPI as an example of the sensorimotor gating abnormalities in schizophrenia patients, extensive studies of the neurobiology and pharmacology of PPI have been conducted in animals. This work has taken advantage of the fact that the cross-species nature of the startle response and PPI enables the use of animal models to investigate behavioral phenomena that are extremely similar to the deficits seen in schizophrenia. Although this research area is little more than a decade old, considerable progress has been made. Beginning with the initial demonstrations of the ability of dopamine (DA) agonists to disrupt PPI in rats (Mansbach et al., 1988; Swerdlow et al., 1986), the basic rodent "PPI model" has evolved into at least four distinct "models," differentiated by the manipulations used to mimic the disruption of PPI seen in schizophrenia.

The Dopamine Prepulse Inhibition Model

The DA hypothesis of schizophrenia has dominated the field for the past two decades, largely supported by the evidence that antagonism of central DA receptors is responsible for the clinical efficacy of typical antipsychotics. The D2 family of DA receptors has been the focus of most psychopharmacological studies related to schizophrenia, by virtue of the strong relationship between D2 receptor affinity and clinical efficacy of typical antipsychotic drugs. Experience with atypical antipsychotics such as clozapine, however, suggests that some patients with schizophrenia can be treated successfully even though they have failed to respond to antagonists at D2 and D3 DA receptors.

In rats, disruptions in PPI very similar to those seen in schizophrenia were first reproduced by the administration of direct or indirect dopamine agonists, such as apomorphine or d-amphetamine (Mansbach et al., 1988; Swerdlow et al., 1991; Swerdlow and Geyer, 1993). These effects are reversed by DA receptor antagonists (Mansbach et al., 1988; Swerdlow et al., 1991). Indeed, the effects of apomorphine are reliably prevented by virtually all antipsychotics that have appreciable affinity for dopamine D2 receptors. In addition to a wide range of typical antipsychotics, atypical antipsychotics, including clozapine, have been demonstrated to prevent the effects of apomorphine or other dopamine agonists on PPI (Swerdlow et al., 1991, 1994; Swerdlow and Geyer, 1993). One exception to this finding (Varty and Higgins, 1995a) was shown subsequently to be due to the use of Wistar rather than Sprague-Dawley rats (Swerdlow et al., 1998). Nevertheless, some newer putative antipsychotics, (such as M100907 and LU111995) are ineffective in blocking the effects of apomorphine on PPI (Geyer et al., 1999a,b). It remains to be seen, however, whether these compounds will prove to be efficacious antipsychotics.

The D2 receptor appears to mediate the apomorphine-disruption of PPI, because it is blocked by D2 antagonists (Mansbach et al., 1988; Swerdlow et al., 1991). Further support for a role of the D2 receptor, but not the D1 receptor in the modulation of PPI is the finding that PPI is disrupted by the D2 agonist quinpirole, but not by the D1 agonist SKF 38393 (Peng et al., 1990). Putative D4 antagonists also restore PPI in apomorphine-treated rats, despite the fact that they are often inactive in traditional preclinical measures of antipsychotic action (Mansbach et al.,

1998). Thus, converging evidence supports the important involvement of dopaminergic systems, acting via D2-family receptors, in the control of PPI.

Given that few specific ligands at D4 receptors have been identified, the availability of animals with genetic modifications of D4 receptors may provide unique and critical insights into the functional roles of these receptors. D2-like DA receptors, including the D2, D3, and D4 subtypes, have all been implicated in the modulation of PPI via studies of DA agonists and antagonists in rats. Nevertheless, the functional relevance of each receptor subtype remains unclear because these ligands are not specific (Caine et al., 1995). To determine the relevance of each receptor subtype, we used genetically altered strains of "knockout" (KO) mice lacking the DA D2, D3, or D4 receptors. D2 and D4 KO and wild-type (WT) mice from Drs. David Grandy and Malcolm Low at Oregon Health Sciences University were used in studies of acoustic startle and PPI in San Diego. In addition, we studied D3 KO mice obtained from Dr. Marc Caron at Duke University. We tested the effects of each knockout on both the phenotypic expression of PPI as well as the disruption of PPI produced by the indirect DA agonist d-amphetamine. In the D2 receptor mutant mice, amphetamine significantly disrupted PPI in the D2 WT mice, while having no effect in the D2 KO mice (Ralph et al., 1999). After amphetamine treatment, both D3 and D4 receptor WT and KO mice had significant disruptions in PPI. These findings indicate that the amphetamine-induced disruption of PPI is mediated via the DA D2 receptor and not the D3 or D4 receptor subtypes. To the extent that the amphetamine disruption of PPI has predictive validity for the efficacy of antipsychotic drugs, these results also indicate that D2 rather than D3 or D4 mechanisms are most critically involved in the therapeutic effects of antipsychotics.

The Serotonin Prepulse Inhibition Model

The second PPI model derives from the fact that PPI in rats is reduced by systemic treatment with 5-HT releasers (Kehne et al., 1992, 1996; Mansbach et al., 1989; Martinez and Geyer, 1997) and by direct agonists for 5-HT1A, 5-HT1B, or 5-HT2 receptors (Rigdon and Weatherspoon, 1992; Sipes and Geyer, 1994). The PPI-disruptive effects of 5-HT releasers are prevented by pretreatment with the 5-HT reuptake inhibitor fluoxetine, which prevents the drug-induced release of 5-HT from presynaptic terminals (Kehne et al., 1992, 1996; Martinez and Geyer, 1997). The PPI-disruptive effects of hallucinogenic 5-HT2 receptor agonists are blocked by pretreatment with non-specific 5-HT2 antagonists (Sipes and Geyer, 1994) or the selective 5-HT2A antagonist M100907 (Padich et al., 1996), but not by a 5-HT2C antagonist (Sipes and Geyer, 1995) or the DA blocker haloperidol (Padich et al., 1996). Such findings have contributed to the current investigation of M100907 as a putative non-dopaminergic antipsychotic in schizophrenia patients (Geyer, 1998). Although this model is demonstrably sensitive to antipsychotic drugs having 5-HT2A antagonist actions (e.g. risperidone, M100907), it is relatively insensitive to most typical antipsychotics that are more selective dopamine D2 antagonists (Kehne et al., 1996; Padich et al., 1996; Sipes and Geyer, 1994; Varty and Higgins, 1995a). As with the apomorphine-based PPI model, the hallucinogen model is based on the use of a receptor agonist to mimic the PPI deficit seen in schizophrenia and is therefore primarily useful in identifying drugs having antagonist actions at the corresponding receptor.

We have extended this work to include studies of the serotonin-1B (5-HT_{1B}) receptor in modulating startle reactivity, habituation, and PPI by comparing 5-HT_{1B} receptor gene KO (5-HT1BKO) with wild-type 129/Sv mice (Dulawa et al., 1997, 1998). We obtained 5-HT1BKO mice from Dr. Rene Hen at Columbia University. Two phenotypic differences were observed after saline treatment: 5-HT1BKO mice consistently exhibited a small increase in PPI that is sometimes significant, depending upon the sample size; and 5-HT1BKO male mice exhibited robust decreases in startle reactivity. Habituation was disrupted consistently by the 5-$HT_{1A/1B}$ agonist RU24969 in WT but not in 5-HT1BKO mice, while the selective 5-HT_{1A} agonist 8-OH-DPAT did not affect habituation. Consistent with the phenotypic difference in PPI, a high dose of RU24969 significantly and consistently reduced PPI in WT but not in 5-HT1BKO mice. This result further confirms that RU24969 exerts these behavioral effects primarily by acting as a 5-HT_{1B} agonist. 8-OH-DPAT has increased PPI in both WT and 5-HT1BKO mice in every experiment we have conducted, even though it consistently decreases PPI in rats (Rigdon and Weatherspoon, 1992; Sipes and Geyer, 1994). Thus, the knockout of the 5-HT_{1B} receptor gene leads to the predicted loss of the effects of a 5-HT_{1B} agonist without altering the effects of a 5-HT_{1A} agonist. These findings suggest that 5-HT_{1B} receptors modulate startle reactivity, habituation, and PPI in mice. Additionally, a potential species difference may exist in the behavioral effects of 5-HT_{1A} receptor activation on PPI. This experimental approach demonstrates the utility of applying genetic knockout techniques towards understanding the physiological substrates of behaviors and processes such as sensorimotor gating.

The Phencyclidine Prepulse Inhibition Model

The third PPI model of relevance to schizophrenia is the "PCP model". Non-competitive NMDA antagonists (e.g., PCP, dizocilpine, and ketamine) produce robust deficits in PPI in rats (Geyer et al., 1990; Mansbach and Geyer, 1989, 1991), mice (Dulawa and Geyer, 1996), or humans (Karper et al., 1994). Many laboratories using a variety of non-competitive and competitive NMDA antagonists and multiple strains of rodents have reproduced this finding. As with apomorphine or schizophrenia, both intra-modal and cross-modal PPI are sensitive to non-competitive NMDA antagonists (Geyer et al., 1990). The initial studies of the effects of antipsychotics on the PPI-disruptive effects of NMDA antagonists indicated that typical antipsychotics such as haloperidol were ineffective (Geyer et al., 1990; Keith et al., 1991). Subsequent studies with additional typical antipsychotics, additional dosages, and other dopamine antagonists confirmed that the effects of NMDA antagonists in this paradigm are insensitive to the acute effects of these drugs (Bakshi et al., 1994; Johansson et al., 1994; Varty and Higgins, 1995b). These results in rats are consistent with the observations in humans that the psychotic symptoms produced by NMDA antagonists are not reduced by typical antipsychotics (Malhotra et al., 1997). Recent preliminary evidence suggests that chronic administrations of typical antipsychotic drugs might reduce the disruptions in PPI caused by NMDA antagonists in rats (Pietraszek and Ossowska, 1998). Because clinical antipsychotic treatments are administered chronically, further work in this area is warranted to confirm this suggestion.

Interest in the PCP-PPI model intensified with the finding that the atypical antipsychotic clozapine was able to prevent the disruption in PPI produced by

NMDA antagonists (Bakshi et al., 1994). This interaction between clozapine and NMDA antagonists is seen only within a limited dose-range and has been confirmed in some (Bakshi and Geyer, 1999; Swerdlow et al., 1996; Swerdlow et al., 1998) but not all studies (Hoffman et al., 1993; Johansson et al., 1994). Nevertheless, the PPI-disruptive effects of NMDA antagonists are also reduced by other multireceptor antagonist antipsychotics, including olanzapine, quetiapine, remoxipride, and, in some rat strains, risperidone (Bakshi et al., 1994; Bakshi and Geyer, 1995; Johansson et al., 1994; Swerdlow et al., 1996; Varty et al., 1999). Such findings led to the suggestion that the PCP-PPI model might enable the specific identification of atypical rather than typical antipsychotic treatments.

Because these atypical antipsychotics affect multiple receptor subtypes, further studies have examined the possible contributions of each receptor subtype using more selective antagonists. Two major candidates have emerged from these studies. First, the alpha-1 adrenergic antagonist prazosin was found to block the effects of PCP, but not those of apomorphine, on PPI (Bakshi and Geyer, 1997). Because prazosin has not been tested in neuroleptic-resistant schizophrenic patients, it may not constitute a false positive for this model. Second, studies have provided evidence for a specific role for 5-HT_{2A} antagonism in the PPI-disruptive effects of NMDA antagonists (Bakshi et al., 1994; Varty et al., 1999). The mixed serotonin receptor antagonists, ketanserin and risperidone, have inconsistent and strain-dependent effects on the disruption of PPI produced by NMDA antagonists (Bakshi et al., 1994; Swerdlow et al., 1996; Varty and Higgins, 1995b). More impressively, pretreatment with the selective 5-HT_{2A} antagonist M100907 (formerly MDL 100,907) fully blocked the effect of dizocilpine in two rat strains, while pretreatment with the 5-HT_{2C} antagonist SDZ SER 082 did not (Varty et al., 1999). These results provide strong evidence that 5-HT_{2A} antagonist actions may be one of the key aspects that contributes to the unusual clinical efficacy of atypical antipsychotics.

One exception to the indications that the PCP-PPI model is specifically sensitive to atypical rather than typical antipsychotics is chlorpromazine, which is a low-potency typical antipsychotic that reduces the effect of ketamine on PPI in rats (Swerdlow et al., 1998). It remains to be determined whether the alpha-adrenergic antagonist properties or low-potency nature of chlorpromazine contribute to its unusual ability to reduce the effects of ketamine on PPI. Furthermore, because the PCP model has generally focussed on PCP and dizocilpine and the effect of chlorpromazine has only been reported with ketamine, additional studies are needed to determine whether there are important differences in the effects of different NMDA antagonists in this model (e.g. PCP and dizocilpine vs. ketamine).

The interactions between atypical antipsychotics and NMDA antagonists with regard to their effects on PPI are not likely to be mediated by competition for a common receptor, because the NMDA antagonists do not have appreciable affinity for either 5-HT_{2A} or alpha-1 receptors. As in the case of the influences of 5-HT_{2A} agonists and antagonists on the locomotor activity profile produced by NMDA antagonists, the reduction in NMDA antagonist-induced PPI deficits following atypical antipsychotics likely reflect interactions within the complex forebrain circuitry that modulates PPI (Swerdlow et al., 1992). That is, the deficits in PPI produced by NMDA antagonists may depend upon actions within brain regions that differ from but are connected to the sites at which drugs such as clozapine, M100907, or prazosin exert their effects (Bakshi and Geyer, 1998).

In conclusion, insofar as the PPI-disruptive effects of NMDA antagonists appear to be insensitive to high-potency typical antipsychotics and sensitive to atypical antipsychotics, this paradigm may reveal information that is specifically relevant to the responsiveness of some neuroleptic-resistant patients to atypical antipsychotics. Of particular interest in this regard is the recent report that the atypical antipsychotic clozapine, unlike typical antipsychotics, appears to normalize PPI deficits in patients with schizophrenia (Kumari et al., 1999). If confirmed, such results would parallel the effects of antipsychotics seen in the PCP model of PPI deficits in rats. Similarly, the psychosis-like effects of ketamine in humans are insensitive to typical antipsychotics such as haloperidol but are reduced by atypical antipsychotics such as clozapine (Malhotra et al., 1997). In this respect, the PCP-PPI model in rats appears to faithfully mimic the differences between typical and atypical antipsychotics in humans.

The Isolation Rearing Prepulse Inhibition Model

The fourth PPI model that appears to be of value in testing antipsychotic treatments is based on isolation rearing of rats. Although pharmacological approaches that alter PPI help to identify relevant neural substrates, they do not assess environmental or developmental contributions to PPI deficits. Because schizophrenia appears to be in part a neurodevelopmental disorder (e.g., Weinberger, 1987), investigators have incorporated the developmental perspective into animal models of sensorimotor gating deficits in schizophrenia. For example, we demonstrated that rats reared in single housing from weaning through adulthood exhibit deficits in PPI compared to socially reared controls (Geyer et al., 1993). The deficit appears to emerge only at or after puberty, as is commonly seen patients with schizophrenia (Bakshi and Geyer, 1999). Further studies revealed that this effect is developmentally specific in that similar isolation of adult rats had no influence on PPI (Wilkinson et al., 1994). Of potential therapeutic importance, the isolation rearing-induced deficits in PPI are reversed by treatment with either typical or atypical antipsychotics, including olanzapine, clozapine, and the putative antipsychotic M100907 (Bakshi et al., 1998; Geyer et al., 1993, 1999a; Varty and Higgins, 1995a). Thus, the isolation-rearing paradigm may provide a non-pharmacological and developmentally specific method of inducing schizophrenic-like behavioral deficits that has potential utility in the screening of novel antipsychotic drugs. Because the isolation-rearing model does not rely on the administration of a drug to produce the behavior of interest, it may prove to be sensitive to antipsychotic treatments that do not act at any known receptor system.

CONCLUSIONS

The study of sensorimotor gating deficits in schizophrenia and in homologous animal models based on the startle PPI paradigm has already advanced our understanding of possible neurobiological contributions to information processing abnormalities in psychotic disorders. The advantages of focussing on studies of homologous behaviors that can be quantified in both patients and laboratory animals in the development of an animal model (Geyer and Markou, 1995) have facilitated the remarkable maturation of this model in less than two decades. While the particular behavioral abnormalities being studied in PPI paradigms are not unique to schizophrenia, the narrowed focus of this work on a specific behavior coupled with the effort to establish and use homologous measures in animals has enabled rigorous studies of both pharmacological and neurobiological influences on sensorimotor gating in rodents that have already prompted clinical tests of novel antipsychotic drugs.

ACKNOWLEDGMENTS

This work was supported by grants from the National Institute of Mental Health (MH52885, MH42228, MH53484), the National Institute on Drug Abuse (DA02925), and the U.S. Veterans Affairs VISN 22 Mental Illness Research, Education, and Clinical Center.

REFERENCES

Bakshi, V.P. and Geyer, M.A. (1995) Antagonism of phencyclidine-induced deficits in prepulse inhibition by the putative atypical antipsychotic olanzapine. Psychopharmacology 122:198-201.

Bakshi, V.P. and Geyer, M.A. (1997) Phencyclidine-induced deficits in prepulse inhibition of startle are blocked by prazosin, an alpha1 noradrenergic antagonist. J Pharmacol Exp Ther 283:666-674.

Bakshi, V.P. and Geyer, M.A. (1998) Multiple limbic regions mediate the disruption of prepulse inhibition produced in rats by the noncompetitive NMDA antagonist, dizocilpine. J Neuroscience 18:8394-8401.

Bakshi, V.P. and Geyer, M.A. (1999) Ontogeny of isolation rearing-induced deficits in sensorimotor gating in rats. Physiol Behav, 67:385-392.

Bakshi, V.P., Swerdlow, N.R., Braff, D.L., Geyer MA. (1998) Reversal of isolation rearing-induced deficits in prepulse inhibition by Seroquel and olanzapine. Biol. Psychiatry 43:436-445.

Bakshi, V.P., Swerdlow, N.R., Geyer, M.A. (1994) Clozapine antagonizes phencyclidine-induced deficits in sensorimotor gating of the startle response. J Pharmacol Exp Ther 271:787-794.

Bakshi, V.P., Tricklebank, M., Neijt, H.C., Lehmann-Masten, V., and Geyer M.A. (1999) Disruption of prepulse inhibition and increases in locomotor activity by competitive N-methyl-D-aspartate receptor antagonists in rats. J Pharmacol Exp Ther 288:643-652.

Bolino, F., Di Michele, V., Di Cicco, L., Manna, V., Daneluzzo, E., Cassachia, M. (1994) Sensorimotor gating and habituation evoked by electrocutaneous stimulation in schizophrenia. Biol Psychiat 36: 670-679.

Braff, D.L., Geyer, M.A. (1990) Sensorimotor gating and schizophrenia: Human and animal model studies. Arch Gen Psychiatry 47:181-188.

Braff, D.L., Grillon, C., Geyer, M. (1992) Gating and habituation of the startle reflex in schizophrenic patients. Arch Gen Psychiat 49: 206-215.

Braff, D., Stone, C., Callaway, E., Geyer, M., Glick, I., Bali, L. (1978) Prestimulus effects on human startle reflex in normals and schizophrenics. Psychophysiology 15: 339-343.

Cadenhead, K.S., Geyer, M.A., Braff, D.L. (1993) Impaired startle prepulse inhibition and habituation in schizotypal patients. Am J Psychiat 150: 1862-1867.

Caine, S.B., Geyer, M.A., Swerdlow, N.R. (1995) Effects of D3/D2 dopamine receptor agonists and antagonists on prepulse inhibition of acoustic startle in the rat. Neuropsychopharmacol 12:139-145.

Dulawa, S.C. and Geyer, M.A. (1996) Psychopharmacology of prepulse inhibition in mice. Chinese J Physiology 39:139-146.

Dulawa, S.C., Hen, R., Scearce-Levie, K., Geyer, M.A. (1997) Serotonin 1B receptor modulation of startle reactivity, habituation, and prepulse inhibition, in wild-type and serotonin 1B receptor knockout mice. Psychopharmacol, 132:125-134.

Dulawa, S.C., Hen, R., Scearce-Levie, K., Geyer, M.A. (1998) 5-HT$_{1B}$ receptor modulation of prepulse inhibition: Recent findings in wild-type and 5-HT$_{1B}$ knockout mice. In: Advances in Serotonin Receptor Research, Annals of the New York Academy of Sciences, 861:79-84.

Geyer, M.A. (1998) Behavioral studies of hallucinogenic drugs in animals: Implications for schizophrenia research. Pharmacopsychiatry, 31:73-79.

Geyer, M.A. and Braff, D.L. (1987) Startle habituation and sensorimotor gating in schizophrenia and related animal models. Schiz Bull 13: 643-668.

Geyer, M.A., Krebs-Thomson, K., and Varty, G.B. (1999a) The effects of M100907 in pharmacological and developmental animal models of prepulse inhibition deficits in schizophrenia. Neuropsychopharmacology, 21:S134-S142.

Geyer, M.A. and Markou, A. (1995) Animal models of psychiatric disorders. In: Psychopharmacology: The Fourth Generation of Progress (FE Bloom and DJ Kupfer, eds), Raven Press, Ltd, New York, pp. 787-798.

Geyer, M.A., Swerdlow, N.R., Lehmann-Masten, V., Teschendorf, H-J., Traut, M., Gross, G. (1999b) Effects of LU-111995 in three models of disrupted prepulse inhibition in rats. J Pharmacol Exp Ther 290:716-724.

Geyer, M.A., Swerdlow, N.R., Mansbach, R.S., Braff, D.L. (1990) Startle response models of sensorimotor gating and habituation deficits in schizophrenia. Brain Res Bull 25: 485-498.

Geyer, M.A., Wilkinson, L.S., Humby, T., and Robbins, T.W. (1993) Isolation rearing of rats produces a deficit in prepulse inhibition of acoustic startle similar to that in schizophrenia. Biol. Psychiatry 34:361-372.

Grillon, C., Ameli, R., Charney, D.S., Krystal, J., Braff, D.L. (1992) Startle gating deficits occur across prepulse intensities in schizophrenic patients. Biol Psychiat 32: 939-943.

Hamm, A., Weike, A., Bauer, U., Valti, D., Gallhofer, B. (1995) Prepulse inhibition in medicated and unmedicated patients. Soc. Psychophysiol. Res S38.

Hoffman, D.C. and Donovan, H. (1994) D1 and D2 dopamine receptor antagonists reverse prepulse inhibition deficits in an animal model of schizophrenia. Psychopharmacol 115: 447-53.

Hoffman, D.C., Donovan, H., and Cassella, J.V. (1993) The effects of haloperidol and clozapine on the disruption of sensorimotor gating induced by the noncompetitive glutamate antagonist MK-801. Psychopharmacology 111:339-344.

Hoffman, H.S. and Ison, J.R. (1980) Reflex modification in the domain of startle: I. Some empirical findings and their implication for how the nervous system processes sensory input. Psychol Rev 87:175-189.

Johansson, C., Jackson, D.M., Svensson, L. (1994) The atypical antipsychotic, remoxipride, blocks phencyclidine-induced disruption of prepulse inhibition in the rat. Psychopharmacology 116:437-442.

Karper, L.P., Freeman, G.K., Grillon, C., Morgan, C.A. 3rd, Charney, D.S., Krystal, J.H. (1996) Preliminary evidence of an association between sensorimotor gating and distractibility in psychosis. J Neuropsychiatry Clin Neurosci 8:60-66.

Karper, L.P., Grillon, C., Charney, D.S., Krystal, J.H. (1994) The effect of ketamine on pre-pulse inhibition and attention. Proc Am Coll Neuropsychopharmacol 124:

Kehne, J.H., McCloskey, T.C., Taylor, V.L., Black, C.K., Fadayel, G.M., Schmidt, C.T. (1992) Effects of serotonin releasers 3,4 Methylenedioxymethamphetamine (MDMA), 4-chloroamphetamine (PCA) and fenfluramine on acoustic and tactile startle reflexes in rat. J Pharmacol Exp Ther 260: 78-89.

Kehne, J.H., Padich, R.A., McCloskey, T.C., Taylor, V.L., Schmidt, C.J. (1996) 5-HT modulation of auditory and visual sensorimotor gating: I. Effects of 5-HT releasers on sound and light prepulse inhibition in Wistar rats. Psychopharmacology 124: 95-106.

Keith, V.A., Mansbach, R.S., Geyer, M.A. (1991) Failure of haloperidol to block the effects of phencyclidine and dizocilpine on prepulse inhibition of startle. Biol. Psychiatry 30:557-566.

Kumari, V., Soni, W., Sharma, T. (1999) Normalization of information processing deficits in schizophrenia with clozapine. Am J Psychiatry 156:1046-1051.

Malhotra, A.K., Adler, C.M., Kennison, S.D., Elman, I., Pickar, D., Breier, A. (1997) Clozapine blunts N-methyl-D-aspartate antagonist-induced psychosis: a study with ketamine. Biol Psychiatry 42:664-668.

Mansbach, R.S., Braff, D.L., Geyer, M.A. (1989) Prepulse inhibition of the acoustic startle response is disrupted by N-ethyl-3,4-methylenedioxy-amphetamine (MDEA) in the rat. Eur J Pharmacol 167: 49-55.

Mansbach, R.S., Brooks, E.W., Sanner, M.A., Zorn, S.H. (1998) Selective dopamine D_4 receptor antagonists reverse apomorphine-induced blockade of prepulse inhibition. Psychopharmacol 135:194-200.

Mansbach, R.S. and Geyer, M.A. (1989) Effects of phencyclidine and phencyclidine biologs on sensorimotor gating in the rat. Neuropsychopharmacology 2:299-308.

Mansbach, R.S. and Geyer, M.A. (1991) Parametric determinants in pre-stimulus modification of acoustic startle: Interaction with ketamine. Psychopharmacol 105:162-168.

Mansbach, R.S., Geyer, M.A., Braff, D.L. (1988) Dopaminergic stimulation disrupts sensorimotor gating in the rat. Psychopharm 94: 507-514.

Martinez, D.L. and Geyer, M.A. (1997) Characterization of the disruptions of prepulse inhibition and habituation of startle induced by alpha-ethyltryptamine. Neuropsychopharm. 16:246-255.

McGhie, A. and Chapman, J. (1961) Disorders of attention and perception in early schizophrenia. Br J Med Psychol 34: 103-116.

Padich, R.A., McCloskey, T.C., Kehne, J.H. (1996) 5-HT modulation of auditory and visual sensorimotor gating: II. Effects of the 5-HT2A antagonist MDL 100,907 on disruption of sound and light prepulse inhibition produced by 5-HT agonists in Wistar rats. Psychopharmacology 124: 107-116.

Peng, R.Y., Mansbach, R.S., Braff, D.L., Geyer, M.A. (1990) A D2 dopamine receptor agonist disrupts sensorimotor gating in rats: implications for dopaminergic abnormalities in schizophrenia. Neuropsychopharm 3:211-218.

Perry, W., Geyer, M.A., Braff, D.L. (1999) Sensorimotor gating and thought disturbance measured in close temporal proximity in schizophrenic patients. Arch Gen Psychiat 56:277-281.

Pietraszek, M. and Ossowska, K. (1998) Chronic treatment with haloperidol diminishes the phencyclidine-induced sensorimotor gating deficit in rats. Naunyn Schmiedebergs Arch Pharmacol 357:466-471.

Ralph, R.J., Varty, G.B., Kelly, M.A., Wang, Y-M., Caron, M.G., Rubinstein, M., Grandy, D.K., Low, M.J., Geyer, M.A. (1999) The dopamine D_2 but not D_3 or D_4 receptor subtype is essential for the disruption of prepulse inhibition produced by amphetamine in mice. J. Neuroscience, 19:4627-4633.

Rasmussen, K., Gates, M.R., Burger, J.E., Czachura, J.F. (1997) The novel atypical antipsychotic olanzapine, but not the CCK-B antagonist LY288513, blocks apomorphine-induced disruption of pre-pulse inhibition. Neurosci Lett 222:61-64.

Rigdon, G. (1990) Differential effects of apomorphine on prepulse inhibition of acoustic startle reflex in two rat strains. Psychopharm. 102: 419-421.

Rigdon, G.C. and Weatherspoon, J. (1992) 5-HT1A receptor agonists block prepulse inhibition of the acoustic startle reflex. J Pharmacol Exp Ther 263: 486-493.

Sipes, T.A. and Geyer, M.A. (1994) Multiple serotonin receptor subtypes modulate prepulse inhibition of the startle response in rats. Neuropsychopharm 33: 441-448.

Sipes, T.E. and Geyer, M.A. (1995) DOI disruption of prepulse inhibition of startle in the rat is mediated by 5-HT2A and not by 5-HT2C receptors. Behav Pharmacol 6:839-842.

Sipes, T.E. and Geyer, M.A. (1997) DOI disrupts prepulse inhibition of startle in rats via $5\text{-}HT_{2A}$ receptors in the ventral pallidum. Brain Res 761:97-104.

Swerdlow, N.R., Bakshi, V., Geyer, M.A. (1996) Seroquel restores sensorimotor gating in phencyclidine-treated rats. J Pharmacol Exp Ther 279:1290-1299.

Swerdlow, N.R., Bakshi, V.P., Waikar, J., Taaid, N., Geyer, M.A. (1998) Seroquel, clozapine and chlorpromazine restore sensorimotor gating in ketamine-treated rats. Psychopharmacology 140:75-80.

Swerdlow, N.R., Braff, D.L., Geyer, M.A., Koob, G.F. (1986) Central dopamine hyperactivity in rats mimics abnormal sensory gating of the acoustic startle response in schizophrenics. Biol Psychiatry 21:23-33.

Swerdlow, N.R., Braff, D.L., Taaid, N., Geyer, M.A. (1994) Assessing the validity of an animal model of sensorimotor gating deficits in schizophrenic patients. Arch Gen Psychiat 51:139-154.

Swerdlow, N.R., Caine, S.B., Braff, D.L., Geyer, M.A. (1992) Neural substrates of sensorimotor gating of the startle reflex: Preclinical findings and their implications. J Psychopharmacology 6:176-190.

Swerdlow, N.R. and Geyer, M.A. (1993) Clozapine and haloperidol in an animal model of sensorimotor gating deficits in schizophrenia. Pharmacol Biochem Behav 44: 741-744.

Swerdlow, N.R., Keith, V.A., Braff, D.L., Geyer, M.A. (1991) The effects of spiperone, raclopride, SCH 23390 and clozapine on apomorphine-inhibition of sensorimotor gating of the startle response in the rat. J Pharmacol Exp Ther 256: 530-536.

Swerdlow, N.R., Varty, G.B., Geyer, M.A. (1998) Discrepant findings of clozapine effects on prepulse inhibition of startle: Is it the route or the rat? Neuropsychopharmacology 18:50-56.

Varty, G.B., Bakshi, V.P., Geyer, M.A. (1999) M100907, a serotonin $5\text{-}HT_{2A}$ receptor antagonist and putative antipsychotic, blocks dizocilpine-induced prepulse inhibition deficits in Sprague-Dawley and Wistar rats. Neuropsychopharmacology 20:311-321.

Varty, G.B. and Higgins, G.A. (1995a) Examination of drug-induced and isolation-induced disruptions of prepulse inhibition as models to screen antipsychotic drugs. Psychopharmacology 122:15-26.

Varty, G.B. and Higgins, G.A. (1995b) Reversal of a dizocilpine-induced disruption of prepulse inhibition of acoustic startle by the $5\text{-}HT_2$ antagonist ketanserin. Eur J Pharmacol 287:201-205.

Weinberger, D.R. (1987) Implications of normal brain development for the pathogenesis of schizophrenia. Arch Gen Psychiatry 44:660-669.

Wilkinson, L.S., Killcross, S.S., Humby, T., Hall, F.S., Geyer, M.A., Robbins, T.W. (1994) Social isolation in the rat produces developmentally specific deficits in prepulse inhibition of the acoustic startle response without disrupting latent inhibition. Neuropsychopharmacol 10: 61-72.

8 NEURAL SYSTEMS INVOLVED IN FEAR INHIBITION: EXTINCTION AND CONDITIONED INHIBITION

Michael Davis, William A. Falls and Jonathan Gewirtz

INTRODUCTION

"I can't get the memories out of my mind! The images come flooding back in vivid detail, triggered by the most inconsequential things, like a door slamming or the smell of stir-fried pork. Last night, I went to bed, was having a good sleep for a change. Then in the early morning a storm-front passed through and there was a bolt of crackling thunder. I awoke instantly, frozen in fear. I am right back in Viet Nam, in the middle of the monsoon season at my guard post. I am sure I'll get hit in the next volley and convinced I will die. My hands are freezing, yet sweat pours from my entire body. I feel each hair on the back of my neck standing on end. I can't catch my breath and my heart is pounding. I smell a damp sulfur smell. Suddenly I see what's left of my buddy Troy, his head on a bamboo platter, sent back to our camp by the Viet Cong. Propaganda messages are stuffed between his clenched teeth. The next bolt of lightning and clap of thunder makes me jump so much that I fall to the floor....." (Paraphrased from a war veteran's conversations with Dr. R. L. Gelman, Dept. of Psychiatry, Yale University School of Medicine).

Perhaps there are no more vivid memories than those stored in the brains of soldiers who have experienced excruciatingly horrible combat situations. Witness the above account of the 50-year old Viet Nam veteran who cannot hear a clap of thunder, see an Oriental woman, or touch a bamboo placemat without re-experiencing the sight of his decapitated friend. Even though this occurred in a far away place long ago, the memory is still vivid in every detail and continues to produce the same state of hyperarousal and fear as it did on that fateful day.

Once called combat fatigue, war neurosis, or shell shock, it is now clear that intense trauma can produce vivid memories that can last a lifetime. They can be triggered by stimuli associated with the original traumatic event, and in some individuals the memories are so intrusive that normal functioning is no longer possible. Traumatic memories are formed when formerly neutral stimuli (e.g., a bamboo placemat) are paired with aversive events (e.g., the site of a head without a body).

Converging evidence from many different laboratories indicates a brain structure called the amygdala is critically involved in both the formation and expression of aversive memories (Aggleton, 1992). Clinically, however, the major problem in Post Traumatic Stress Syndrome and certain other types of anxiety disorders is an inability to suppress or inhibit these terrible memories. As the Viet Nam veteran stated above "I can't get the memories out of my mind! The images come flooding back in vivid detail, triggered by the most inconsequential things, like a door slamming or the smell of stir-fried pork." Despite the passage of many years and an environment very different from Viet Nam, the fear persists. Hence, an important area of inquiry concerns the way in unwanted memories can be inhibited and why this is so difficult following traumatic fear conditioning.

The present chapter will review selected aspects of the animal literature on two phenomena, extinction and conditioned inhibition, that deal with fear reduction and have considerable relevance to the problems seen in psychiatric disorders such as Post Traumatic Stress Syndrome. It will begin by reviewing data that show that extinction does not result from an erasure of the original memory but instead the development of competing inhibition, a critical distinction for an eventual analysis of brain systems involved in extinction. It will then describe the phenomenon of conditioned inhibition. Finally, brain structures and neurotransmitters involved in extinction and conditioned inhibition will be discussed. Given space limitations, the review will be restricted to Pavlovian fear conditioning and will not cover the extensive literature on extinction related to positive reinforcement or avoidance behavior.

DEFINITION OF EXTINCTION

When Pavlov paired the sound of a bell (the conditioned stimulus - CS) with the sight of food (the unconditioned stimulus - US), his dogs began to salivate (conditioned response) during presentation of the bell alone. When the bell was then presented over and over again without food, salivation to the sound of the bell gradually diminished and finally did not occur at all. This decrease in amplitude or probability of the conditioned response (CR) following presentations of the CS in the absence of the US is known as experimental extinction. Because extinction requires the CS be presented in the absence of the US, it is considered to be an active process. This contrasts with "forgetting," the term commonly used to refer to a loss of responding that results merely from the passage of time without any intervening CS presentations.

In fear conditioning, it is more difficult to directly observe the conditioned response. Because of this, it is generally assumed (cf. McAllister and McAllister, 1971) that during the conditioning phase the aversive stimulus (the sight of a decapitated head) produces a constellation of emotional behaviors (e.g., cold, clammy skin, hair on the back of the neck standing straight up, heightened startle) that collectively define a state of fear. Neutral stimuli (e.g., bamboo place mat) that are directly paired with the aversive stimulus or other stimuli that remind one of the general setting in which the traumatic event took place (e.g., the smell of stir fried pork, the site of a oriental women) now can elicit the same state of fear. In this instance, extinction would be defined as a loss of this fear reaction when these conditioned stimuli were presented over and over again without being paired with the original fear provoking stimulus.

DATA SUPPORTING THE VIEW THAT EXTINCTION DOES NOT RESULT FROM AN ERASURE OF ORIGINAL LEARNING

Demonstrations of spontaneous recovery, reinstatement and context specificity of extinction collectively support the idea that extinction fails to erase all of the original excitatory associations.

Spontaneous Recovery

Pavlov (1927) observed that an extinguished conditioned response would "spontaneously regenerate" with the passage of time. In one experiment three non-reinforced presentations of a well-trained CS at a 10-minute inter-trial interval resulted in complete extinction of the conditioned response (from 8 drops of saliva to 0). After an interval of 20 minutes, the CS was again presented and a complete recovery of the conditioned response was observed (7 drops of saliva). This effect was termed "spontaneous recovery" and was taken as evidence that the original excitatory conditioning had not been lost but simply overlaid with inhibition. However, as argued by Estes (1955) and Skinner (1950), extinction may still involve an erasure of many excitatory associations. Because the conditions of original training are not identical to conditions during extinction, enough connections may still be intact to support spontaneous recovery. In fact, few theorists now accept spontaneous recovery as evidence for inhibition in extinction (see Bouton, 1993 for an explanation of spontaneous recovery based on changes in the temporal context). Instead, it is viewed as one example of a class of phenomena to indicate that excitation is not completely lost following non-reinforced CS presentations.

Reinstatement

Both Pavlov (1927) and Konorski (1948) reported that presentation of a US alone was sufficient to renew responding to an extinguished CS. An example of this is exemplified by a study of Rescorla and Heth (1975). Using a conditioned emotional response procedure (suppression of bar pressing in the presence of a cue previously paired with shock) groups of rats were first given either explicitly paired or unpaired presentations of a tone and footshock. All groups were then given non-reinforced presentations of the tone. Next, half of each of the paired and unpaired groups was given a single "reminder" footshock identical to the US used in training. Twenty four hours later all animals were tested for conditioned suppression of bar pressing to the tone. The results showed that after non-reinforced tone presentations, both the paired and unpaired groups showed the same lack of conditioned suppression to the tone, i.e., the paired group was extinguished. However, at testing, the paired group that received the reminder shock 24 hours earlier showed renewed suppression to the tone. Groups that did not receive a reminder shock as well as the unpaired group that did receive a reminder shock, did not show renewed suppression to the tone. The failure to see a "reinstatement-like" effect in the unpaired group indicates that reinstatement was not the result of sensitization but instead worked through an associative process.

Rescorla and Heth (1975) assumed that extinction decreases not only the strength or number of CS-US associations, but also the strength of the representation of the US. A reminder shock reinstates the full value of the US representation of shock, therefore allowing it to be fully activated by the remaining excitatory CS - US connections. Several experiments support this idea.

In contrast, Bouton and colleagues have emphasized context dependent mechanisms over a US memory renewal mechanism as underlying reinstatement (Bouton and Bolles, 1979b; Bouton and Bolles, 1985). For example, reinstatement occurred only when the rats were tested in the context in which they received the reinstating shocks, and extinguishing the context in which reminder shocks were given prevented reinstatement in that context (Bouton and Bolles, 1979b). One mechanism by which contextual cues could mediate reinstatement is through a summation of contextual excitation with residual excitation of the extinguished CS. Alternatively, as will be described below, context might "gate" suppression of conditioned responding, such that suppression only occurs in the context in which the CS was not paired with shock. According to this account, reinstatement occurs because shock presentation in the extinction context makes the context a less effective retrieval cue for the CS – no shock association. This would be consistent with the putative role of context in conditioned inhibition (see below). Regardless of which account one uses, the phenomenon of reinstatement indicates that extinction does not completely erase excitatory CS - US connections, although it does not clearly support an active inhibitory account.

Context Specific Extinction

In an impressive series of experiments, Bouton and colleagues have shown that extinction may be specific to the experimental context in which non-reinforcement occurs. For example, Bouton and Bolles (1979b) used four groups of rats that were first given tone - foot shock pairings in a training chamber. After conditioning, two groups received non-reinforced tone presentations in context B and two groups in context C. Two of the four groups were subsequently tested for extinction in the same context in which non-reinforcement occurred and the other two in the alternate context. Although all four groups showed extinction in the contexts where they were non-reinforced, rats subsequently tested in a context different from the one in which they were extinguished showed renewed suppression to the tone, a phenomenon Bouton terms renewal. Control animals tested and extinguished in the same context did not show renewed fear. The data clearly show that under circumstances in which the rat can discriminate contexts, extinction performance can come under the control of contextual cues (for a critique of context specific effects, see Lovibond et al., 1984).

The context specific extinction effect argues strongly against an erasure hypothesis of extinction. The rat was fully capable of performing the conditioned response in a context other than the one in which it was non-reinforced. To explain these data it is necessary to invoke an associative mechanism of extinction. One approach is to adopt the language of Konorski (1967) that stimuli present during non-reinforcement acquire inhibitory CS - US connections that summate with existing excitatory CS - US connections. In the presence of those stimuli, the

gap between the inhibitor and CS or with the offset of the inhibitor coincident with the onset of the CS. Holland and colleagues (Holland, 1985) have shown that in some circumstances the temporal arrangement of inhibitor and CS dictates the nature of the inhibitory learning. In their conditioning preparations, the inhibition produced by an inhibitor trained in a serial compound shows little or no transfer to a separately trained CS and does not show retardation. Holland (1985) has argued that simultaneous compounds favor the development of conditioned inhibition in which the inhibitor acquires inhibitory associations that compete with the CS's excitatory associations. Thus, inhibitors trained in a simultaneous compound show both transfer and retardation (as discussed above). Serial compounds, on the other hand, favor the development of "negative occasion setting" in which the CS is stored in a conditional memory system in which its conditional value (e.g., inhibition) is determined by the presence or absence of the inhibitor. In other words, following serial training the inhibitor acquires the ability to set the occasion for non-reinforcement of the particular CS it was trained with. Thus an occasion setter will not show transfer or retardation.

However, in a series of experiments using the fear-potentiated startle paradigm we showed that serial compound training can lead to the development of traditional conditioned inhibition (Falls and Davis, 1997). Rats were given training in which a light was paired with shock and a serial noise and light compound was presented in the absence of shock. The noise not only inhibited fear-potentiated startle to the light, it also inhibited fear-potentiated startle to a separately trained tactile stimulus (i.e., transfer). More importantly, the serially trained inhibitor also showed retardation. However, retardation was only evident after training in which the shock US was presented after the offset of the noise (i.e., a trace conditioning procedure). Standard delay conditioning, in which the inhibitor and shock coterminate, did not produce retardation.

This result can be explained by assuming that as a consequence of the serial noise and light compound, the noise acquired inhibitory associations that were tied to the offset of the inhibitor. This is consistent with theories of conditioning that assume that inhibitory associations develop at the time when the expectancy of the US is maximal. In a serial inhibitor and CS compound the expectation of the US is maximal after the offset of the inhibitor during the presentation of the excitatory CS. Thus inhibition accrues to the offset of the inhibitor. This result is important in two respects. It suggests that a serial procedure does not always lead to the inhibitor acquiring occasion setting properties and it suggests that the temporal aspects of inhibitory conditioning must also be considered when evaluating the nature of the inhibition.

Importantly, the conditioned inhibition procedure does not differ substantially from the normal extinction procedure. Both involve non-reinforcement in the presence of an otherwise excitatory CS, and in both, a decrement in conditioned responses is observed over repeated non-reinforced trials. In fact, because extinction is context specific, it could be argued the context acts like a conditioned inhibitor, signaling that the tone will not be followed by shock. However, if this were true, one would expect to see transfer of context dependent extinction, a phenomenon that has not been demonstrated. For example, Bouton and King (1983) used a summation test where rats previously trained to be fearful of a light in another distinctive context were now tested in the one where extinction to a tone had taken place. If the extinction context were generally inhibitory, one would expect less fear of the light in this context compared to one where extinction had not taken place. However, Bouton and King (1983) failed to detect inhibition by the extinction context with this summation technique. Because of this, these investigators abandoned a contextual inhibition hypothesis (Bouton and Bolles, 1985; Bouton and King, 1986) and suggested that some other contextually controlled mechanism was at work. As in the case of extinction, they suggested that the context may retrieve a specific memory of non-reinforcement, such as, *the tone is not followed by shock in this place* (italics ours). However, this memory is rather specific and does <u>not</u> generalize to an idea such as, *because the tone is not reinforced in this place the light also will not be reinforced.*

CLINICAL IMPLICATIONS

Because psychotherapy often involves procedures to rid patients of unwanted fear memories, a behavioral analysis of extinction has a number of clinical implications, as suggested by Bouton and Swartzentruber (1991). As they point out, "performance after extinction is inherently unstable" (p 128). Phenomena such as spontaneous recovery and reinstatement may explain why conditioned fears and phobias in humans sometimes seem to return spontaneously without any obvious cause. The renewal effect may explain why fears reduced successfully in the therapist's office reappear when the patient returns to his home or his job. If a drug is used as an adjunct to therapy, renewal of fear could occur when the fearful stimulus is encountered in the absence of the drug. In fact, animal experiments show that when benzodiazepines are given during extinction, fear of the CS returns when testing occurs in the absence of the drug (Bouton et al., 1990).

An analysis of conditioned inhibition may also have a great deal of clinical relevance. For example, one of our colleagues told us about a particular patient suffering from Post Traumatic Stress Disorder. This patient had had excruciating combat trauma in Viet Nam and later spent many years in treatment. Eventually, however, he was doing much better and got married. It was a June wedding and he was wearing a white tuxedo with a pink carnation in the lapel. It happened to be a rainy day. As he and his new bride were walking down the steps of the church a car passed by and backfired. The veteran instantly dove into a nearby patch of muddy bushes, ruining his white tuxedo and pink carnation.

This is a poignant example illustrating a profound failure of conditioned inhibition. There were many cues that should have served as safety signals on this June morning. The veteran was in the United States, not in Viet Nam. He was wearing a white tuxedo, not battle fatigues. And he was walking out of a church with his new bride. Nevertheless, when he heard the sound of a car backfiring reminiscent of mortar fire, none of the safety signals could prevent the formerly adaptive behavior of driving for cover. Because this inappropriate behavior seemed to involve an inability to inhibit traumatic fear memories, understanding the neural basis of extinction and conditioned inhibition should eventually lead to better treatments for these types of anxiety disorders.

NEURAL SYSTEMS INVOLVED IN EXTINCTION

Sensory Cortex

Assuming that extinction results from active inhibition (see above) one might expect that lesions of various brain areas would disrupt either the development or expression of extinction. LeDoux, Romanski and Xagoraris (1989) performed bilateral ablations of visual cortex or sham operations on rats prior to giving them repeated light-footshock pairings. Ablated and sham controls acquired conditioned fear responses at similar rates as assessed by the light's ability to suppress licking of a water tube. However, with repeated non-reinforced light presentations, visual cortex-ablated rats failed to show extinction of lick suppression relative to sham controls over days. In a similar study employing heart rate conditioning in the rabbit, Teich et al. (1989) showed that although bilateral lesions of either auditory or visual cortex did not disrupt acquisition to a tone CS, auditory cortex lesions, but not visual cortex lesions, blocked extinction of conditioned heart rate. Based on known anatomical connections between sensory cortex and thalamic structures, the authors of both experiments concluded that during extinction sensory cortices exert a modality specific inhibition of the thalamic structures important for the performance of conditioned responses.

However, we found no effect of complete visual cortex lesions on extinction of fear potentiated startle using a visual CS when the lesions were made either prior to light-shock pairings or following light-shock pairings and extinction (Falls and Davis, 1994). Figure 1 shows the level of fear potentiated startle in the sham and visual cortex ablation groups on an initial test prior to extinction and then on subsequent weekly test sessions following 60 CS alone presentations between test sessions 1 and 2. Fear potentiated startle is defined by the difference in the amplitude of the acoustic startle reflex elicited in the presence of a light previously paired with footshock compared to startle amplitude in the dark. Visual cortex ablation did not alter either the acquisition or extinction of fear potentiated startle. A control experiment showed that the decrease in conditioned fear over test sessions was not due to forgetting. In another experiment, rats were trained, then extinguished and then given visual cortex ablations or sham ablations. Post-extinction lesions failed to disrupt prior extinction, as would be expected if the visual cortex was required for the expression of extinction. These data clearly indicate that extinction to a visual CS can still occur without visual cortex.

There were procedural differences between these two reports, including the measure of conditioned fear, the post-operative recovery time, the quality of the visual conditioned stimulus, the number of conditioning and extinction trials and the degree of dissimilarity between the conditioning and testing contexts. Although these differences may account for the failure of visual cortex aspirations to prevent extinction in these experiments, the conclusion that sensory cortex is universally involved in extinction of conditioned fear is not supported.

Frontal cortex

Rats with lesions of the ventral medial prefrontal cortex made prior to fear conditioning required more days to reach an extinction criterion using an auditory CS and freezing as the measure of fear (Morgan et al., 1993). However, in these

122

Lesions of visual cortex do not block extinction of fear-potentiated startle

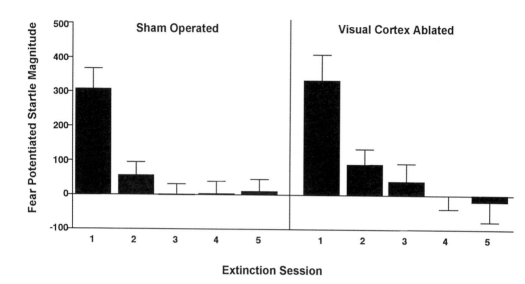

Figure 1. Visual cortex aspirations do not prevent extinction of fear-potentiated startle to a visual conditioned stimulus. Following surgery, rats were given light-footshock training trials followed by five fear-potentiated startle test sessions. Shown are the mean startle difference scores (light-noise minus noise alone amplitude) for the first three test trials of each sessions. Error bars represent 1 standard error of the mean.

same animals, extinction of conditioned fear to contextual cues was not impaired, suggesting that the role of the medial prefrontal cortex in fear inhibition may be highly specific. However, in an extensive series of experiments, we found normal rates of extinction to both explicit and contextual cues after total removal of the ventral medial prefrontal cortex using both freezing and fear-potentiated startle as measures of conditioned fear (Gewirtz et al., 1997). In these studies, training, extinction and testing occurred in the same test boxes. Figure 2 shows that pre-training lesions of the medial prefrontal cortex failed to alter the rate of extinction across days using an auditory CS and the fear-potentiated startle test. Figure 3 shows comparable data measuring cage activity shortly after onset of the auditory CS, which correlated highly with observer rated levels of freezing. Figure 3 indicates that across sessions there was a gradual increase in cage activity measured after onset of the auditory CS, indicative of extinction of freezing over days, which, like fear-potentiated startle, was not affected by lesions of the medial prefrontal cortex. It is presently unclear why different effects were found in our study and in Morgan et al. (1993), especially given that the lesions were similar in the two studies (Morgan and LeDoux, personal communication).

However, because the lesions in the Morgan et al. (1993) study were performed before fear conditioning, the apparent blockade of extinction following ventral medial prefrontal cortex lesions may have resulted from an increase in the strength of original fear conditioning, rather than by interfering with the process of

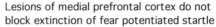

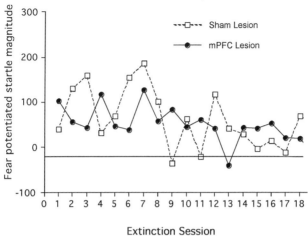

Figure 2. Fear-potentiated startle over extinction for sham and mPFC lesioned rats. Fear-potentiated startle was calculated as the difference between mean startle amplitudes on startle stimulus alone trials and auditory CS test trials. There were no differences in the rate of extinction of fear-potentiated startle between the two groups.

extinction. Although the two groups did not differ significantly in their level of freezing before the initiation of the extinction sessions, freezing to explicit cues often becomes maximal after a very few training trials so that "ceiling effects" might well have been operating. Because rate of extinction can be a more sensitive index of the strength of original conditioning than the terminal level of performance prior to the initiation of extinction (e.g., Annau and Kamin, 1961), the slower rate of extinction in the lesioned animals may have reflected a stronger degree of original learning. The fact that the lesions had no effect on the rate of extinction of context conditioning, which clearly was not at the ceiling of the freezing scale, is consistent with this interpretation. We also did not find any effect of pre-training ventral prefrontal cortex lesions on extinction of contextual fear potentiated startle or freezing (Gewirtz et al., 1997). In addition, we did not find any effect of ventral medial prefrontal cortex lesions on extinction when lesions were made after fear conditioning but before extinction (Gewirtz et al., 1997). Morgan and LeDoux (1996) also found no effect on the rate of extinction when ventral prefrontal cortex lesions were made after fear conditioning, but before extinction. If the frontal cortex is required for the development of extinction or for the inhibition of fear after extinction, one would expect lesions to block the development of extinction, irrespective of whether the lesions were made before or after the initial phase of fear conditioning.

More recently, Morgan and LeDoux (1999) reported that lesions of the ventrolateral prefrontal cortex had no effect on extinction although acquisition of contextual fear conditioning was retarded. In contrast, lesions of the dorsal medial prefrontal cortex increased the amount of freezing to both the CS and US during acquisition as well as the number of days to reach extinction criteria (Morgan and LeDoux, 1995). In that case they concluded that the delay in extinction was attributable to greater fear conditioning in the lesions rats and estimated that these

Lesions of medial prefrontal cortex do not block extinction of freezin

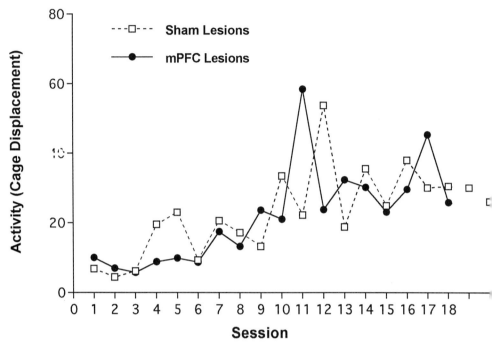

Figure 3. Changes in activity over extinction for sham and mPFC lesioned rats. Following fear conditioning, activity levels after CS exposure were at low levels (freezing) but then gradually increased (less freezing) over days. There were no differences in the rate of extinction of freezing between the two groups.

animals were more often at the ceiling of their measurement system. In the same analysis, however, they reported that the animals with ventral medial prefrontal cortex lesions in the Morgan et al. (1993) study were not at ceiling based on a similar criteria. However, the activity burst that occurs after shocks are delivered may interfere with the true measurement of conditioning freezing during acquisition (Fanselow, 1986a). In fact, it is often the case that the levels of freezing at the beginning of an extinction test are substantially higher than those seen at the end of training (e.g., Harris and Westbrook, 1998a and see below). In sum, therefore, designing studies in which lesions are made before original fear conditioning leaves open the possibility that the lesions indirectly alter extinction by affecting original acquisition. Hence, to make inferences about whether a brain area is involved in extinction it would appear preferable to manipulate that brain area after original fear conditioning.

Similarly complex effects on extinction have been reported regarding depletion of dopamine in the prefrontal cortex (Morrow et al., 1999b). Pre-conditioning lesions of dopamine terminals in the medial prefrontal cortex retarded the rate of extinction when a 0.8 mA shock was used but not when a 0.4 mA shock was used. Inspection of the results strongly suggests that the 0.8 mA group was at the ceiling of the measurement scale at the beginning of the extinction session (approximately 90% of the time spent freezing) compared to their terminal level during acquisition of about 60%. In contrast, the 0.4 mA group clearly was not at ceiling at the beginning of the extinction session (approximately 50% of the time spent freezing) compared to their terminal level during acquisition of about 30%. Thus, even though the terminal level of freezing in the 6-OHDA and sham groups trained with 0.8 mA shocks did not differ at the end of acquisition, ceiling effects might well have been operating during the extinction test. In fact, these same authors found that infusion into the prefrontal cortex of c-fos antisense vs. sense oligonucleotides 12 hrs. prior to fear conditioning produced a dramatic decrease in the levels of freezing measured 72 hrs. later, despite the fact that both groups had equivalent levels of freezing at the end of acquisition (Morrow et al., 1999a). Hence, manipulations of frontal cortex prior to training can have effects on subsequent performance in the absence of effects measured during fear acquisition. Once again, this indicates that pretraining manipulations can lead to changes in the magnitude of original acquisition that can complicate the interpretation of later changes in extinction. On the other hand, post-conditioning 6-OHDA lesions of the frontal cortex substantially retarded extinction following 0.8 mA tone-shock pairings, an effect that cannot be ascribed to a change in the level of original conditioning given that the lesions were made after fear conditioning (Morrow et al., 1999b). Thus, it is possible that dopamine levels in the prefrontal cortex are important for extinction when conditioning has produced high, but not more moderate levels of fear. Alternatively, it is possible that these lesions might have affected extinction indirectly by generally disinhibiting fear. To test this possibility, it would be informative to include a group trained with a moderate shock intensity but not given extinction. If post-training 6-0HDA lesions increased the level of fear in this group as well, then the effects of the lesion would be attributable to a general disinhibition of fear, rather than to a disruption of extinction.

Quirk et al. (1998) found that pre-training lesions of the ventral medial prefrontal cortex did not block the development of conditioned freezing or the rate of within session extinction. However, the lesioned rats showed much more spontaneous recovery measured 24 hrs later. Similar results were found using systemic administration of an NMDA antagonist (Quirk et al., 1999). In contrast, we found no change in the rate or final level of extinction, measured with fear-potentiated startle and freezing, when extinction was assessed over 18 daily sessions using a small number of CS presentations each day (Figures 2 and 3). Also, there were no differences in the degree of spontaneous recovery measured 5 days later or in shock-induced reinstatement measured 24 hrs after a single footshock. Hence, the Quirk et al. (1998; 1999) findings may depend critically on the use of a relatively small amount extinction training.

Overall, these results indicate that the medial prefrontal cortex is not generally essential for the inhibition of fear, but may be important in highly constrained circumstances. Some, but not all of the effects on extinction may be accounted for by a change in the acquisition of conditioned fear, even if this change is not always apparent at the end of conditioning. More work clearly needs to be done, using multiple measures, to examine the limits of the role of the prefrontal cortex in extinction of conditioned fear, including the significance of the level of original fear conditioning, pre- versus post-training lesions, and the exact location within prefrontal cortex where lesions are made.

Hippocampus

Although a complete review of the hippocampal literature is well beyond the scope of this chapter, this brain area has received a great deal of experimental attention and was once widely believed to be involved in extinction. Theories of extinction confront the problem of designing a mechanism capable of discriminating occasions of reinforcement from non-reinforcement. For example, Konorski (1948) proposed that the strengthening of inhibitory connections during extinction would occur when activation of a CS center coincided with the fall in activation of the US center, which was presumed to occur when the US was omitted. Later, he proposed that inhibition resulted from the strengthening of excitatory connections from the CS center to a no-US center which in turn had hard-wired inhibitory connections to the US center (Konorski, 1967). In both instances some mechanism for detecting the absence of the US following CS presentation would be required. In fact, Douglas (1972) suggested that the hippocampus is a non-reinforcement detector providing the organism with the means to "tune out" information that is of no motivational consequence. It is possible that the hippocampus recognizes that the CS is no longer followed by the US and feeds forward inhibition to relevant sensory or conditioned response production centers. For example, hippocampal lesions prevent discrimination reversals, where a stimulus previously reinforced is now non-reinforced and vice versa (Buchanan and Powell, 1980; Berger et al., 1986). Furthermore, although the hippocampus is not always required for simple contextual conditioning (McNish et al., 1997), it appears to be required for more complex, context-dependent retrieval phenomena (Good et al., 1998). For example, lesions or chemical inactivation of the dorsal hippocampus abolished the context specificity of latent inhibition (Honey and Good, 1993; Holt and Maren, 1999). Given the role of contextual cues in retrieval of memories of extinction, one might expect hippocampal manipulations to impair extinction as well.

A variety of conditioning paradigms have been used to assess this question including the rabbit nictitating membrane response (Schmaltz and Theiosus, 1972; Solomon, 1977; Berger et al., 1986), conditioned heart rate (Buchanan and Powell, 1980) and conditioned suppression (Leaton and Borszcz, 1990; Wilson et al., 1995; Frohardt et al., 1999). While some of these experiments have found that hippocampal lesions attenuate extinction (Schmaltz and Theiosus, 1972) others have found no effect (e.g., Solomon, 1977) and still another has shown facilitated extinction (Leaton and Borszcz, 1990). Once again, some of these studies used pre-training lesions which themselves may have increased rates of original fear conditioning (e.g., Schmaltz and Theiosus, 1972), thereby altering subsequent rates of extinction (e.g., Annau and Kamin, 1961).

Because extinction is context specific (see above) one might expect that lesions of the hippocampus would disrupt this contextual control of extinction. However, direct tests of this hypothesis have not found a disruption of context specific extinction using pre-training lesions. Hence, neither fimbria-fornix lesions (Wilson et al., 1995) nor excitotoxic lesions of the entire hippocampus (Frohardt et al., 1999) had any effect on the rate of extinction or on renewal of conditioned fear, although both types of lesions disrupted reinstatement. In contrast, large hippocampal lesions do not disrupt reinstatement of appetitively conditioned behavior (Fox and Holland, 1998). These findings suggest that the role of the hippocampus in extinction is much more constrained than was once thought to be the case.

NEUROTRANSMITTERS INVOLVED IN EXTINCTION

The Role of NMDA Receptors in the Amygdala in Extinction

As mentioned earlier, there is broad agreement that the amygdala is critically involved in the formation and retention of aversive memories (cf. Aggleton, 1992). CS and US information converges at the amygdala which projects to brainstem and hypothalamic target areas involved in specific signs of fear and anxiety. Accumulating data suggest that the amygdala is the actual site of plasticity for conditioned fear. For example, local infusion of NMDA antagonists directly into the amygdala blocks the acquisition of conditioned fear (cf. Davis et al., 1994). One might expect, therefore, that a site important for the acquisition and performance of conditioned fear also would be important for the extinction of conditioned fear. Assessing this is difficult, however, because unlike visual or frontal cortex, the amygdala is essential for both acquisition or expression of conditioned fear,. Therefore, a reversible lesion occurring at the time of non-reinforced CS presentations is necessary to allow one to assess the role of the amygdala in extinction. Furthermore, if one assumes that extinction is a form of new learning, it might be affected by pharmacological treatments that block learning.

Reasoning along these lines, we wondered whether local infusion of NMDA antagonists into the amygdala would block the development of long-term extinction (Falls et al., 1992). Rats were implanted with bilateral cannulas in the basolateral nucleus of the amygdala. Following two sessions of light-shock pairings the initial level of conditioned fear was measured and rats were matched into two groups with equivalent levels of fear on this test. On each of the next two days, all animals were presented with 30 light alone trials 5 min after infusion of either the NMDA antagonist DL-2-amino-5-phosphonovaleric acid (AP5) or artificial cerebrospinal fluid (ACSF). Twenty four hours later the rats were again tested for potentiated startle. Figure 4 shows that rats infused with ACSF during non-reinforced CS presentations showed near complete extinction of potentiated startle compared to their initial levels. However, rats receiving AP5 did not show extinction. These data suggest that activity at NMDA receptors in the amygdala during non-reinforced CS presentations is essential for extinction of fear potentiated startle using a visual CS. Intra-amygdala infusion of AP5 also blocked extinction using an auditory CS and freezing as a measure of conditioned fear (Lee and Kim, 1998).

Unlike the sensory cortex and the hippocampus, the amygdala is thought to be critical for the acquisition and performance of fear conditioning, which leads to several explanations of these data. Perhaps the amygdala detects the occurrence of the CS and provides this information to other structures that are responsible for detecting non-reinforcement and then in turn feed inhibition either back to the amygdala or to one of its afferent or efferent structures. Alternatively, because the amygdala is thought to be a convergent zone of CS and US information, it may detect the absence of reinforcement and signal other structures to inhibit the amygdala or one of its afferent or efferent structures. Lastly, perhaps the amygdala is critical for extinction because the plasticity associated with extinction occurs in the amygdala itself.

Effects of Systemic Administration of NMDA Antagonists on Extinction

It should be acknowledged, however, that Falls et al., (1992) did not include a control for context specific extinction produced by a change in drug state from extinction training to extinction testing (e.g., Bouton et al., 1990), which might account for these results. However, if this were true, the "drug context" would have to be that produced by local blockade of excitatory amino acid transmission in the amygdala. Whether this would be a sufficient cue to signal non-reinforcement remains to be tested. Furthermore, several studies using systemic administration of NMDA antagonists also have reported deficits in extinction. In some cases these effects could not be explained by state-dependent learning deficits. For example, Cox and Westbrook (1994) exposed six groups of rats to a hot-plate to produce conditioned analgesia, a reliable measure of conditioned fear (Bolles and Fanselow, 1980; Fanselow, 1986b; Helmstetter, 1992). Four groups were exposed to a non-heated plate on each of the next 6 days, to produce extinction. The other two groups remained in the colony room. Next, all groups were re-exposed to the hot plate on Day 7 and the latency to retract their paw was recorded. A 2 x 2 design was used for the extinguished groups in which they received either saline or the NMDA antagonist MK-801 before either extinction or testing. The non-extinguished groups were tested with either saline or MK-801. The results showed that MK-801 did not significantly alter the magnitude of conditioned analgesia measured on Day 7. Exposure to the non-heated plate for 6 days produced significant extinction in the groups extinguished under saline, but not the groups extinguished under MK-801, regardless of the drug condition during testing. In fact, the magnitude of the conditioned response in testing for the groups extinguished under MK-801 was similar to that of the control groups not given any extinction trials, indicating a full blockade of extinction by MK-801, that could not be explained by state-dependent learning. A similar blockade of extinction was reported using a lick-suppression CER paradigm that also could not be explained by state-dependent learning (Baker and Azorlosa, 1996) as well as extinction of the rabbit nictitating membrane preparation (Kehoe et al., 1996). In the later case, the authors suggest that this resulted from a decrease in CS processing during extinction because MK-801 significantly reduced the conditioned response during extinction. However, this could not explain the decrease in extinction of fear potentiated startle after local infusion of AP5 into the amygdala (Falls et al., 1992), because this treatment does not decrease the expression of fear potentiated startle (Miserendino et al., 1990; Campeau et al., 1992; Gewirtz and Davis, 1997). Moreover, MK-801 also failed to block latent inhibition of rabbit eyeblink conditioning (Robinson et al., 1993), which might be expected if it decreased CS processing. Taken together, these data indicate that NMDA antagonists can block the development of extinction measured on subsequent test sessions. This may even occur under conditions where the antagonist does not block the development of short-term extinction. Thus, systemic injection of the NMDA antagonist CPP prior to extinction blocked the expression of conditioned freezing by about 40% but did not block the development of extinction. However, the CPP group showed substantial recovery of conditioned freezing measured 24 hrs later suggesting that CPP blocked the long-term development of extinction. (Quirk et al., 1999). Interestingly, this group found a similar effect with pre-conditioning lesions of the ventral prefrontal cortex, although the connection between these two sets of data remains to be made.

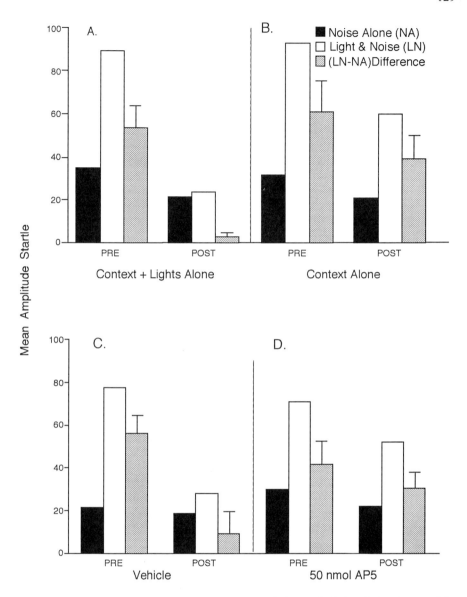

Figure 4. The amplitude of fear-potentiated startle before and after manipulations designed to reveal the relative contributions of light-alone presentations, context exposure and the passage of time on the extinction of conditioned fear. Shown is the amplitude of startle in the presence (light and noise (LN)) and absence (noise alone (NA)) of the light conditioned stimulus and the difference between the two trial types (LN-NA difference; + S.E.M.). The LN-NA difference score represents the magnitude of conditioned fear. A. The group that received context plus lights-alone showed a significant reduction in the magnitude of fear-potentiated startle from the pre-test to the post-test. B. In contrast, exposure to the context alone did not significantly reduce fear-potentiated startle. Hence, these groups showed significant fear-potentiated startle during both the pre-extinction and the post-extinction tests. C. Infusions of artificial cerebral spinal fluid (ACSF) vehicle immediately before light-alone presentations showed a significant reduction in fear-potentiated startle from the pre-extinction test. In contrast, rats that received the NMDA antagonist, AP5 did not show a significant reduction in fear-potentiated startle and had significant fear-potentiated startle during the post-extinction test. This data indicate that local infusion of an NMDA antagonist into the amygdala blocked the development of extinction.

The Role of GABA in Extinction

Several studies have suggested that GABA agonists given prior to non-reinforced CS presentations interfere with the development of extinction (cf. Bouton et al., 1990; Falls and Davis, 1995a). However, many of these effects may be attributable to state dependent learning rather than a blockade of learning during non-reinforced CS exposure. For example, Bouton (1990), using lick suppression as a measure of fear, showed a blockade of extinction when rats were given chordiazepoxide during non-reinforced CS presentations and then tested in the absence of the drug. However, when chordiazepoxide also was given prior to testing, extinction was still evident. This suggests that the benzodiazepine did not actually block the learning that was occurring during extinction but instead the change in drug state between extinction and testing produced produced renewal (e.g., Bouton and Bolles, 1979a).

Interestingly, Harris and Westbrook have found similar, situationally-dependent effects with the amnestic effects of benzodiazepines on excitatory conditioning as well. For example, rats given fear conditioning after injection with benzodiazepines showed an impairment in conditioned freezing measured 24 hrs later in the same context compared to rats trained under the drug but tested in different context (Harris and Westbrook, 1999) or rats given a stressor prior to testing (Harris and Westbrook, 1998a). Thus, the benzodiazepines did not actually prevent original learning, but instead produced a state during conditioning that interfered with retrieval during testing.

Hence, it would seem that GABA agonists do not directly interfere with either excitatory or inhibitory learning, but instead act powerfully on processes that are important for retrieval of prior learning. However, if extinction is a form of active inhibition, it is possible that GABA might be one of the neurotransmitters necessary for the expression of extinction. In fact, in an elegant set of experiments, Harris and Westbrook (1998b) provide evidence that extinction is mediated by GABA release. Systemic administration of the inverse agonist FG 7142, which decreases GABA transmission, blocked both the development and expression of extinction to an auditory CS paired with footshock using freezing as a measure. This effect could not be ascribed to state dependency because animals injected with the compound before both extinction training and extinction testing still displayed more freezing than animals given vehicle on both occasions. The drug did not affect the level of freezing when rats were placed in the context where conditioning took place, leading the authors to conclude that the decrease in the rate of extinction to the tone could not be attributed to a ceiling effect. Pretest administration of FG 7142 reinstated freezing when assessed in the context where extinction took place, but not in a novel context, which itself reinstated freezing and the two effects were not additive statistically. Finally, FG 7142 did not affect the low levels of freezing that developed after CS pre-exposure (latent inhibition) even though this also was context specific. This last experiment lends further support to the conclusion that latent inhibition does not involve an active inhibitory process (e.g., Reiss and Wagner, 1972) as well as showing that the FG 7142-induced disruption of extinction was not due to state-dependency (e.g., by causing an change in context between CS pre-exposure and CS testing). Harris and Westbrook conclude that "extinction of fear involves the acquisition of a context-gated inhibitory association between the conditioned stimulus and noxious unconditioned stimulus, and this inhibitory association is mediated by GABA binding to GABA-A receptors"

(1998b, p. 114). They further speculate that GABA may be acting in the basolateral amygdala to mediate extinction, although there is as yet little evidence to firmly support this conclusion. On several occasions, we have tried to test whether local infusion of GABA-A antagonists into the amygdala would reverse extinction or conditioned inhibition, but we have not been able to carry out these experiments because of seizure activity (Gewirtz and Davis, unpublished observations). Finally, Harris and Westbrook point out that the disruption of extinction by FG 7142 is not complete, leaving open the possibility that other mechanisms and neurotransmitters also may be involved.

Interestingly, however, disruption of GABA transmission shortly following non-reinforced CS exposure may actually facilitate extinction (McGaugh et al., 1990). In this experiment with mice, a tone was paired 20 times with footshock on Day 1 and then presented 20 times without shock on Day 2. Immediately after Day 2 extinction the mice were injected with either saline or the GABA antagonist picrotoxin and then tested the next day in the absence of the drug. Control groups were injected with either saline or picrotoxin but not extinguished. Post-extinction injection of picrotoxin facilitated extinction measured by the number of arm entries in a Y-maze that could not be explained by a performance effect of picrotoxin given 24 hrs prior to testing. The authors considered this to be another example where GABAergic systems are important for the consolidation of recently acquired memories, similar to their effects on excitatory conditioning (cf. McGaugh et al., 1995). Taken together with the findings of Harris and Westbrook (1998b) outlined above, the data suggest that pre-extinction vs. post-extinction manipulations of GABA transmission may have opposite effects on the development of extinction. Because of this, pre-extinction drug treatments that last into the consolidation period could have complex, or unexpected effects on subsequent test performance. Clearly a systematic evaluation of the role of GABA-related compounds during the development and consolidation of extinction is warranted.

The Role of Dopamine in Extinction

As described above, 6-OHDA-induced lesions of monoaminergic, and primarily dopaminergic neurons in the medial prefrontal cortex blocked within-session extinction of fear conditioned with strong (0.8-mA) shocks. This suggests a role of dopaminergic neurons in the prefrontal cortex in the development of within-session extinction.

The dopaminergic system also has been implicated in extinction of fear conditioning by studies in which dopamine agonists have been administered systemically. An initial study showed that a high dose of cocaine (40 mg/kg) blocked extinction of fear-potentiated startle when the drug was injected prior to each of seven extinction sessions comprised of 30 unpaired presentations of a light CS (Willick and Kokkinides, 1995). State-dependency could not account for the effect, because the blockade was observed regardless of whether subjects were tested in the cocaine or drug-free state. A subsequent study demonstrated a similar blockade of extinction when cocaine, amphetamine, or the specific D1 agonist SKF 38393 were injected prior to a single extinction session comprised of 120 unpaired presentations of the CS (Borowski and Kokkinides, 1998). Moreover, a single injection of cocaine or SKF 38393 reinstated fear-potentiated startle in rats that had been given two sessions of extinction.

These data suggest that D_1 receptor stimulation interferes with extinction. At first sight, this might appear to be inconsistent with the blockade of extinction seen after lesions of dopaminergic neurons in the prefrontal cortex. However, the studies differed in that the effects of lesions were observed within a single extinction session whereas the systemic drug effects were observed primarily when subjects were tested one or more days after extinction training. Thus, this may be further evidence that short- and long-term extinction involve different receptor mechanisms. Furthermore, depletion of dopaminergic neurons in medial prefrontal cortex may enhance responses of subcortical dopamine neurons (Deutch et al., 1990; King et al., 1997). Although Morrow et al. (1999b) found no effect of the lesions on dopamine metabolism in the nucleus accumbens during extinction, it is possible that the lesions still elevated dopamine release in other structures, such as the basolateral complex of the amygdala. In fact, dopamine release in the amygdala is especially sensitive to stress (Coco et al., 1992) and local infusion of dopamine D1 agonists into the amygdala increase levels of conditioned fear (e.g., Guarraci et al., 1999). Thus, treatments that increase dopamine transmission in the amygdala either directly (e.g., systemic administration of dopamine agonist) or indirectly (e.g., depletion of prefrontal dopamine) may block extinction via an increase in conditioned fear.

Clearly, further research is required to ascertain the location of the D1 receptors mediating extinction effects. However, it is tempting to speculate that D_1 receptors in the basloateral complex of the amygdala may be involved. This would be consistent with the finding that local infusion of the D_1 antagonist SCH 23390 reduces expression of conditioned fear (Nader and LeDoux, 1999).

The Role of ACTH and Vasopressin in Extinction

Work by DeWied, Van Wiersima, Izquierdo and Richardson and their co-workers indicates that administration of various peptides such as adrenocorticotropic hormone (ACTH) or vasopressin either before or after extinction training attenuates subsequent extinction performance. Because most of these experiments involve active avoidance, these very interesting observations will not be reviewed here (for review see Falls and Davis, 1995a).

NEURAL SYSTEMS INVOLVED IN CONDITIONED INHIBITION

Conditioned inhibition offers experimental advantages for understanding the neural basis of fear inhibition. In this paradigm it is possible to measure the magnitude of excitatory conditioning and its reduction in the presence of the conditioned inhibitor in the same animal in the same test session. Because of this, it is possible to measure whether various treatments alter the level of excitatory conditioning or, instead, the amount of inhibition. Despite its inherent advantages compared to extinction, very little is known about the neural mechanisms of conditioned inhibition, although three general classes of studies have begun to address this fascinating problem.

Where Does a Conditioned Inhibitor Act to Inhibit Fear?

One kind of study asks "at what point within the neural circuitry known to produce a fear response does a conditioned inhibitor act so as to inhibit fear?" Elsewhere (Figure 5 in Falls and Davis, 1995b) we have outlined possible points where a conditioned inhibitor might act to decrease fear potentiated startle, based on the neural circuitry we believe is necessary for this measure of fear as well as on certain known properties of conditioned inhibition (i.e., stimulus and response transfer, retardation and "superconditioning"). Although this analysis suggested that inhibition might be exerted at either the perirhinal cortex or central nucleus of the amygdala, lesions of neither structure blocked the expression of conditioned inhibition (Falls and Davis, 1995b; Falls et al., 1997). In these studies, we faced the difficulty that fear-potentiated startle itself is abolished by lesions of either structure, thereby preventing the measurement of conditioned inhibition. To circumvent this problem, we took advantage of the finding that fear-potentiated startle can be re-established after lesions of the central nucleus of the amygdala or perirhinal cortex if additional training is given after surgery (Campeau and Davis, 1992b; Kim and Davis, 1993). Thus, rats were first given light-shock and tone-light-no shock training, followed by lesions of either structure, followed by retraining. It is important to note that retraining comprised further light-shock pairings, but no further tone-light-no shock pairings. When then tested in the presence of the conditioned inhibitor, robust conditioned inhibition still occurred after lesions of either structure.

A second approach to answering this question is to compare neural activity in pathways that mediate conditioned fear, when conditioned fear is induced in the presence versus the absence of a conditioned inhibitor. Using fluorodeoxyglucose autoradiography to measure neural activity, Mcintosh and Gonzalez-Lima (1995) compared region-specific activity in parallel auditory pathways in two groups presented with a tone-light compound. In both groups the tone was a fear-eliciting CS. The groups differed with respect to the significance of the light, which had been trained as a conditioned inhibitor in one group, and as a neutral stimulus in the other. Thus, the experiment allowed for an analysis of whether a conditioned inhibitor modulates activity in sensory areas normally activated by an auditory fear-eliciting CS. Interestingly, in only one area, the ventral medial geniculate nucleus, was there a significant difference in activation between the two groups. This structure showed less activation in the conditioned inhibition group, suggesting that a conditioned inhibitor may act at this locus in the auditory pathway to inhibit conditioned fear normally produced by an auditory CS.

What Sensory Structures are Involved in Conditioned Inhibition?

Another kind of study asks "what brain structures are required for a conditioned inhibitor to inhibit fear?" For example, an auditory conditioned inhibitor must be processed by auditory structures in the brain. Identification of these auditory structures will, by definition, identify the "sensory limb" of the conditioned inhibition circuit and provide an anchor point for identifying the remaining portion of the circuitry. Work in the Falls laboratory began to explore this question by testing the effects of lesions of auditory structures on conditioned inhibition using an auditory stimulus as a conditioned inhibitor. As expected, electrolytic lesions of the inferior colliculus, that included damage to the dorsal nucleus of the lateral lemniscus, eliminated conditioned inhibition (Heldt and Falls, 1999, unpublished data, Auditory pathways mediating conditioned inhibition of fear to an auditory conditioned inhibitor, The University of Vermont). Because the auditory thalamus is the major recipient of ascending collicular efferents, we then examined the effect of medial geniculate lesions on conditioned inhibition (Heldt and Falls, 1998). Remarkably, lesions of the medial geniculate that included bilateral destruction of the dorsal, ventral and medial divisions of the medial geniculate and the suprageniculate nucleus, did not affect conditioned inhibition. However, consistent with other data (LeDoux et al., 1986; LeDoux et al., 1986a; Campeau and Davis, 1995) these same animals failed to show conditioned fear reactions to an auditory CS when it was later paired with shock.

These data suggest that the inferior colliculus, but not the medial geniculate, is part of the neural circuit for conditioned inhibition activated by an auditory conditioned inhibitor. Because of the well-documented role of the medial geniculate in the expression of conditioned fear, these data suggest that the neural circuit for the acquisition and expression of conditioned fear is segregated from the neural circuit involved in conditioned inhibition of fear. Moreover, because the medial geniculate is the primary source of auditory projections to auditory, these data suggest that the auditory cortex may not be involved in conditioned inhibition. Although the medial geniculate is the primary target of ascending inferior colliculus projections, it also projects to the posterior intralaminar nucleus and the lateral subparafasicular nucleus which lie ventral to the medial geniculate. These nuclei project to other thalamic nuclei, cortex and the amygdala and may be part of the neural circuit mediating conditioned inhibition to an auditory conditioned inhibitor.

Alternatively, the deep and intermediate layers of the superior colliculus also receive auditory input. A subset of these projections originate in the inferior colliculus, although most originate in the dorsal nucleus of the lateral lemniscus. Because lesions of the inferior colliculus that blocked conditioned inhibition included significant damage to the dorsal nucleus of the lateral lemniscus, it is possible that the sensory limb of the neural circuit for conditioned inhibition involves projections from the inferior colliculus and dorsal nucleus of the lateral lemniscus to the superior colliculus. Interestingly, using c-fos as a marker for neuronal activation during conditioned inhibition, we found significant increases in c-fos in the dorsal nucleus of the lateral lemniscus and the inferior colliculus in the presence of an auditory conditioned inhibitor (Campeau et al., 1997). Furthermore, preliminary results suggest that post-training excitotoxic lesions of the superficial and intermediate layers of the superior colliculus interfere with conditioned inhibition using an auditory conditioned inhibitor (Falls, Wadell and Pistel ,unpublished data, Post-training excititotoxic lesions of the superior colliculus interfere with conditioned inhibition of fear, The University of Vermont). Although this effect needs to be verified, it is interesting to note that the ascending thalamic projections of the superior colliculus terminate in the vicinity of neurons that project to the lateral nucleus of the amygdala (Linke et al., 1999). This may provide a means for the conditioned inhibitor to affect the expression of conditioned fear.

What Brain Areas are Involved in Conditioned Inhibition?

Another approach to identifying the circuitry underlying conditioned inhibition would be to examine the role of brain areas that have been implicated in extinction (e.g., frontal cortex, hippocampus), or more generally in emotionality (e.g., the septal area). In addition, brain areas involved in positive affect (e.g., nucleus accumbens) might be relevant, because a conditioned inhibitor of fear operationally can serve as a conditioned reinforcer (Dickinson and Pearce, 1977).

We have found normal conditioned inhibition of fear potentiated startle, using a visual excitatory stimulus and an auditory conditioned inhibitor following lesions of either the medial prefrontal cortex (Gewirtz et al., 1997) or the nucleus accumbens (Falls et al., 1998). In addition, local infusion into the nucleus accumbens of either amphetamine or glutamate antagonists did not alter the magnitude of conditioned inhibition, as they alter responding to conditioned reinforcers trained in an operant situation (Taylor and Robbins, 1984; Burns et al., 1994).

Recently, in an appetitive learning situation, Holland et al. (1999) reported that lesions of the hippocampus appeared to block feature negative conditional discrimination, a phenomenon closely related to conditioned inhibition. Although space does not allow a thorough discussion of this interesting, but complex, paper, the data seem to differ from an earlier report where lesions of the hippocampus did not block conditioned inhibition using aversive eyeblink conditioning in rabbits (Solomon, 1977). Based on the results of a transfer test and the use of serial vs. simultaneous compound stimuli, Holland et al. (1999) point out that the form of inhibitory learning they were studying was more like negative occasion setting than simple conditioned inhibition, which Solomon (1977) was studying. Thus, it would be important to evaluate the role of the hippocampus in these different types of inhibitory learning using Pavlovian fear conditioning.

Several studies suggest that the lateral septum may play an important role in conditioned inhibition. Using Pavlovian discriminative fear conditioning, single unit firing rates in the dorsal lateral septal nucleus increased in the presence of a conditioned inhibitor and decreased in the presence of a conditioned excitor (Yadin and Thomas, 1981; Thomas et al., 1991). This was not seen when recordings were made in the medial septal nucleus (Yadin, 1989). More recently, Yadin and Thomas (1996) reported that stimulation of the same area of dorsolateral septal nucleus inhibited restraint stress-induced ulcers. Using c-fos mRNA as a measured of neuronal activation, we found a somewhat unique increase in c-fos in a ventral part of the lateral septum, the so-called septohypothalamic nucleus when a conditioned inhibitor of fear was presented (Campeau et al., 1997). Curiously, however, lesions of the lateral septal nucleus did not block the expression of conditioned inhibition in preliminary pilot studies, although further work certainly is required to evaluate the role of the lateral septum, perhaps using acute inactivation techniques rather than lesions.

A recent study suggests that the dorsal central gray may play an important role in conditioned inhibition of fear. Fendt (1998) reported that post-test infusions of 5 ng of picrotoxin (a GABA chloride channel blocker) into the dorsal central gray, but not the lateral or ventrolateral central gray, reduced the expression of conditioned inhibition without affecting the expression of conditioned fear. While this result is complicated by the fact that neither 2.5 nor 10 ng doses affected conditioned inhibition, it raises the intriguing possibility that a conditioned inhibitor of fear releases GABA into the dorsal central gray. Alternatively, because low doses of picrotoxin would be expected to activate the dorsal central gray by removing tonic inhibition, these results could be interpreted as indicating that the dorsal central gray is involved in inhibiting an unknown brain structure mediating conditioned inhibition (Fendt, 1998). Given the prominent role of the central gray in the expression of fear (Fanselow, 1991; Graeff et al., 1993; Bandler and Shipley, 1994; Helmstetter and Tershner, 1994; Fendt et al., 1996; Walker et al., 1997; DeOca et al., 1998), more work is needed to investigate the role of the dorsal central gray in conditioned inhibition of fear.

SUMMARY AND CONCLUSIONS

At the behavioral level, a great deal is now known about extinction, whereby presentation of a CS in the absence of the US with which it was formerly paired leads to a reduction in the magnitude or probability of a conditioned response. Although a CS may no longer elicit a conditioned response following extinction, it is clear that original CS-US associations still exist so that the original memory has not be erased. Phenomena seen after extinction such as spontaneous recovery (recovery of a conditioned response with the passage of time); reinstatement (recovery of a conditioned response following presentation of a US) or renewal (recovery of a conditioned response when testing takes place in a context different from the one used in extinction) all demonstrate this. Although data such as these suggest that extinction results from an active inhibitory process, this has been difficult to demonstrate experimentally. On the other hand, a closely related phenomenon, conditioned inhibition, clearly seems to result from an inhibitory process. Typically, conditioned inhibition is produced when one stimulus, such as a light, is paired with shock whereas another stimulus, such as a tone, when placed in compound with the light, is not followed by shock. One can show that the tone in this example will reduce fear in the presence of the light, (summation) or a novel fearful stimulus (transfer). Moreover, if a US is then paired with the tone, fear will develop more slowly to that tone following such training compared to a condition in which the tone has not been trained as a conditioned inhibitor (retardation).

In contrast to the rich behavioral literature on extinction and conditioned inhibition, much less is known about the neural mechanisms involved in these phenomena. Although sensory cortex, medial prefrontal cortex, and the hippocampus have been implicated, extinction certainly can occur after lesions of each of these structures. NMDA receptor activation in the amygdala, and perhaps elsewhere, seems critical for the development of extinction. Furthermore, recent studies suggest that extinction is mediated by release of GABA.

Structures involved in conditioned inhibition appear to include the lateral septum, based on unit recording, electrical stimulation and measurement of c-fos mRNA. In contrast, conditioned inhibition is not disrupted by lesions of two other candidate structures, the medial prefrontal cortex and nucleus accumbens. An auditory conditioned inhibitor seems to require the inferior colliculus but not the medial geniculate nucleus. However, it is still unclear how a conditioned inhibitor inhibits conditioned fear. Elucidation of this issue could provide important insights into the pathophysiology and treatment of anxiety.

REFERENCES

Aggleton, J.P. (1992) The amygdala. Neurochemical aspects of emotion, memory, and mental dysfunction. New York: John Wiley-Liss and Sons.

Annau, Z. and Kamin, L.J. (1961) The conditioned emotional response as a function of US intensity. Journal of Comparative and Physiological Psychology 54: 428-432.

Baker, J.D. and Azorlosa, J.L. (1996) The NMDA antagonist MK-801 blocks the extinction of Pavlovian fear conditioning. Behav Neurosci 110: 618-620.

Bandler, R. and Shipley, M.T. (1994) Columnar organization in the midbrain periaqueductal gray: modules for emotional expression? TINS 17: 379-389.

Berger, T.W., Weiker,t C.L., Basset, J.L., Orr, W.B. (1986) Lesions of the retrosplinal cortex produce deficits in reversal learning of the rabbit nictitating membrane response: implications for potential interactions between hippocampal and cerebellar brain systems. Behav Neurosci 100: 802-809.

Bolles, R.C. and Fanselow, M.S. (1980) A perceptual-defensive-recuperative model of fear and pain. The behavioral and brain sciences 3: 281-323.

Borowski, T.B. and Kokkinides, L. (1998) The effects of cocaine, amphetamine, and the dopamine D1 receptor agonist SKF 38393 on fear extinction as measured with potentiated startle: Implications for psychomotor stimulant psychosis. Behav Neurosci 112: 952-965.

Bouton, M.D. and Bolles, R.C. (1979a) Role of contextual stimuli in reinstatement of extinguished fear. J Exp Psychol:Animal Behav Process 5: 368-378.

Bouton, M.E. (1993) Context, time and memory retrieval in the interference paradigms of Pavlovian conditioning. Psychological Bulletin 114: 80-99.

Bouton, M.E. and Bolles, R.C. (1979b) Contextual control of the extinction of conditioned fear. Learn and Motiv 10: 455-466.

Bouton, M.E. and Bolles, R.C. (1985) Context, event-memories, and extinction. Hillsdale, NJ: Lawrence Erlbaum Associates.

Bouton, M.E. and Brooks, D.C. (1993) Time and context effects on performance in a Pavlovian discrimination reversal. Behav Neurosci 19: 165-179.

Bouton, M.E., Kenney, F.A., Rosengard, C. (1990) State-dependent fear extinction with two benzodiazepine tranquilizers. Behav Neurosci 104: 44-55.

Bouton, M.E. and King, D.A. (1983) Contextual control of conditioned fear: tests for the associative value of the context. J Exp Psychol:Animal Behav Process 9: 248-256.

Bouton, M.E. and King, D.A. (1986) Effect of context with mixed histories of reinforcement and nonreinforcement. J Exp Psychol:Animal Behav Process 12: 4-15.

Bouton, M.E. and Nelson, J.B. (1994) Context specificity of target versus feature inhibition in a feature-negative discrimination. J Exp Psychol:Animal Behav Process 20: 51-65.

Bouton, M.E. and Swartzentruber, D. (1991) Sources of relapse after extinction in Pavlovian instrumental learning. Clinical Psychological Review 11: 123-140.

Buchanan, S.L. and Powell, D.A. (1980) Divergencies in Pavlovian conditioned heart rate and eyeblink responses produced by hippocampectomy in the rabbit (Oryctolagus cuniculus). Behav Neural Biol 30: 20-38.

Burns, L.H., Everitt, B.J., Kelly, A.E., Robbins, T.W. (1994) Glutamate-dopamine interactions in the ventral striatum: role in locomotor activity and responding with conditioned reinforcement. Psychopharmacology 115: 516-528.

Campeau, S. and Davis, M. (1992b) Involvement of the lateral amygdala and perirhinal cortex in fear potentiated startle to acoustic and visual conditioned stimuli. Soc Neurosci Abst 18: 1562.

Campeau, S. and Davis, M. (1995) Involvement of subcortical and cortical afferents to the lateral nucleus of the amygdala in fear conditioning measured with fear-potentiated startle in rats trained concurrently with auditory and visual conditioned stimuli. J Neurosci 15: 2312-2327.

Campeau, S,. Falls, W.A., Cullinan, W.E., Helmreich, D.L., Davis, M,. and Watson, S.J. (1997) Elicitation and reduction of fear: behavioral and neuroendocrine indices and brain induction of the immediate-early gene c-fos. Neuroscience 78: 1087-1104.

Campeau, S., Miserendino, M.J.D., Davis, M. (1992) Intra-amygdala infusion of the N-methyl-D-Aspartate receptor antagonist AP5 blocks acquisition but not expression of fear-potentiated startle to an auditory conditioned stimulus. Behav Neurosci 106: 569-574.

Coco, M.L., Kuhn, C.M., Ely, T.D., Kilts, C.D. (1992) Selective activation of mesoamygdaloid dopamine neurons by conditioned stress: attenuation by diazepam. Brain Res 590: 39-47.

Cox, J. and Westbrook, R.F. (1994) The NMDA receptor antagonist MK-801 blocks acquisition and extinction of conditioned hypoalgesia responses in the rat. Quarterly Journal of Experimental Psychology 47B: 187-210.

Davis, M,. Rainnie, D., Cassell, M. (1994) Neurotransmission in the rat amygdala related to fear and anxiety. Trends in Neuroscience 17: 208-214.

138

DeOca, B.M., DeCola, J.P., Maren, S., Fanselow, M.S. (1998) Distinct regions of the periaqueductal gray are involved in the acquisition and expression of defensive responses. The Journal of Neuroscience: 3426-3432.

Deutch, A.Y., Clark, W.A., Roth, R.H. (1990) Prefrontal cortical dopamine depletion enhances the responsiveness of mesolimbic dopamine neurons to stress. Brain Res 521: 311-315.

Dickinson, A. and Pearce, J.M. (1977) Inhibitory interactions between appetitive and aversive stimuli. Psychologcal Bulletin 84: 690-711.

Douglas, R.J. (1972) Inhibition and learning. Pavlovian conditioning in the brain. London: Academic Press.

Estes, W. (1955) Statistical theory of spontaneous recovery and regression. Psychology Review 62: 145-154.

Falls, W.A., Bakken, S., and Heldt, S.A. (1997) Lesions of the perirhinal cortex block conditioned excitation but not conditioned inhibition of fear. Behav Neurosci 111: 476-486.

Falls, A. and Davis, M. (1995a) Behavioral and physiological analysis of fear inhibition. In: M. J. Friedman, Charney D. S. and Deutch A. Y., eds. Neurobiological and clinical consequences of stress: From normal adaptation to PTSD. Philadelphia: Lippincott-Raven Publishers.

Falls, W.A. and Davis, M, (1995b) Lesions of the central nucleus of the amygdala block conditioned excitation, but not conditioned inhibition of fear as measured with the fear-potentiated startle effect. Behav Neurosci 109: 379-387.

Falls, W.A. and Davis, M.J. (1997) Inhibition of fear-potentiated startle can be detected after the offset of a feature trained in a serial feature negative discrimination. Journal of Experimental Psychology: Animal Behavioral Processes 23: 1-14.

Falls, W.A., Josselyn, S.A., Gewirtz, J.C., Pistell, P., and Davis, M. (1998) The nucleus accumbens if not critical for condtioned inhibition of fear as measured with fear-potentiated startle. Soc Neurosci Abst 28: .

Falls, W.A., Miserendino, M.J.D., and Davis, M. (1992) Extinction of fear-potentiated startle: blockade by infusion of an NMDA antagonist into the amygdala. J Neurosci 12: 854-863.

Falls, W.F. and Davis, M. (1994) Visual cortex ablations do not prevent extinction of fear-potentiated startle using a visual conditioned stimulus. Behav Neural Biol 60: 259-270.

Fanselow, M.S. (1986a) Associative vs. topographical accounts of the immediate shock freezing deficit in rats: Implications for the response selection rules governing species-specific defensive reactions. Learn and Motiv 17: 16-39.

Fanselow, M.S. (1986b) Conditioned fear-induced analgesia: A competing motivational state theory of stress-analgesia. Annuals of the New York Academy of Science 467: 40-54.

Fanselow, M.S. (1991) The midbrain periaqueductal gray as a coordinator of action in response to fear and anxiety. In: A. Depaulis and Bandler R., eds. The Midbrain Periaqueductal Gray Matter: Functional, Anatomical and Neurochemical Organization. New York: Plenum Publishing Co.

Fendt, M. (1998) Different regions of the periaqueductal grey are involved differently in the expression and conditioned inhibition of fear-potentiated startle. European Journal of Neuroscience 10: 3876-84.

Fendt, M., Koch, M., Schnitzler, H.-U. (1996) Lesions of the central gray block conditioned fear as measured with the potentiated startle paradigm. Behavioural Brain Research 74: 127-134.

Fox, G.D. and Holland, P.C. (1998) Neurotoxic hippocampal lesions fail to impair reinstatement of an appetitively conditioned response. Behav Neurosci 112: 255-260.

Frohardt, R., Guarraci, F.A., Bouton, M.E. (1999) The effects of neurotoxic hippocampal lesions on two effects of context following fear extinction. Behav Neurosci In press: .

Gewirtz, J. and Davis, M. (1997) Second order fear conditioning prevented by blocking NMDA receptors in the amygdala. Nature 388: 471-474.

Gewirtz, J.C., Falls, W.A., Davis, M. (1997) Normal conditioned inhibition and extinction of freezing and fear potentiated startle following electrolytic lesions of medial prefrontal cortex. Behav Neurosci 111: 712-726.

Good, M., deHoz, L., Morris, R.G.M. (1998) Contingent versus incidental context processing during conditioning: Dissociation after excitotoxic hippocampal plus dentate gyrus lesions. Hippocampus 8: 147-159.

Graeff, F.G., Silveira, M.C.L., Nogueira, R.L., Audi, E.A., Oliveira, R.M.W. (1993) Role of the amygdala and periaqueductal gray in anxiety and panic. Behav Brain Res 58: 123-131.

Guarraci, F.A. and Frohardt, R.J. (1999) Amygdaloid D1 dopamine receptor involvement in Pavlovian fear conditioning. Brain Res 827: 28-40.

Harris, J.A. and Westbrook, R.F. (1998a) Benzodiazepine-induced amnesia in rats: reinstatement of conditioned performance by noxious stimulation on test. Behav Neurosci 112: 183-192.

Harris, J.A. and Westbrook, R.F. (1998b) Evidence that GABA transmission mediates context-specific extinction of learned fear. Psychopharmacology 140: 105-115.

Harris, J.A. and Westbrook, R.F. (1999) The benzodiazepine midazolam does not impair Pavlovian fear conditioning but regulates when and where fear is expressed. Journal of experimental psychology: Animal behavioral processes 25: 236-246.

Hearst, E. (1972) Some persistent problems in the analysis of conditioned inhibition. In: R. A. Boakes and Halliday M. S., eds. Inhibition and Learning. New York: Academic Press.

Heldt, S.A. and Falls, W.A. (1998) Destruction of the auditory thalamus disrupts the production of fear but not the inhibition of fear conditioned to an auditory stimulus. Brain Res 813: 274-282.

Helmstetter, F.J. (1992) The amygdala is essential for the expression of conditioned hypoalgesia. Behav Neurosci 106: 518-528.

Helmstetter, F.J. and Tershner ,S.A. (1994) Lesions of the periaqueductal gray and rostral ventromedial medulla disrupt antinociceptive but not cardiovascular aversive conditional responses. The Journal of Neuroscience 14: 7099-7108.

Holland, P.C. (1985) The nature of conditioned inhibition in serial and simultaneous feature negative discriminations. In: R. R. Miller and Spear N. E., eds. Information Processing in Animals: Conditioned Inhibition. Hillsdale, N.J.: Lawrence Erlbaum Associates.

Holland, P.C., Lamoureux, J.A., Han, J.-S., Gallagher, M. (1999) Hippocampal lesions interfere with Pavlovian negative ossasion setting. Hippocampus 9: 143-157.

Holt, W. and Maren, S. (1999) Muscimol inactivation of the dorsal hippocampus impairs contextual retrieval of fear memory. J Neurosci 19: 9054-9062.

Honey, R.C. and Good, M. (1993) Selective hippocampal lesions abolish the context specificity of latent inhibition and conditioning. Behav Neurosci 107: 23-33.

Kehoe, E.J., Macrae, M., Hutchinson, C.L. (1996) MK-801 protects conditioned response from extinction in the rabbit nictitating membrane preparation. Psychobiology 24: 127-135.

Kim, M. and Davis, M. (1993) Electrolytic lesions of the amygdala block acquisition and expression of fear-potentiated startle even with extensive training, but do not prevent re-acquisition. Behav Neurosci 107: 580-595.

King, D., Zigmond, M.J., and Finlay, J.M. (1997) Effects of dopamine depletion in the medial prefrontal cortex on the stress-induced increase in extracellular dopamine in the nucleus accumbens core and shell. Neuroscience 77: 141-153.

Konorski, J. (1948) Conditioned reflexes and neuronal organization. London: Cambridge University Press.

Konorski, J. (1967) Integrative activity of the brain: An interdisciplinary approach. Chicago: The University of Chicago Press.

Leaton, R.N. and Borszcz, G.S. (1990) Hippocampal lesions and temporally chained conditioned stimuli in a conditioned suppression paradigm. Psychobiology 18: 81-88.

LeDoux, J.E., Romanski, L., Xagoraris, A. (1989) Indelibility of subcortical memories. J Cogn Neurosci 1: 238-243.

LeDoux, J.E., Sakaguchi, A., Iwata, J., Reis, D.J. (1986a) Interruption of projections from the medial geniculate body to an archi-neostriatal field disrupts the classical conditioning of emotional responses to acoustic stimuli. Neuroscience 17: 615-627.

LeDoux, J.E., Sakaguchi, A., Reis, D.J. (1986) Interuption of projections from the medial geniculate mediate emotional responses conditioned to acoustic stimuli. J Neurosci 17: 615-627.

Lee, H. and Kim, J. (1998) Amygdalar NMDA receptors are critical for new fear learning in previously fear-conditioned rats. Journal ofNeuroscience 18: 8444-8454.

Linke, R., De Lima, A.D., Schwegler, H., Pape, H.C. (1999) Direct synaptic connections of axons from superior colliculus with identified thalamo-amygadloid projection neurons in the rat: Possible substrates of a subcortical visual pathway to the amygdala. The Journal of Comparative Neurology 403: 158-170.

Lovibond, P.F., Preston, G.C., and Mackintosh, N.J. (1984) Context specificity of conditioning, extinction and latent inhibition. Journal of Experimental Psychology: Animal Behavioral Processes 10: 360-375.

Lubow, R.E. (1989) Latent inhibition and conditioned attention theory. New York: Cambridge University Press.

Mackintosh, N.J. (1974) The psychology of animal learning. New York: Academic Press.

McAllister, W.R. and McAllister, D.E. (1971) Behavioral measurement of conditioned fear. In: F. R. Brush, ed Aversive Conditioning and Learning. New York: Academic Press.

McGaugh ,J., Cahill, L., Parent, M.B., Mesches, M.H., Coleman-Mesches, K., Salinas, J.A. (1995) Involvement of the amygdala in the regulation of memory storage. In: J. McGaugh, Bermudez-Rattoni F. and Praco-Alcala R. A., eds. Plasticity in the Central Nervous System. Hillsdale, NJ: Lawrence Erlbaum Associates.

McGaugh, J.L., Castellano, C., and Brioni, J. (1990) Picrotoxin enhances latent extinction of conditioned fear. Behvioral Neuroscience 104: 264-267.

McIntosh, A.R. and Gonzalez-Lima, F. (1995) Functional network interactions between parallel auditory pathways during Pavlovian conditioned inhibition. Brain Res 683: 228-241.

McNish, K.A., Gewirtz, J.C. and Davis, M. (1997) Evidence of contextual fear conditioning following lesions of the hippocampus: A disruption of freezing but not fear-potentiated startle. J Neurosci 17: 9353-9360.

Miserendino, M.J.D., Sananes ,C.B., Melia, K.R., Davis, M. (1990) Blocking of acquisition but not expression of conditioned fear-potentiated startle by NMDA antagonists in the amygdala. Nature 345: 716-718.

Morgan, M.A. and LeDoux, J.E. (1995) Differential contribution of dorsal and ventral medial prefrontal cortex to the acquisition and extinction of conditioned fear in rats. Behav Neurosci 109: 681-688.

Morgan, M.A. and LeDoux, J.E. (1996) Medial prefrontal cortex (mPFC) and the extinction of fear: Differential effecs of pre- or post-training lesions. Soc Neurosci Abst 22: 1116.

Morgan, M.A. and LeDoux JE (1999) Contribution of ventrolateral prefrontal cortex to the acquistion and extinction of conditioned fear in rats. Neurobiol Learn Memory 72: 244-251.

Morgan, M.A., Romanski, L.M., LeDoux, J.E. (1993) Extinction of emotional learning: contribution of medial prefrontal cortex. Neurosci Letts 163: 109-113.

Morrow, B.A., Elsworth, J.D., Inglis, F.M., Roth, R.H. (1999a) An antisense oligonucleotide reverses the footshock-induced expression of Fos in the rat medial prefrontal cortex and the subsequent expression of conditioned fear-induced immobility. J Neurosci 19: 5666-5673.

Morrow, B.A., Elsworth, J.D., Rasmusson, A.M., Roth, R.H. (1999b) The role of mesoprefrontal dopamine neurons in the acquisition and expression of conditioned fear in the rat. Neuroscience 92: 553-564.

Nader, K. and LeDoux, J.E. (1999) Inhibition of the mesoamygdala dopaminergic pathway impairs the retrieval of conditioned fear associations. Behav Neurosci 113: 891-901.

Papini, M.R. and Bitterman, M.E. (1993) The two-test strategy in the study of inhibitory conditioning. Journal of Experimental Psychology: Animal Behavior Processes 19: 342-352.

Pavlov, I.P. (1927) Conditioned Reflexes. Oxford University Press: Oxford University Press.

Quirk, G.J., Kohanski, G.J., Ayala, O. (1998) Lesions of medial prefrontal cortex retard extinction of fear conditioning between sessions, but not within a session. Soc Neurosci Abst 28: 1683.

Quirk, G.J., Rosaly, E., Romero, R.V., Santini, E., Muller, R.U. (1999) NMDA receptors are required for long-term but not short-term memory of extinction learning. Soc Neurosci Abst 25: 1620.

Reiss, S. and Wagner, A.R. (1972) CS habituation produces a "latent inhibition effect" but no active "conditioned inhibition." Learning & Motivation 3: 237-245.

Rescorla, R.A. (1969) Pavlovian conditioned inhibition. Psychological Bulletin 72: 77-94.

Rescorla, R.A. and Heth, C.D. (1975) Reinstatement of fear to an extinguished conditioned stimulus. Journal of Experimental Psychlogy: Animal Behavior Processes 1: 88-96.

Robinson, G.B., Port, R.L., Stillwell, E.J. (1993) Latent inhibition of the classically conditioned rabbit nictitating membrane response is unaffected by the NMDA antagonist MK801. Psychobiology: 120-124.

Schmaltz, L.W. and Theiosus, J. (1972) Acquisition and extinction of a classically conditioned response in hippocampectomized rabbits (oryctolagus cuniculus). J Comp Physiol Psychol 79: 328-333.

Skinner, B. F. (1950) Are theories of learning necessary? Psychology Review 57: 193-216.

Skinner, B.F. (1938) Behavior of Organisms. New York: Appleton-Century-Crofts.

Solomon, P.R. (1977) Role of hippocampus in blocking and conditioned inhibition of the rabbit's nictitating membrane response. Journal of Comparative Physiological Psychiatry 91: 407-417.

Taylor, J.R. and Robbins, T.W. (1984) Enhanced behavioral control by conditioned reinforcers following microinjections of d-amphetamine into the nucleus accumbens. Psychopharmacology 84: 405-412.

Teich, A.H., McCabe, P.M., Gentile, C.C., Schneiderman, L.S., Winters, R.W., Liskosky, D.R., Schneiderman, N. (1989) Auditory cortex lesions prevent the extinction of heart rate conditioning to tonal stimuli in rabbits. Brain Res 480: 210-218.

Thomas, E., Yadin, E., Strickland, C.E. (1991) Septal unit activity during classical conditioning: A regional comparison. Brain Res 547: 303-308.

Walker, D.L., Cassella, J.V., Lee, Y., de Lima, T.C.M., Davis, M. (1997) Opposing roles of the amygdala and dorsolateral periaqueductal gray in fear-potentiated startle. Brain Res Bull 111: 692-702.

Williams, D.A., Overmier, J.B., LoLordo, V.M. (1992) A reevaluation of Rescorla's early dictums about Pavlovian Conditioned Inhibition. Psychological Bulletin 111: 275-290.

Willick, M.L. and Kokkinides, L. (1995) Cocaine enhances the expression of fear-potentiated startle: Evaluation of state-dependent extinction and the shock-sensitization of acoustic startle. Behav Neurosci 109: 929-938.

Wilson, A., Brooks, D., and Bouton, M.E. (1995) The role of the rat hippocampal system in several effects of context extincition. Behav Neurosci 109: 828-836.

Yadin, E. (1989) Unit activity in the medial septum during differential appetitive conditioning. Behavioural Brain Research 33: 45-50.

Yadin, E. and Thomas, E. (1981) Septal correlates of conditioned inhibition. J Comp Physiol Psychol 95: 331-340.

Yadin, E. and Thomas, E. (1996) Stimulation of the lateral septum attenuates immobilization-induced stress ulcers. Physiol Behav 59: 883-886.

9 BRAIN LATERALITY AS A SOURCE OF INDIVIDUAL DIFFERENCES IN BEHAVIOR: ANIMAL MODELS OF DEPRESSION AND SUBSTANCE ABUSE

Jeffrey N. Carlson, Isabelle M. Maisonneuve and Stanley D. Glick

INTRODUCTION

Functional and anatomical laterality of the human brain has been studied since the early neurologist Broca reported that lesions of the left cerebral hemisphere resulted in language disorders. His findings suggested a specialized role for this hemisphere in controlling speech (Broca, 1861). Since these early reports, numerous differences between the left and right hemispheres of the human brain have been reported. Many hemispheric asymmetries have been shown to involve dominance where one hemisphere plays a greater role in control of a specific behavior (Corballis, 1991; Hellige, 1993). It has been shown, for example, that while the human left hemisphere is specialized for the processing of language, the right hemisphere has a dominant role for the processing of musical, visuospatial and emotional information (Springer and Deutsch, 1981). Lateralization of brain function often indicates that the two hemispheres are differentially proficient in controlling various behavioral activities. Differential degrees of brain lateralization appear to occur within the population. Variation in human functional brain asymmetry is associated with differences in handedness (Annett, 1985; Bryden, 1982), cognitive ability (O'Boyle and Hellige, 1989), emotional function (Davidson, 1992) and psychopathology (Flor Henry, 1986).

Research conducted in this as well as in other laboratories indicates that brain asymmetry also determines behavioral variation in the rodent. Behavioral differences in rats are accompanied by distinct neurochemical and morphologic differences in brain regions controlling particular behaviors. Animal models of human behavioral function and psychopathology have been used in our laboratory to allow for the more precise study of relationships between chemical and morphological asymmetries and differences in behavior. Using these systems, differences in brain asymmetry have been linked to differences in spatial behavior, stress reactivity, susceptibility to stress-related pathology such as depression, and vulnerability to drug and ethanol abuse. In this chapter we will review the evidence that brain laterality in animals is in many respects analogous to that in humans. and should be considered in animal models of psychopathology.

TURNING BEHAVIOR, DOPAMINE AND NIGROSTRIATAL ASYMMETRY

Afferent neurons of the dopamine system play a role in the control of motor behavior. In the early 1970s the discovery of l-dopa's efficacy in treating the symptoms of nigrostriatal loss in Parkinson's disease (Cotzias et al., 1967) led to a search for animal models for the evaluation of new and potentially more useful agents for this disorder. A well investigated experimental technique was to create a neurochemical asymmetry of the nigrostriatal pathways by performing unilateral lesions with the dopamine neurotoxin 6-hydroxydopamine (6OHDA) (Ungerstedt, 1971). The efficacy of various dopaminergic drugs such as d-amphetamine (d-A) could then be evaluated by monitoring changes in the direction and intensity of rats turning or circling behavior. During this period it was found that d-A also induced circling, at lower rates, in rats that were not lesioned (Jerussi and Glick, 1974, 1976). Subsequent studies demonstrated that, as with lesioned rats, the rotation of unlesioned rats was consistent in direction and correlated in magnitude upon repeated testing. Some rats rotated consistently to the left while others rotated to the right. Furthermore, unilateral 6OHDA lesions of the striata of rats caused more rotation if the lesion was made ipsilateral rather than contralateral to the preoperative direction of circling (Jerussi and Glick, 1975). It was suggested that the directional preference for motor behavior as expressed in circling represented a manifestation of an endogenous asymmetry of nigrostriatal DA pathways. This hypothesis was supported by data showing that d-A enhanced T maze side preferences in a direction that is consistent with that of circling preference (Glick, 1973; Glick and Jerussi, 1974). The validity of circling behavior as an index of brain asymmetry was extended when it was shown that drug naive rats also rotate spontaneously at night, the active part of their diurnal cycle. For individual rats, the direction of nocturnal rotation was usually the same as that induced by d-A and correlated in magnitude (Glick et al., 1986; Glick and Cox, 1978; Glick et al., 1976, 1977).

It was known that rotational behavior in lesioned rats was caused by a large unilateral loss of nigrostriatal dopaminergic neurons. It was thus hypothesized that circling behavior in normal rats was caused by a smaller endogenous asymmetry occurring in these same cells (Glick et al., 1974; Jerussi and Glick, 1976). This prediction was confirmed. Endogenous biochemical asymmetries in the striatum were identified for DA content (Zimmerberg et al., 1974), DA release and DA metabolism (Glick et al., 1988a), DA-stimulated adenylate cyclase activity (Jerussi et al., 1977) and DA receptors (Drew et al., 1986; Glick et al., 1988b). The strength and direction of chemical asymmetry is related to the magnitude and direction of behavioral asymmetries other than circling. For example, intrinsic side preferences, as indicated by choice behavior in a T maze (Zimmerberg et al., 1974), were related to differences in asymmetries in striatal DA content.

CORTICAL ASYMMETRY AND ITS MODULATION OF NIGROSTRIATAL ASYMMETRY

A number of functional and morphologic asymmetries are also found in the rat cortex. Differential effects on behavior are brought about by unilateral damage to opposing sides of this structure (Kubos et al., 1985; Robinson, 1985; Starkstein et al., 1988), indicating that the two sides influence behavior differently. The rat left cortex is morphologically thicker than the right cortex (Diamond et al., 1981, 1983) and DA is asymmetrically distributed across the two sides. The direction of cortical DA asymmetry varies among strains of rats with some strains showing a left > right asymmetry (Carlson et al., 1988; Slopsema et al., 1982) and others a right > left asymmetry (Rosen et al., 1984). There is a left > right asymmetry of frontal cortical energy metabolism in the rat as evidenced by measures of labeled 2-deoxyglucose uptake (2DG) (Glick et al., 1979; Ross et al., 1981). Cortical asymmetry also appears to influence the direction and amount of turning behavior. Turning preferences are stronger if 2DG uptake is greater in the cortex contralateral rather than ipsilateral to the preferred rotational direction. Right-turning rats with greater 2DG activity in the left cortex have stronger turning preferences than left-turning rats (Glick and Ross, 1981). Bilateral cortical lesions alter behavioral asymmetry by decreasing right-turns and increasing left-turns (Ross and Glick, 1981). This body of data thus indicates that the cortex exerts an asymmetric effect on the output of the nigrostriatal system as evidenced by turning behavior.

CORTICAL ASYMMETRY, EMOTIONAL BEHAVIOR, AND ANIMAL MODELS OF PSYCHOPATHOLOGY

Human Cortical Asymmetry and Depression

Besides modifying the output of the nigrostriatal system, the cortex is also involved in modifying the function of other brain regions. Considerable evidence concerning the cortex's role in regulating centers controlling emotional behavior has been found in studies with humans. The two sides of the human cortex are differentially involved in controlling an individual's mood. For example, activation of the left cortex is associated with positive emotion and approach-related behavior. Increased neuronal activity in the corresponding right cortex accompanies negative mood and withdrawal-related behavior (Davidson, 1995). Personality differences have also been attributed to cortical asymmetry. An individual's emotional reactivity, mood and temperament can be predicted on the basis of relative amounts of electrical activity in the left and right sides of the anterior cortex (Tomarken et al., 1992). Cortical asymmetry is also involved in the genesis of a number of psychopathologic states (Cutting, 1990). Electroencephalographic studies have found abnormalities of the left hemisphere, particularly the left temporal cortex, in patients with schizophrenia (Gur, 1978; Suddath et al., 1989). These functional differences are related to left to right differences in concentrations of the neurotransmitters dopamine and glutamate (Deakin et al., 1989; Reynolds, 1983). Cortical asymmetry also appears to play a role in depression. Studies by Robinson and colleagues (Robinson and Chait, 1985) have shown that damage to the left but not the right frontal lobe results in symptoms of clinical depression. Clinically depressed individuals have been shown to have a left > right asymmetry in frontal cortical serotonin (5HT2) receptors (D'haenen et al., 1992). Prefrontal cortical blood flow is greater in the right hemisphere of patients that exhibit symptoms of unipolar depression (Drevets et al., 1992).

Cortical Asymmetry in an Animal Model of Depression

Since we knew that the rat cortex is also lateralized, we wondered whether it functioned similarly to the human cortex during depression-like behavioral states. We investigated this issue by looking at the degree to which cortical asymmetry accompanies depressed behavior in the Learned Helplessness (LH) animal model. LH is a behavioral state that occurs after animals are exposed to stressors that can not be controlled (Maier and Seligman, 1976). LH animals become passive, appear to "give up" and fail to maintain active responding in the face of new stressors. The model thus duplicates many of the important symptomatic aspects of human clinical depression. The clinical relevance of the model is supported by data showing that symptoms of LH are reversed by chronic treatment with antidepressant drugs (Willner, 1983a,b).

Stress Control and Turning Behavior

A number of studies indicate that stressors, similar to those used in the LH model, selectively activate DA neurons projecting to the PFC (Abercrombie et al., 1989; Carlson et al., 1987a; Herman et al., 1982; Thierry et al., 1976). Our own data showed that mild stressors such as foot shock, (Carlson et al., 1987b) and food deprivation (Carlson et al., 1988), changed the direction of d-A-induced and nocturnal turning behavior. Because other evidence showed that the cortex exerted an asymmetric effect on turning (Glick and Greenstein, 1973; Ross and Glick, 1981), we sought to determine whether stressors evoked behavioral changes through their actions on asymmetric brain cortical systems. We hypothesized that, as in human depression, LH effects are mediated by cortical asymmetry in the rat. To test this hypothesis we evaluated the effects of foot shock stress on turning behavior (Carlson et al., 1987b). The direction of d-A induced turning was determined before and again following either uncontrollable foot shock stress, identical controllable foot shock or no stress. Uncontrollable foot shock stress increased rightward turning in male rats. Identical foot shock that could be turned off (controlled) by a bar-press response, however, preferentially increased left turns. Thus, the experience of a lack of control over stress, when compared to that of controlling identical stress, exerted an opposite effect on functional brain asymmetry as indicated by turning behavior.

Individual Differences in Stress-induced Behavioral Deficits

Most individuals experience uncontrollable stressful events, yet relatively few of them become depressed. The LH model has been criticized in that it relies upon the use of 'normal' animals where no defined bias toward LH susceptibility has been established (Jesberger and Richardson, 1985). Studies using the LH model have, however, been quite variable in their reported effects. All rats do not become "depressed." Besides reports of failures to replicate the phenomenon (Beatty, 1979; Henn et al., 1985), various other (Henn et al., 1985; Kelsey, 1983) laboratories have reported that as few as 5-20 % of rats tested exhibit the LH phenomenon. Mice (Anisman et al., 1979) and rats (Henn et al., 1985; Scott et al., 1996) may be selectively bred to be vulnerable to the phenomenon. It has also been shown that differences in susceptibility to LH are found among rats obtained from different stocks and suppliers (Wieland et al., 1986). Apparently, LH susceptibility is a specific behavioral trait that is variably expressed within populations of rats.

Variability in intrinsic turning preferences in rats is associated with variability in a number of other behavioral traits. In response to d-A, right-turning rats are more active and have stronger side preferences than left-turning rats (Glick and Ross, 1981). Left and right turning rats also respond differently to stress. When exposed to a controllable stressor, left turners engage in more escape-related activity (Carlson et al., 1990) and show greater levels of stress-induced plasma ACTH and norepinephrine (LaHoste et al., 1988a,b) than right-turners. Though right-turning rats are initially less active when confronted with foot shock stress, they learn to escape controllable foot shock better than left-turning rats (Carlson and Glick, 1991, 1992). Since we knew that left- and right-turning rats differed in cortical asymmetry, we assessed whether they also differed in susceptibility to the effects of LH. Rats that differed in the direction of d-A-induced turning behavior were exposed to the LH treatment. A differential susceptibility to LH was associated with turning differences. Following the LH treatment, non-turning and right-turning rats had more difficulty escaping foot shock stress than left-turning rats (Carlson and Glick, 1989).

Stress and Individual Differences in PFC DA Metabolism

Further studies explored potential neurochemical differences among rats differing in LH susceptibility. In other studies, we had obtained evidence indicating that stress-induced activation of DA projections to the medial prefrontal cortex (PFC) is asymmetrical. Food deprivation (Carlson et al., 1988) and physical restraint (Carlson et al., 1991; Sullivan and Szechtman, 1995) as well as foot shock (Carlson et al., 1990) all altered PFC DA utilization asymmetrically across the two hemispheres. It also was also found that the two sides of the PFC responded differently to stress over time. When rats are first exposed to an uncontrollable stressor (such as being restrained) they engage in vigorous behavior to control or "cope" with the stressor. This behavior is accompanied by a greater activation of DA (as indicated by increased metabolite levels) on the left side of the PFC. However, at later time points, when coping behavior has ceased (e.g., when a restrained rat has stopped struggling), there is more DA metabolism on the right side of the PFC (Carlson et al., 1991). Experiments were then designed to assess potential asymmetric PFC DA function that might accompany individual differences in LH effects (Carlson et al., 1993). We found that LH effects (decreased stress coping) in right turning rats is accompanied by a greater metabolic activation of DA in the right PFC. Successful stress coping, as seen in left turning rats, is accompanied by a similar change in the left PFC.

PFC DA, Stress and Subcortical DA Function

The PFC controls anticipatory behaviors that are involved with coping with stress (Claustre et al., 1986; LeMoal and Simon, 1991). As part of this function it also inhibits output from limbic brain regions. PFC DA appears to play a role in this process. When DA is released in the PFC it inhibits the firing of pyramidal neurons and dampens their firing activity. These neurons form the origin of the PFC's primary efferent system which projects back to the VTA as well as to subcortical regions such as the nucleus accumbens (NAS) and striatum (Carter and Pycock, 1980; Glick and Greenstein, 1973; Ross and Glick, 1981). DA-mediated neuronal inhibition from the PFC takes place through this efferent pathway. It limits the activity of neurons in the NAS. The net effect of activity in this pathway is to keep NAS DA release under tonic inhibitory control. Altering DA function in the PFC thus affects neuronal activity in the NAS. Disruption of PFC DA function with 6OHDA lesions increases DA activity in the NAS in response to stress (Deutch et al., 1990).

We had evidence to suggest that there is asymmetrical control of subcortical DA utilization during the behavioral response to stressors. We hypothesized that left > right PFC DA activation inhibited NAS DA utilization to a greater extent than right > left PFC DA activation. In order to test this hypothesis we performed left, right or sham lesions of the PFC using 6OHDA (Carlson et al., 1996). We then exposed all animals to a series of mild foot shocks. The effects of foot shock stress on NAS DA utilization were greater following left 6OHDA PFC lesions than following right and sham lesions. Left turning rats significantly increased their circling behavior following right sided lesions and showed disrupted foot shock escape behavior following left sided lesions. The data thus indicated that an intrinsic asymmetry in brain DA systems interacts with left- and right-PFC lesions to differentially determine sub-cortical DA function as well as turning and stress responsive behaviors that it subserves. The data indicated that the PFC DA system on the left side may be the predominant cortical influence in inhibiting NAS neuronal activity during the behavioral response to stressors.

In further work (Nielsen et al., 1996), we showed that asymmetric cortical inhibition may be D_1 receptor mediated. Experiments with the D_1 antagonist drug SCH-23390 assessed hypothesized differential effects of intra-cortical drug infusion on the two sides of the PFC. Different groups of rats received unilateral intra-PFC injections of SCH-23390 (0.25 µg/side) or saline. They were then given a shock escape test in a shuttle box. We found that SCH-23390 injections in the left PFC caused a greater disruption of shuttle box foot shock escape responding than injections on the right side. Presumably, PFC DA acts on D_1 receptors in the PFC to inhibit corticofugal neurons projecting to the NAS and VTA. These findings are in accord with those obtained with 6OHDA lesions of the PFC and further suggest a lateralized contribution of PFC D_1 receptors in governing the behavioral response to stress. They are also consistent with observations showing a lateral asymmetry of the D_1 receptor-associated DA regulated phosphoprotein DARPP-32 (Toomim et al., 1992) in various cingulate cortical areas including the PFC.

Antidepressant Drug Treatment, Turning Behavior and PFC DA

If part of the etiological basis for depression lies in lateralized PFC function, then a reasonable approach to therapy would involve altering this function through a pharmacological intervention. Among the neurotransmitters located within the PFC, 5HT appears to play the most clearly delineated role in depression both in human studies (Agren and Reibring, 1994; Petty et al., 1996) and in animal models (Espejo and Minano, 1999; Petty et al., 1994). While lateralized PFC function has been repeatedly shown to play a major role in human depression, a role for DA is far from clear (Willner, 1983a,b,c). It is known that acute administration of antidepressant (AD) drugs increases extracellular DA concentrations in the PFC (Carboni et al., 1990; Tanda et al., 1994) but little is known about the effects of chronic treatment.

Various uncontrolled stressors, similar to those used in the LH model, have been shown to asymmetrically alter the PFC DA system (Carlson et al., 1988, 1991). For example, brief physical restraint stress induces an asymmetric increase in PFC DA function (Carlson et al., 1991). To assess the potential of AD drugs to alter stress-induced PFC DA changes, and potentially LH effects, we assessed chronic antidepressant effects on the DA response of the PFC to a brief period of restraint stress. The effects of chronic administration of desipramine (DMI), nortryptiline (NOR) and paroxetine (PAR) (10 mg/kg/day, 21 days) on changes in turning (circling) behavior and on DA in the PFC were evaluated. All three drugs eliminated turning biases in right turning rats. All drugs also increased DA concentrations in the PFC and increased the magnitude of a normal left > right DA asymmetry in that region. The drugs thus reduced a turning bias that is associated with LH susceptibility and enhanced a neurochemical asymmetry that is associated with LH resistance. Right turning rats express an increased vulnerability to stress-induced LH effects. Depressive- like effects within the LH model have been associated with uncontrollable stress-induced right > left alterations in PFC. Perhaps part of the mechanism by which AD drugs eliminate LH effects is by restoring or maintaining "normal" PFC asymmetry. The findings suggest that chronic antidepressant drug treatment increases the capacity of the PFC to release DA during the stress response (e.g., by increasing synthesis) and prevents its depletion. LH effects involve an asymmetric reduction of PFC DA function. Antidepressant drugs may prevent behavioral deficits by ameliorating this loss.

PFC Asymmetry and Depression in an Animal Model of Psychopathology

The results of the above studies show that DA systems projecting to the PFC are activated asymmetrically in response to uncontrolled stressors. The direction of this asymmetrical activation differs between left and right turning rats. Right PFC activation is associated with depression-like effects in the LH model. Results of studies using asymmetric 6OHDA lesions show that the left PFC exerts a greater amount of inhibition on NAS DA activation than does the right PFC during the response to stress. Pharmacologic studies show that D_1 antagonists injected into the left PFC cause a greater disruption of active behavioral responding that is aimed at terminating a stressor. Taken together these findings suggest that adequate behavioral responding to stressors is associated with left > right asymmetry of PFC DA systems. Furthermore, the findings suggest that decrements in responding to stressors, occurring when right > left asymmetry is present, may be the result of a failure of the PFC to adequately inhibit sub-cortical (NAS) neuronal activity. Studies with antidepressant drugs suggest that part of their action may be to maintain left > right asymmetry of PFC DA systems and thereby "protect" behavior from the deleterious effects of right > left PFC activation.

CORTICAL ASYMMETRY, STRESS AND AN ANIMAL MODEL OF HUMAN COCAINE ABUSE

Human Cortical Asymmetry and Cocaine Abuse

Vulnerability to stimulant addiction is associated with a number of stress-related traits. Hyperactivity, impulsiveness, aggressiveness and emotionality in stressful situations have been identified as antecedent conditions to stimulant misuse (Tarter et al., 1995). A number of studies have focused on the human prefrontal, cingulate and temporal cortices as biological substrates that govern these stress and drug related behaviors (Majewska, 1996; Tarter and Hegedus, 1985). Low levels of electrical activity in the left prefrontal cortex predicts the onset of substance seeking behavior in adolescents (Deckel et al., 1995). Similar processes may operate for cocaine. Chronic cocaine abuse has been linked to dysfunction of specific prefrontal brain regions (Bolla et al., 1998). Functional MRI studies have shown specific activation of subregions of the right cingulate cortex during a cocaine "rush" (Breiter et al., 1997). Cocaine abusers exhibit a specific metabolic activation of the right orbito-frontal and prefrontal cortices during stimulant-induced craving (Volkow et al., 1999). Similar asymmetric variation in the activity of the cortices is also a predictor of individual differences in sensation seeking, obsessive-compulsive disorders (Insel, 1992) and the behavioral response to stress (Davidson and Sutton, 1995).

The PFC and the Rewarding Effects of Cocaine

Modern theories of drug abuse emphasize the idea that drugs are abused because they interact with brain regions that govern reinforcement or reward (Koob, 1992; Koob et al., 1998; Robinson and Berridge, 1993; Wise, 1978). DA transmission in the NAS has been repeatedly described as the major brain process involved in determining the rewarding effects of abused drugs. A variety of experimental findings (Hoebel et al., 1983; Lyness et al., 1979; Phillips et al., 1994; Roberts et al., 1977; Yokel and Wise, 1975) using diverse techniques have supported this conclusion. Thus the addictive effects of stimulants such as amphetamine and cocaine have been attributed to their ability to elevate extracellular concentrations of DA in the NAS. Indeed, many drugs of abuse, including morphine (Olds, 1982), amphetamine (Phillips et al., 1994) and ethanol (McBride et al., 1993), are reliably self-administered directly into the NAS. Rats will similarly self-administer dopamine itself (Guerin et al., 1984). However, cocaine appears to be somewhat different from the agents listed above. Though experimenter-controlled intra-NAS cocaine infusions elevate local DA levels (Hernandez and Hoebel, 1988; Nomikos et al., 1990), rats do not self-administer intra-NAS cocaine (Carlezon et al., 1995; Goeders and Smith, 1983).

Evidence indicates that the PFC plays a unique role in the regulation of the rewarding effects of cocaine. Unlike the stimulants listed above, rats will self-administer cocaine directly into the PFC (Goeders and Smith, 1983). During intra-PFC self-administration, dopamine turnover increases in the NAS (Goeders and Smith, 1993). There appears to be a more subtle role for PFC DA in regulating systemic cocaine self-administration. When the PFC is lesioned with 6OHDA, rats respond reliably for lower systemic doses of cocaine than do intact sham rats (Schenk et al., 1991). Nonetheless, response rates for higher doses of cocaine appear to be unaffected (Martin-Iverson et al., 1986). Similarly, with low dose cocaine infusions, 6OHDA PFC lesions cause a significant *increase* in break point on a progressive-ratio schedule (i.e., the number of responses made to obtain the last reinforcement of a self-administration session; a higher number indicates greater reward) (McGregor et al., 1996). Similar lesions of the NAS *lower* the break point (Koob et al., 1987).The progressive-ratio paradigm is considered a reliable model of drug craving (Markou et al., 1993). These findings are therefore consistent with the idea that neuronal activity in the PFC plays a role in "adjusting" the rewarding effects (incentive value) of cocaine by modulating DA activity in the NAS. The PFC appears to limit the extent to which animals will seek cocaine.

Brain asymmetry, reward thresholds and the effects of cocaine

Asymmetry of Reward Thresholds

A series of studies performed some years ago in this laboratory provided evidence that some of cocaine's effects on reward are different from those of other drugs of abuse. A well-investigated approach to evaluating the rewarding effects of drugs is an assessment of the degree to which they change current thresholds for reinforcing lateral hypothalamic stimulation (ICSS) (Kornetsky and Esposito, 1979; van Wolfswinkel and van Ree, 1985; Schaefer and Michael, 1988; Maldonado-Irizarry et al., 1994). We have known for a number of years that the two sides of the rat brain are differentially sensitive to ICSS. Thresholds are lower on the side contralateral to the preferred turning direction for female rats and on the ipsilateral side for male rats (Glick et al., 1980). Drugs that rats self-administer also lower ICSS thresholds. Different agents act predominantly on different sides of the brain (Fromm and Schopflocher, 1984; Glick et al., 1981; ; Glick and Badalamenti, 1986). As an example, stimulants like amphetamine preferentially affect the lower current threshold (more rewarding) side of the brain while the opioid morphine preferentially affects the high threshold side. Furthermore, these asymmetric effects depend on the direction of the individual rat's spontaneous turning behavior. For amphetamine, the shift in reward threshold occurs more for the side contralateral to animal's turning direction while for morphine, the shift is greater on the ipsilateral side. The above data indicated to us that individual differences in the tendency to self-administer different classes of drugs might be in part related to differences in lateralized functioning of specific brain systems. By knowing an animal's rotational asymmetry, which is a manifestation of asymmetry of nigrostriatal DA, we were able to predict the side of the brain that was more sensitive to ICSS.

Asymmetric effect of cocaine on reward thresholds

When we tested cocaine for its effects on ICSS thresholds a very different pattern was found. Before cocaine, all rats had asymmetries in ICSS thresholds that corresponded, as before, to their preferred turning direction. They were lower on the ipsilateral side of male rats and on the contralateral side of females. However, In both sexes, cocaine acted predominantly on the contralateral side: that is, cocaine lowered the thresholds and shifted the rate-intensity functions to the left on both sides of the brain, but the effects were much greater on the side of the brain contralateral to the preferred direction of rotation. When compared to baseline parameters, cocaine enhanced the asymmetry of self-stimulation in female rats, but reduced or reversed the asymmetry of self-stimulation in male rats. These data suggested that a separate lateralized system, distinct from the nigrostriatal pathways, mediated cocaine's effects on self-stimulation of the lateral hypothalamus. They showed that the relative importance of these systems differs between the sexes and that cocaine selectively affects one of these systems. Since the time of these early studies, a number of experimental results have pointed to the PFC as the second asymmetric system. In more recent studies we have continued to investigate the hypothesis that individual differences in cocaine intake can be predicted on the basis of lateralized differences in PFC DA systems.

Asymmetric Participation of the PFC in Drug Self-administration

Cocaine, DA Asymmetry and Turning Behavior

Results from a number of studies indicate that stimulant drugs such as amphetamine and morphine induce turning behavior in non-lesioned rats (Glick et al., 1974; Jerussi and Glick, 1976). Generally the direction of spontaneous and stimulant-induced circling are the same except that the rate of turning differs (Glick and Cox, 1978). Drugs such as d-A and morphine also have equivalent effects on increasing the turning behavior of left- and right-turning rats. Pronounced differences between rats that normally turn to the left and those that turn to the right were observed, however, following an acute injection of cocaine (Glick et al., 1983). Left-rotating male rats rotated more than right rotators, and female right rotators much more than left rotators. These findings were in sharp contrast to those obtained with d-A where no significant differences between left- and right-turning rats were found. In light of data indicating asymmetric structure and function in the frontal cortex, we attributed this effect to cocaine's preferential effect on PFC neurons. We then hypothesized that cocaine-like effects on rotational behavior would be produced by d-A when we activated PFC neurons with stress. This hypothesis was supported by studies demonstrating that foot shock stress exerted an effect on d-A induced rotational behavior to resemble turning induced by cocaine (Carlson et al., 1987b). We subsequently found that cocaine exhibits a number of other properties that distinguish it from other stimulants. As with other locomotor behavior, stimulant-induced turning undergoes sensitization. We found that single-dose sensitization occurred more readily to cocaine-induced turning behavior than to d-A-induced turning (Glick and Hinds, 1984). Brief food deprivation, which activates PFC DA like as a mild stressor (Carlson et al., 1987a), caused d-A to mimic the asymmetric effects of cocaine on turning behavior (Carlson et al., 1988). Finally, food deprivation stress enhanced the self-administration of cocaine more than that of d-A(Glick et al., 1987). The data indicated that a part of cocaine's brain action involved an effect on asymmetric stress-responsive systems of the PFC.

We then sought to evaluate whether cocaine's apparent unique asymmetric actions in the PFC could be distinguished neurochemically. We assessed the effects of behaviorally equivalent doses of d-A and cocaine on extracellular levels of DA in the PFC using the in vivo microdialysis technique. Each drug increased extracellular

PFC DA levels and, in each case, the effects were greater in the left than in the right side of the brain. The data also seemed to indicate that, contrary to some previous reports, d-A and cocaine did not differ substantially with regard to their effects on DA neurotransmission in the PFC (Maisonneuve et al., 1990). However, when we compared d-A and cocaine's effects across structures, we saw an important way in which the drugs differed. It was found that d-A caused greater increases in extracellular levels of DA in the striatum and NAS, whereas cocaine caused a greater increase in extracellular levels of DA in the PFC (Carboni et al., 1989; Kuczenski et al., 1991; Maisonneuve et al., 1992; Maisonneuve and Glick, 1992).

Maximum increases (% of baseline) in DA levels induced by d-A were approximately 1250% in the striatum, 800% in NAS, and 1000% in PFC; for cocaine the values were approximately 350% in STR, 400% in NAC and 800% in PFC. Thus, contrary to our original hypothesis, cocaine and d-A may not differ in their actions in the PFC in an absolute sense but they do appear to differ in their relative actions in different brain regions. The data indicated that with regard to relative magnitudes of response, PFC DA may thus indeed be a more important substrate for cocaine's effects than for d-A's effects.

PFC DA Asymmetry and Cocaine Self-administration

We performed a series of studies to assess whether subjects having neurochemical differences in PFC DA function also differed in the acquisition of cocaine self-administration. To help distinguish cocaine from other agents, we conducted similar experiments with morphine. Extracellular levels of DA and its metabolites were thus measured bilaterally in the PFC of naive rats that were subsequently trained to self-administer morphine or cocaine intravenously. It was found that asymmetric patterns of DA activity were related to the dynamics of responding for these drugs. For morphine, DOPAC and HVA levels in the right but not in the left side of the PFC were positively correlated with self-administration rates (Glick et al., 1992). For cocaine, self-administration rates were positively correlated with the magnitude of the left to right ratio of DOPAC and HVA levels on the two sides of the PFC (Glick et al., 1994). Thus, animals whose pre-drug rates of DA metabolism were greater on the left side of the PFC displayed a greater predisposition to self-administer cocaine.

Extracellular DA levels in the PFC decrease as rats become sensitized to cocaine (Karoum et al., 1990; Sorg et al., 1997; Meiergerd et al., 1997). DA activity in the PFC limits NAS DA release (Deutch et al., 1990; Karreman and Moghaddam, 1996; Murase et al., 1993; Rosin et al., 1992). A diminished PFC DA response with continued stimulant intake is thus consistent with the development of increased responding during the acquisition of stimulant self-administration. Individual rats whose rates of DA metabolism are greater on the left side might show a more rapidly or more sensitized (diminished) DA response in the left PFC during the acquisition of cocaine self-administration and self-administer greater amounts.

The above observations have led us to the hypothesis that animals showing a greater basal and stress-induced level of DA metabolism in the left PFC administer more cocaine because their left PFC DA response sensitizes (diminishes) more rapidly during cocaine acquisition. In the future we plan to perform additional experiments to fully elaborate this hypothesis as an animal model of cocaine abuse.

CORTICAL ASYMMETRY, STRESS AND AN ANIMAL MODEL OF HUMAN ETHANOL ABUSE

Human Cortical Asymmetry and Ethanol Abuse

Vulnerability to alcohol abuse in humans is associated with several behavioral characteristics. Hyperactivity, impulsiveness, aggressiveness and emotionality in stressful situations have been identified as conditions antecedent to problem drinking (Tarter and Ryan, 1983). A number of human studies have focused on the prefrontal cortex as the biological substrate governing these behaviors (Tarter and Hegedus, 1985). A deficiency of electrical activity in the left prefrontal cortex has been found to be a predictor of impulsive, aggressive behavior and the tendency to consume alcohol (Deckel et al., 1995). Asymmetric variation in the activity of the human prefrontal cortex also predicts differences in the behavioral response to stress (Davidson and Sutton, 1995).

The PFC and the Response to Ethanol

Evidence from animal studies shows that the PFC plays a role in determining the rewarding effects of ethanol As we already discussed, efferent projections from the PFC DA system mediate positive reinforcement by modulating DA activity in the NAS (Di Chiara and Imperato, 1988; Wise, 1978). A number of studies show that individual variability in the reinforcing effects of ethanol may be related to the strength of this PFC modulation. For example, in the selectively-bred alcohol-preferring P line of rats, cortical regulation of NAS function appears to be less prominent (McBride et al., 1993) than in the alcohol-non-preferring (NP) line. The P line rat's PFC contains a lower content of DA and fewer D2 receptors as compared to the NP line of rat. When PFC D2 receptors are blocked with antagonists, rats' responding for ethanol increases (Hodge et al., 1996). The findings thus indicate a participation of DA in the PFC in ethanol's role as a reinforcer.

Ethanol's interaction with PFC DA may be modulated by a system of lateralized GABA interneurons (Ticku, 1989). Drugs that affect benzodiazepine (BDZ), GABA-gated chloride channel receptors (Deutch et al., 1989; Lavielle et al., 1979) alter PFC DA release in response to stress (Fadda et al., 1978). Radioligand binding studies indicate that there are more channel controlling receptors on the left than on the right side of the PFC. The magnitude of this receptor asymmetry changes with increased exposure to stress (McIntyre et al., 1988). The pharmacological effects of ethanol are mediated in part through an alteration of BZD/GABA-gated chloride channel function in the PFC. Not all BDZ/GABA complex receptors are affected equally in all brain regions by ethanol, however (Reynolds et al., 1992; Soldo et al., 1994). These differences have been attributed to variation in subunit composition in different brain regions (Breese et al., 1993; Criswell et al., 1993). Stressors modify the subunit composition and therefore the pharmacologic properties of the PFC BDZ/GABA receptor complex (Korpi and Luddens, 1993; Orchinik et al., 1994). The asymmetric receptor change induced by stress may thus result from a change in subunit composition. The relevance of changes in receptor subunit composition during stress to changes in ethanol consumption is supported by findings showing that exposure to stress differentially alters benzodiazepine binding in long sleep (LS) and short sleep (SS) mice. These animals are specifically bred for differences in response to ethanol (Bowers and Wehner, 1992). A number of studies (Doherty and Gratton, 1999; Westerink et al., 1998) have shown that GABA interneurons play an important role in regulating PFC DA activity. Part of ethanol's action in the PFC may be brought about through an interaction with this system of lateralized GABA interneurons.

Ethanol and PFC DA

The effects of ethanol in the PFC differ depending on the endpoint that is measured. Low doses (0.25 g/kg) increase rates of 2-[14C] deoxyglucose incorporation (an index of neuronal activity) but higher doses do not (Williams-Hemby and Porrino, 1994). Ethanol at moderate doses (0.5-1.0 g/kg), blocks the increase in PFC DOPAC normally seen with restraint stress (Matsuguchi et al., 1994). Following stress, however, (Hegarty and Vogel, 1993) ethanol exerts a potentiating effect on stress-induced PFC DOPAC concentrations. Even higher (2g/kg) doses of ethanol (Fadda et al., 1985) potentiate foot shock-induced increases of the DA metabolite HVA. Clearly, ethanol alters the function of PFC neurons and also interacts with the DA response that these neurons make to stress. These processes may have relevance for the variable effects seen in animal models of stress-induced ethanol drinking (Anisman and Waller, 1974; Bond, 1978; Caplan and Puglisi, 1986; Ng Cheong Ton et al., 1983).

Stress, Individual Differences in Ethanol Drinking and Brain Asymmetry

The amount of ethanol drinking in response to stress is not the same for all rats. Experiments performed in different laboratories using different stocks and strains of inbred and outbred rats have found variable effects of stress on ethanol consumption (Anisman and Waller, 1974; Bond, 1978; Caplan and Puglisi, 1986; Ng Cheong Ton et al., 1983). A number of findings have also shown that the degree of brain asymmetry, as well as the relative incidence of left- and right-turning preference, varies among strains and stocks of rats (Brass and Glick, 1981; Carlson and Glick, 1989; Glick et al., 1986). Stock and strain differences have also been reported in the susceptibility of rats to the effects of stress (Chisari et al., 1995; Dhabhar et al., 1997; Gomez et al., 1998). Finally, the work we have reviewed indicates that brain and behavior changes caused by stress vary with turning direction and the lateralized functioning of the stress responsive PFC.

In light of these considerations, we performed experiments to test whether much of the reported variance in stress-induced ethanol drinking is attributable to inter-animal variation in PFC function. We felt that much of the apparent complexity and contradiction in the stress-induced ethanol literature might be accounted for by the failure to consider differences in PFC DA function. Human (Deckel et al., 1995) and animal (Deckel et al., 1996; Shoemaker et al., 1996) show that some aspects of alcohol abuse are related to PFC asymmetry. Variation in the function of this area appears to be important in the development of alcohol-related behavior. Although hypotheses relating cortical asymmetry to ethanol abuse have been made previously (Backon, 1989), they have never been adequately tested under laboratory conditions. We thus initiated a series of studies to test the hypothesis that individual differences in ethanol seeking behavior are associated with functional, morphological and biochemical differences in PFC asymmetry .

Turning Behavior and Ethanol Drinking

We sought to determine whether left and right turning rats differed in their levels of ethanol consumption in a simple 2-bottle choice situation. We identified rats as being either left rotators, right rotators or non-rotators in our "nocturnal test" of rotational behavior. Over 5 days of continuous 24-hr access to water and to 10% ethanol in the home cage, right-turning rats on average drank approximately 25% more ethanol than left-turning rats (Nielsen et al., 1999a). There were no differences in average total fluid (water plus ethanol) intake between left- and right-turning rats. We also looked at correlations between the amount of ethanol ingestion and the amount of turning behavior. Positive correlations were seen between the number of right turns and the amount of drinking for right-turning rats while negative correlations were seen for left turns in left rotators. The greater the number of turns to the right the higher the ethanol preference. Right-turning rats, that have been shown to have greater difficulty coping with stressors in the LH model of depression, also drank more ethanol and the amount of this drinking was correlated with their degree of right sidedness as shown by turning behavior. The analyses indicated that turning bias accounts for approximately 48 % of the variance in drinking.

Ethanol and Asymmetric PFC DA Metabolism

We have also assessed potential neurochemical substrates for ethanol-related behavioral differences between left- and right-turning rats. Differences in brain chemistry that are similar to differences that we observed following stress exposure have been observed. Rats were injected with a moderate (0.5 g/kg) dose of ethanol 15 minutes before sacrifice. PFC homogenates were subsequently assayed for DA and its metabolites. Following ethanol injection, left-turning rats displayed a significant increase in DA metabolism in the left PFC and right turners a predominant increase on the right side (Nielsen et al., 1999b). These data suggest that experimenter-administered (uncontrolled) ethanol intake, like uncontrolled stress, asymmetrically activates DA systems projecting to the PFC. The effect is consistent with the hypothesis that left- and right-turning rats differ in ethanol consumption because ethanol differentially activates DA systems on the left and right sides of the PFC.

Ethanol Drinking and Asymmetric PFC DA Function

In subsequent studies we focused on the evaluation of a mechanistic role for PFC in controlling ethanol intake. Our previous work indicated that DA in the left and right PFC differentially controls drug intake (Glick et al., 1992, 1994) and responding during stress (Carlson et al., 1996; Nielsen et al., 1996). In light of our neurochemical findings showing a stress-like asymmetric effect of ethanol in the

PFC, we hypothesized a differential role of the left and right PFC in controlling ethanol intake. As we did in our experiments with stress, we used 6OHDA to damage DA terminals in the PFC and deplete DA on the left or right side. Our hypothesis was that lesions on the left side of the PFC would increase ethanol drinking. A well documented effect of ethanol as well as other abused substances is to increase DA utilization in the NAS (Di Chiara and Imperato, 1988); in fact, this increase has been suggested to be a general property of rewarding stimuli (Wise, 1978). We hypothesized that the effects of left lesions would be similar to those seen in our experiments with stress. Lesions of the left PFC would disinhibit DA utilization in the NAS, cause ethanol to be "more rewarding" and increase ethanol drinking. The obtained data supported the hypothesis. Lesions of the left PFC caused a significant increase in ethanol preference during continuous access to water and 10% ethanol. The data also showed that lesions of the right PFC decreased ethanol ingestion. Thus, when left to right PFC DA asymmetry is augmented with lesions, an even greater difference in spontaneous ethanol intake over that seen in rats with intrinsic asymmetry is obtained (Nielsen et al., 1999c).

The data indicated that an important factor in the regulation of ethanol intake is a balance between left and right PFC DA. When DA activity on the right is eliminated with a lesion, there is proportionally more activity on the left. In fact, earlier studies from this laboratory (Carlson et al., 1996) showed that a significant *increase* in DA concentration is found on the contralateral (left) side 3-4 weeks following a right 6OHDA lesion. Thus a right lesion increases left > right DA asymmetry not only by lowering DA concentrations on the right side but by also raising them on the left.

The results of the foregoing studies indicate that differences in rats turning preference also predict differences in amounts of spontaneous voluntary ethanol ingestion. Differences in stress responsiveness and in ethanol consumption appear to be similarly determined, in part, by asymmetric variation in the organization of dopamine neurons projecting to the PFC.

CONCLUSIONS

We have reviewed a body of research conducted in this as well as in other laboratories that indicates that, as with humans, brain asymmetry determines behavioral variation in the rodent. Behavioral differences in rats are accompanied by distinct neurochemical and morphologic differences in brain regions controlling particular behaviors. We have reviewed findings to show that this is particularly true for the PFC, which regulates the stress response. We have shown how differences in brain asymmetry have been linked to differences in susceptibility to stress-related pathology such as depression and in vulnerability to drug and ethanol abuse. This evidence strongly suggests that brain laterality in animals is in many respects analogous to that in humans and should be considered in animal models of psychopathology.

REFERENCES

Abercrombie, E.D., Keefe, K.A., DiFrischia, D.S., Zigmond, M.J. (1989) Differential effect of stress on in vivo dopamine release in striatum, nucleus accumbens, and medial frontal cortex. J.Neurochem. 52:1655-1658.

Agren, H. and Reibring, L. (1994) PET studies of presynaptic monoamine metabolism in depressed patients and healthy volunteers. Pharmacopsychiatry 27:2-6.

Anisman, H., Grimmer, J., Irwin, J., Remington, G., Sklar, L.S. (1979) Escape performance after inescapable shock in selectively bred lines of mice: response maintenance and catecholamine activity. J.Comp.Physiol.Psychol. 93:229-241.

Anisman, H. and Waller, T.G. (1974) Effects of inescapable shock and shock-produced conflict on self selection of alcohol in rats. Pharmacology, Biochemistry and Behavior 2:27-33.

Annett, M. (1985) Left, right, hand and brain: The right shift theory. Erlbaum, Hillsdale, NJ.

Backon, J. (1989) Etiology of alcoholism: relevance of prenatal hormonal influences on the brain, anomalous dominance, and neurochemical and pharmacological brain asymmetry. [Review]. Medical Hypotheses 29:59-63.

Beatty, W.W. (1979) Failure to observe learned helplessness in rats exposed to inescapable footshock. Bull.Psychonom.Soc. 13:272-273.

Bolla, K.I., Cadet, J.L., London, E.D. (1998) The neuropsychiatry of chronic cocaine abuse. [Review] [82 refs]. Journal of Neuropsychiatry & Clinical Neurosciences 10:280-289.

Bond, N.W. (1978) Shock induced alcohol consumption in rats: role of initial preference. Pharmacology, Biochemistry & Behavior 9:39-42.

Bowers, B.J. and Wehner J.M. (1992) Adrenalectomy and stress modulate GABAA receptor function in LS and SS mice. Brain Research 576:80-88.

Brass, C.A. and Glick S.D. (1981) Sex differences in drug-induced rotation in two strains of rats. Brain Res. 223:229-234.

Breese, G.R., Morrow, A.L., Simson, P.E., Criswell, H.E., McCown, T.J., Duncan, G.E., Keir, W.J. (1993) The neuroanatomical specificity of ethanol action on ligand-gated ion channels: a hypothesis. [Review]. Alcohol & Alcoholism Supplement. 2:309-313.

Breiter, H.C., Gollub, R.L., Weisskoff, R.M., Kennedy, D.N., Makris, N., Berke, J.D., Goodman, J.M., Kantor, H.L., Gastfriend, D.R., Riorden, J.P., Mathew, R.T., Rosen, B.R., Hyman, S.E. (1997) Acute effects of cocaine on human brain activity and emotion. Neuron 19:591-611.

Broca, P. (1861) Remarques sur le siege de la faculte du langage articule. Bull Soc d'Anthropol Paris,2nd series, 6:398-407.

Bryden, M.H. (1982) Laterality, functional asymmetry in the intact brain. Academic Press, New York.

Caplan, M.A. and Puglisi, K. (1986) Stress and conflict conditions leading to and maintaining voluntary alcohol consumption in rats. Pharmacology, Biochemistry & Behavior 24:271-280.

Carboni, E., Imperato, A., Perezzani, L., Di Chiara, G. (1989) Amphetamine, cocaine, phencyclidine and nomifensine increase extracellular dopamine concentrations preferentially in the nucleus accumbens of freely moving rats. Neuroscience 28:653-661.

Carboni, E., Tanda, G.L., Frau, R., Di Chiara, G. (1990) Blockade of the noradrenaline carrier increases extracellular dopamine concentrations in the prefrontal cortex: evidence that dopamine is taken up in vivo by noradrenergic terminals. Journal of Neurochemistry 55 :1067-1070.

Carlezon, W.A. Jr., Devine, D.P., Wise, R.A. (1995) Habit-forming actions of nomifensine in nucleus accumbens. Psychopharmacology (Berl) 122:194-197.

Carlson, J.N., Fitzgerald, L.W., Keller, R.W. Jr., Glick, S.D. (1991) Side and region dependent changes in dopamine activation with various durations of restraint stress. Brain Res. 550:313-318.

Carlson, J.N., Fitzgerald, L.W., Keller, R.W. Jr., Glick, S.D. (1993) Lateralized changes in prefrontal cortical dopamine activity induced by controllable and uncontrollable stress in the rat. Brain Res. 630:178-187.

Carlson, J.N. and Glick, S.D. (1989) Cerebral lateralization as a source of interindividual differences in behavior. Experientia 45:788-798.

Carlson, J.N. and Glick, S.D. (1991) Brain laterality as a determinant of susceptibility to depression in an animal model. Brain Res. 550:324-328.

Carlson, J.N. and Glick, S.D. (1992) Behavioral laterality as a determinant of individual differences in behavioral function and dysfunction, in Genetically Defined Animal Models of Neurobehavioral Dysfunctions (Driscoll P ed) pp 189-216, Birkhauser, Boston.

Carlson, J.N., Glick, S.D., Hinds, P.A. (1987b) Changes in d-amphetamine elicited rotational behavior in rats exposed to uncontrollable footshock stress. Pharmacol.Biochem.Behav. 26:17-21.

Carlson, J.N., Glick, S.D., Hinds, P.A., Baird, J.L. (1988) Food deprivation alters dopamine utilization in the rat prefrontal cortex and asymmetrically alters amphetamine- induced rotational behavior. Brain Res. 454:373-377.

Carlson, J.N., Herrick, K.F., Baird, J.L., Glick, S.D. (1987a) Selective enhancement of dopamine utilization in the rat prefrontal cortex by food deprivation. Brain Res. 400:200-203.

Carlson, J.N., Keller, R.W., Glick, S.D. (1990) Individual differences in the behavioral effects of stressors attributable to lateralized differences in mesocortical dopamine systems. Society for Neuroscience abstracts 16.233

Carlson, J.N., Visker, K.E., Keller, R.W. Jr., Glick, S.D. (1996) Left and right 6-hydroxydopamine lesions of the medial prefrontal cortex differentially alter subcortical dopamine utilization and the behavioral response to stress. Brain Research 711:1-9.

Carter, C.J. and Pycock, C.J. (1980) Behavioral and neurochemical effects of dopamine and noradrenaline depletion within the medial prefrontal cortex of the rat. Brain Res. 192:163-176.

Chisari, A., Carino, M., Perone, M., Gaillard, R.C., Spinedi, E. (1995) Sex and strain variability in the rat hypothalamo-pituitary-adrenal (HPA) axis function. J of Endocrinological Investigation 18:25-33.

Claustre, Y., Rivy, J.P., Dennis, T., Scatton, B. (1986) Pharmacological studies on stress-induced increase in frontal cortical dopamine metabolism in the rat. J.Pharmacol.Exp.Ther. 238:693-700.

Corballis, M.C. (1991) The Lopsided Ape. Oxford University Press, Oxford.

Cotzias, G.C., Van Woert, M.H., Schiffer, L.M. (1967) Aromatic amino acids and modification of parkinsonism. New Engl.J.Med. 276:374-379.

Criswell, H.E., Simson, P.E., Duncan, G.E., McCown, T.J., Herbert, J.S., Morrow, A.L., Breese, G.R. (1993) Molecular basis for regionally specific action of ethanol on gamma-aminobutyric acidA receptors: generalization to other ligand-gated ion channels. Journal of Pharmacology & Experimental Therapeutics 267:522-537.

Cutting, J. (1990) The right cerebral hemisphere and psychiatric disorders. Oxford University Press, Oxford.

D'haenen, H., Bossuyt, A., Mertens, J., Bossuyt-Piron, C., Gijsemans, M., Kaufman, L. (1992) SPECT imaging of serotonin2 receptors in depression. Psychiatry Research: Neuroimaging 45:227-237.

Davidson, R.J. (1992) Anterior cerebral asymmetry and the nature of emotion. Brain Cogn. 20:125-151.

Davidson, R.J. (1995) Cerebral asymmetry, emotion and affective style, in Brain Asymmetry (Davidson RJ and Hugdahl K eds) pp 362-387, MIT Press, Cambridge, MA.

Davidson, R.J. and Sutton, S.K. (1995) Affective neuroscience: the emergence of a discipline. [Review]. Curr.Opin.Neurobiol. 5:217-224.

Deakin, J.F., Slater, P., Simpson, M.D., Gilchrist, A.C., Skan, W.J., Royston, M.C., Reynolds, G.P., Cross, A.J. (1989) Frontal cortical and left temporal glutamatergic dysfunction in schizophrenia. J.Neurochem. 52:1781-1786.

Deckel, A.W., Bauer, L., Hesselbrock, V. (1995) Anterior brain dysfunctioning as a risk factor in alcoholic behaviors. Addiction 90:1323-1334.

Deutch, A.Y., Gruen, R.J., Roth, R.H. (1989) The effects of perinatal diazepam exposure on stress-induced activation of the mesotelencephalic dopamine system. Neuropsychopharmacology 2: 105-114.

Deckel, A.W., Shoemaker, W.J., Arky, L. (1996) Dorsal lesions of the prefrontal cortex: Effects on alcohol consumption and subcortical monoaminergic systems. Brain Research 723:70-76.

Deutch, A.Y., Clark, W.A., Roth, R.H. (1990) Prefrontal cortical dopamine depletion enhances the responsiveness of mesolimbic dopamine neurons to stress. Brain.Res. 521:311-315.

Dhabhar, F.S., McEwen, B.S., Spencer, R.L. (1997) Adaptation to prolonged or repeated stress--comparison between rat strains showing intrinsic differences in reactivity to acute stress. Neuroendocrinology 65:360-368.

Di Chiara, G. and Imperato, A. (1988) Drugs abused by humans preferentially increase synaptic dopamine concentrations in the mesolimbic system of freely moving rats. Proceedings of the National Academy of Sciences of the United States of America 85:5274-5278.

Diamond, M.C., Dowling, G.A., Johnson, R.E. (1981) Morphological cerebral cortical asymmetry in male and female rats. Exper.Neurol. 71:261-268.

Diamond, M.C., Johnson, R.E., Young, D., Sukhwinder Singh, S. (1983) Age-related morphologic differences in the rat cortex and hippocampus: male-female; right-left. Exper.Neurol. 81:1-13.

Doherty, M.D. and Gratton, A. (1999) Effects of medial prefrontal cortical injections of GABA receptor agonists and antagonists on the local and nucleus accumbens dopamine responses to stress. Synapse 32:288-300.

Drevets, W.C., Videen, T.O., Price, J.L., Preskorn, S.H., Carmichael, S.T., Raichle, M.E. (1992) A functional anatomical study of unipolar depression. Journal of Neuroscience 12:3628-3641.

Drew, K.L., Lyon, R.A., Titeler, M., Glick, S.D. (1986) Asymmetry in D-2 binding in female rat striata. Brain Res. 363:192-195.

Espejo, E.F. and Minano, F.J. (1999) Prefrontocortical dopamine depletion induces antidepressant-like effects in rats and alters the profile of desipramine during Porsolt's test. Neuroscience 88:609-615.

160

Fadda, F., Argiolas, A., Melis, M.R., Tissari, A.H., Onali, P.L., Gessa, G.L. (1978) Stress-induced increase in 3,4-dihydroxyphenylacetic acid (DOPAC) levels in the cerebral cortex and in n. accumbens: reversal by diazepam. Life.Sci. 23:2219-2224.

Fadda, F., Mosca, E., Meloni, R., Gessa, G.L. (1985) Ethanol-stress interaction on dopamine metabolism in the medial prefrontal cortex. Alcohol & Drug Research 6:449-454.

Flor Henry, P. (1986) Observations, reflections and speculations on the cerebral determinants of mood and on the bilaterally asymmetrical distributions of the major neurotransmitter systems. Acta Neurol.Scand.Suppl. 109P75-89.:75-89.

Fromm, D. and Schopflocher, D. (1984) Neuropsychological test performance in depressed patients before and after drug therapy. Biol.Psychiatry 19:55-72.

Glick, S.D. (1973) Enhancement of spatial preferences by (+) -amphetamine. Neuropharmacol. 12:43-47.

Glick, S.D. and Badalamenti, J.I. (1986) Sex difference in reward asymmetry and effects of cocaine. Neuropharmacology. 25:633-637.

Glick, S.D., Carlson, J.N., Baird, J.L., Maisonneuve, I.M., Bullock, A.E. (1988a) Basal and amphetamine-induced asymmetries in striatal dopamine release and metabolism: bilateral in vivo microdialysis in normal rats. Brain Res. 473:161-164.

Glick, S.D., Cox, F.D., Jerussi, T.P., Greenstein, S. (1977) Normal and amphetamine-induced rotation of rats on a flat surface. J.Pharm.Pharmacol. 29:51-52.

Glick, S.D. and Cox, R.D. (1978) Nocturnal rotation in normal rats: correlation with amphetamine-induced rotation and effects of nigrostriatal lesions. Brain Res. 150:149-161.

Glick, S.D. and Greenstein, S. (1973) Possible modulating influence of frontal cortex on nigro- striatal function. Br.J.Pharmacol. 49:316-321.

Glick, S.D. and Hinds, P.A. (1984) Sex-differences in sensitization to cocaine-induced rotation. Eur.J.Pharmacol. 99:119-121.

Glick, S.D., Hinds, P.A., Carlson, J.N. (1987) Food deprivation and stimulant self-administration in rats: Differences between cocaine and d-amphetamine. Psychopharmacol. 91:372-374.

Glick, S.D., Hinds, P.A., Shapiro, R.M. (1983) Cocaine-induced rotation: Sex-dependent differences between left- and right-sided rats. Science 221:775-777.

Glick, S.D. and Jerussi, T.P. (1974) Spatial and paw preferences in rats: their relationship to rate-dependent effects of d-amphetamine. Journ.Pharmacol.Exper.Theraput. 188:714-725.

Glick, S.D., Jerussi, T.P., Water, D.H., Green, J.P. (1974) Amphetamine-induced changes in striatal dopamine and acetylcholine levels and relationship to rotation (circling behavior) in rats. Biochem.Pharmacol. 23:3223-3225.

Glick, S.D., Lyon, R.A., Hinds, P.A., Sowek, C., Titeler, M. (1988b) Correlated asymmetries in striatal D1 and D2 binding: relationship to apomorphine-induced rotation. Brain Res. 455:43-48.

Glick, S.D., Meibach, R.C., Cox, R.D., Maayani, S. (1979) Multiple and interrelated functional asymmetries in rat brain. Life Sci. 25:395-400.

Glick, S.D., Merski, C., Steindorf, S., Wang, S., Keller, R.W., Carlson, J.N. (1992) Neurochemical predisposition to self administer morphine in rats. Brain Res. 578:215-220.

Glick, S.D., Raucci, J., Wang, S., Keller, R,W. Jr., Carlson, J.N. (1994) Neurochemical predisposition to self-administer cocaine in rats: Individual differences in dopamine and its metabolites . Brain Research 653:148-154.

Glick, S.D. and Ross, D.A. (1981) Right-sided population bias and lateralization of activity in normal rats. Brain Res. 205:222-225.

Glick, S.D., Shapiro, R.M., Drew, K.L., Hinds, P.A., Carlson, J.N. (1986) Differences in spontaneous and amphetamine-induced rotational behavior, and in sensitization to amphetamine, among Sprague-Dawley derived rats from different sources. Physiol.Behav. 38:67-70.

Glick, S.D., Weaver, L.M., Meibach, R.C. (1980) Lateralization of reward in rats: differences in reinforcing thresholds. Science 207:1093-1095.

Glick, S.D., Weaver, L.M., Meibach, R.C. (1981) Amphetamine enhancement of reward asymmetry. Psychopharmacol. 73:323-327.

Glick, S.D., Zimmerberg, B., Greenstein, S. (1976) Individual differences among rats in normal and amphetamine-enhanced locomotor activity: Relationship to behavioral indicies of striatal asymmetry. Brain Res. 105:362-364.

Goeders, N.E. and Smith, J.E. (1983) Cortical dopaminergic involvement in cocaine reinforcement. Science 221:773-775.

Goeders, N.E. and Smith, J.E. (1993) Intracranial cocaine self-administration into the medial prefrontal cortex increases dopamine turnover in the nucleus accumbens. Journal of Pharmacology & Experimental Therapeutics 265:592-600.

Gomez, F., de Kloet, E.R., Armario, A. (1998) Glucocorticoid negative feedback on the HPA axis in five inbred rat strains. American Journal of Physiology 274:R420-R427.

Guerin, G. F., Goeders, N. E., Dworkin, S. I., Smith, J. E. (1984) Intracranial self-administration of dopamine into the nucleus accumbens. Soc.Neurosci.Abst. 10, 1072. Ref Type: Abstract

Gur, R.E. (1978) Left hemisphere dysfunction and left hemisphere overactivation in schizophrenia. Journal of Abnormal Psychology 87:226-238.

Hegarty, A.A. and Vogel, W.H. (1993) Modulation of the stress response by ethanol in the rat frontal cortex. Pharmacology, Biochemistry & Behavior 45:327-334.

Hellige, J.B. (1993) Hemispheric asymmetry: What's right and what's left. Harvard University Press, Cambridge, MA.

Henn, F.A., Johnson, J., Edwards, E., Anderson, D. (1985) Melancholia in rodents: neurobiology and pharmacology. Psychopharmacol.Bull. 21:443-446.

Herman, J.P., Guillonneau, D., Dantzer, R., Scatton, B., Semerdjian Rouquier, L., Le Moal, M. (1982) Differential effects of inescapable footshocks and of stimuli previously paired with inescapable footshocks on dopamine turnover in cortical and limbic areas of the rat. Life Sci. 30:2207-2214.

Hernandez, L. and Hoebel, B.G. (1988) Food reward and cocaine increase extracellular dopamine in the nucleus accumbens as measured by microdialysis. Life Sciences 42:1705-1712.

Hodge, C.W., Chappelle, A.M., Samson, H.H. (1996) Dopamine receptors in the medial prefrontal cortex influence ethanol and sucrose reinforced responding. Alcohol.Clin.Exp.Res. 20:1631-1638.

Hoebel, B.G., Monaco, A.P., Hernandez, L., Aulisi, E.F., Stanley, B.G., Lenard, L. (1983) Self-injection of amphetamine directly into the brain. Psychopharmacology (Berl) 81:158-163.

Insel, T.R. (1992) Toward a neuroanatomy of obsessive-compulsive disorder [see comments]. [Review] [57 refs]. Archives of General Psychiatry 49:739-744.

Jerussi, T.P. and Glick, S.D. (1974) Amphetamine-induced rotation in rats without lesions. Neuropharmacology. 13:283-286.

Jerussi, T.P. and Glick, S.D. (1975) Apomorphine-induced rotation in normal rats and interaction with unilateral caudate lesions. Psychopharmacologia. 40:329-334.

Jerussi, T.P. and Glick, S.D. (1976) Drug-induced rotation in rats without lesions: behavioral and neurochemical indices of a normal asymmetry in nigro-striatal function. Psychopharmacology.(Berlin.) 47:249-260.

Jerussi, T.P., Glick, S.D., Johnson, C.L. (1977) Reciprocity of pre- and postsynaptic mechanisms involved in rotation as revealed by dopamine metabolism and adenylate cyclase stimulation. Brain Res. 129:385-388.

Jesberger, J.A. and Richardson, J.S. (1985) Animal models of depression: parallels and correlates to severe depression in humans. Biol.Psychiatry 20:764-785.

Karoum, F., Suddath, R.L., Wyatt, R.J. (1990) Chronic cocaine and rat brain catecholamines: long-term reduction in hypothalamic and frontal cortex dopamine metabolism. European Journal of Pharmacology 186:1-8.

Karreman, M. and Moghaddam, B. (1996) The prefrontal cortex regulates the basal release of dopamine in the limbic striatum: an effect mediated by ventral tegmental area. Journal of Neurochemistry 66:589-598.

Kelsey, J.E. (1983) The role of norepinephrine and acetylcholine in mediating escape deficits produced by inescapable shocks. Behavioral & Neural Biology 37:326-331.

Koob, G.F. (1992) Neural mechanisms of drug reinforcement. [Review] [97 refs]. Annals of the New York Academy of Sciences 654:171-191.

Koob, G.F., Roberts, A.J., Schulteis, G., Parsons, L.H., Heyser, C.J., Hyytia, P., Merlo-Pich, E., Weiss, F. (1998) Neurocircuitry targets in ethanol reward and dependence. [Review] [42 refs]. Alcoholism: Clinical & Experimental Research 22:3-9.

Koob, G.F., Vaccarino, F.J., Amalric, M., Bloom, F.E. (1987) Positive reinforcment properties of drugs: search for neural substrates, in Brain Reward Systems and Abuse (Engel J and Oreland L eds) pp 35-50, Raven, New York.

Kornetsky, C. and Esposito, R.U. (1979) Euphorigenic drugs: effects on the reward pathways of the brain. Federation Proceedings 38:2473-2476.

Korpi, E.R. and Luddens, H. (1993) Regional gamma-aminobutyric acid sensitivity of t-butylbicyclophosphoro[35S]thionate binding depends on gamma- aminobutyric acidA receptor alpha subunit. Molecular Pharmacology 44:87-92.

Kubos, K.L., Brady, J.V., Moran, T.H., Smith, C.H., Robinson, R.G. (1985) Asymmetrical effect of unilateral cortical lesions and amphetamine on DRL-20: a time-loss analysis. Pharmacology, Biochemistry & Behavior 22:1001-1006.

Kuczenski, R., Segal, D.S., Aizenstein, M.L. (1991) Amphetamine, cocaine, and fencamfamine: relationship between locomotor and stereotypy response profiles and caudate and accumbens dopamine dynamics. Journal of Neuroscience 11:2703-2712.

LaHoste, G.J., Mormede, P., Rivet, J.M., Le Moal, M. (1988a) Differential sensitization to amphetamine and stress responsivity as a function of inherent laterality. Brain Research 453:381-384.

LaHoste, G.J., Mormede, P., Rivet, J.M., Le Moal, M. (1988b) New evidence for distinct patterns of brain organization in rats differentiated on the basis of inherent laterality. Brain Research 474:296-308.

Lavielle, S., Tassin, J.P., Thierry, A.M., Blanc, G., Herve, D., Barthelemy, C., Glowinski, J. (1979) Blockade by benzodiazepines of the selective high increase in dopamine turnover induced by stress in mesocortical dopaminergic neurons of the rat. Brain Res. 168:585-594.

LeMoal, M. and Simon, H. (1991) Mesocorticolimbic dopaminergic network: functional and regulatory roles. Physio Rev 71:155-234.

Lyness, W.H., Friedle, N.M., Moore, K.E. (1979) Destruction of dopaminergic nerve terminals in nucleus accumbens: effect on d-amphetamine self-administration. Pharmacology, Biochemistry & Behavior 11:553-556.

Maier, S.F. and Seligman, M.E.P. (1976) Learned helplessness: Theory and evidence. Journ.Exper.Psychol.: Gen. 105:3-46.

Maisonneuve, I.M. and Glick, S.D. (1992) Interactions between ibogaine and cocaine in rats: in vivo microdialysis and motor behavior. European Journal of Pharmacology 212:263-266.

Maisonneuve, I.M., Keller, R.W., Glick, S.D. (1990) Similar effects of D-amphetamine and cocaine on extracellular dopamine levels in medial prefrontal cortex of rats. Brain Research 535:221-226.

Maisonneuve, I.M., Keller, R.W, Jr., Glick, S.D. (1992) Interactions of ibogaine and D-amphetamine: in vivo microdialysis and motor behavior in rats. Brain Research 579:87-92.

Majewska, M.D. (1996) Cocaine addiction as a neurological disorder: implications for treatment. [Review] [124 refs]. NIDA Research Monograph 163:1-26.

Maldonado-Irizarry, C.S., Stellar, J.R., Kelley, A.E. (1994) Effects of cocaine and GBR-12909 on brain stimulation reward. Pharmacology, Biochemistry & Behavior 48:915-920.

Markou, A., Weiss, F., Gold, L.H., Caine, S.B., Schulteis, G., Koob, G.F. (1993) Animal models of drug craving. [Review]. Psychopharmacology (Berl) 112:163-182.

Martin-Iverson, M.T., Szostak, C., Fibiger, H.C. (1986) 6-Hydroxydopamine lesions of the medial prefrontal cortex fail to influence intravenous self-administration of cocaine. Psychopharmacology (Berl) 88:310-314.

Matsuguchi, N., Ida, Y., Shirao, I., Tsujimaru, S. (1994) Blocking effects of ethanol on stress-induced activation of rat mesoprefrontal dopamine neurons. Pharmacology, Biochemistry & Behavior 48:297-299.

McBride, W.J., Murphy, J.M., Gatto, G.J., Levy, A.D., Yoshimoto, K., Lumeng, L., Li, TK. (1993) CNS mechanisms of alcohol self-administration. Alcohol & Alcoholism Supplement. 2:463-467.

McGregor, A., Baker, G., Roberts, D.C. (1996) Effect of 6-hydroxydopamine lesions of the medial prefrontal cortex on intravenous cocaine self-administration under a progressive ratio schedule of reinforcement. Pharmacology, Biochemistry & Behavior 53:5-9.

McIntyre, T.D., Trullas, R., Skolnick, P. (1988) Asymmetrical activation of GABA-gated chloride channels in cerebral cortex. Pharmacol.Biochem.Behav. 30:911-916.

Meiergerd, S.M., Schenk, J.O., Sorg, B.A. (1997) Repeated cocaine and stress increase dopamine clearance in the rat medial prefrontal cortex. Brain Research 773:203-207.

Murase, S., Grenhoff, J., Chouvet, G., Gonon, F.G., Svensson, T.H. (1993) Prefrontal cortex regulates burst firing and transmitter release in rat mesolimbic dopamine neurons studied in vivo. Neuroscience Letters 157:53-56.

Ng Cheong Ton, M.J., Brown, Z., Michalakeas, A., Amit, Z. (1983) Stress induced suppression of maintenance but not of acquisition of ethanol consumption in rats. Pharmacology, Biochemistry & Behavior 18:141-144.

Nielsen, D.M., Crosley, K.J., Keller, R.W. Jr., Glick, S.D., Carlson, J.N. (1999c) Left and Right 6-Hydroxydopamine Lesions of the Medial Prefrontal Cortex Differentially Affect Voluntary Ethanol Consumption. Brain Research 823:59-66.

Nielsen, D.M., Crosley, K.J., Keller, R.W. Jr., Glick, S.D., Carlson, J.N. (1999a) Rotation, Locomotor Activity and Individual Differences in Voluntary Ethanol Consumption. Brain Research 823:59-66.

Nielsen, D.M., Crosley, K.J., Keller, R.W. Jr., Glick, S.D., Carlson, J.N. (1999b) Ethanol induced differences in medial prefrontal cortex dopamine asymmetry and in nucleus accumbens dopamine metabolism in left- and right-turning rats. Brain Research 823:207-212.

Nielsen., D.M., Keller, R.W. Jr., Glick, S.D., Carlson, J.N. (1996) Microinjection of the D1 antagonist SCH23390 into the left or right medial prefrontal cortex differentially alters the behavioral and neurochemical responses to footshock stress. Soc.Neurosci.Abst. 22: 161.

Nomikos, G.G., Damsma, G., Wenkstern, D., Fibiger, H.C. (1990) In vivo characterization of locally applied dopamine uptake inhibitors by striatal microdialysis. Synapse 6:106-112.

O'Boyle, M.W. and Hellige, J.B. (1989) Cerebral hemisphere asymmetry and individual differences in cognition. Learning and Individual Differences 1:7-35.

Olds, M.E. (1982) Reinforcing effects of morphine in the nucleus accumbens. Brain Research 237:429-440.

Orchinik, M., Weiland, N.G., McEwen, B.S. (1994) Adrenalectomy selectively regulates GABAA receptor subunit expression in the hippocampus. Molecular & Cellular Neurosciences 5:451-458.

Petty, F., Davis, L.L., Kabel, D., Kramer, G.L. (1996) Serotonin dysfunction disorders: a behavioral neurochemistry perspective. [Review] [24 refs]. Journal of Clinical Psychiatry 57 Suppl 8:11-16.

Petty, F., Kramer, G., Moeller, M. (1994) Does learned helplessness induction by haloperidol involve serotonin mediation? Pharmacology, Biochemistry & Behavior 48:671-676.

Phillips, G.D., Robbins, T.W., Everitt, B.J. (1994) Bilateral intra-accumbens self-administration of d-amphetamine: antagonism with intra-accumbens SCH-23390 and sulpiride. Psychopharmacology (Berl) 114:477-485.

Reynolds, G.P. (1983) Increased concentrations and lateral asymmetry of amygdala dopamine in schizophrenia. Nature 305:527-529.

Roberts DC, Corcoran ME, Fibiger HC (1977) On the role of ascending catecholaminergic systems in intravenous self-administration of cocaine. Pharmacology, Biochemistry & Behavior 6:615-620.

Robinson, R.G. (1985) Lateralized behavioral and neurochemical consequences of unilateral brain injury in rats., in Cerebral Lateralization in Nonhuman Species. (Glick SD ed) pp 135-156, Academic Press, Orlando, Fl.

Robinson, R.G. and Chait, R.M. (1985) Emotional correlates of structural brain inj2Pharmacology, Biochemistry & Behavior 6:615-620.

Robinson, R.G. (1985) Lateralized behavioral and neurochemical consequences of unilateral brain injury in rats., in Cerebral Lateralization in Nonhuman Species. (Glick SD ed) pp 135-156, Academic Press, Orlando, Fl.

Robinson, R.G. and Chait, R.M. (1985) Emotional correlates of structural brain injury with particular emphasis on post-stroke mood disorders. CRC.Crit.Rev.Clin.Neurobiol. 1:285-318.

Robinson, T.E. and Berridge, K.C. (1993) The neural basis of drug craving: an incentive-sensitization theory of addiction. [Review]. Brain Research - Brain Research Reviews 18:247-291.

Rosen, G.D., Finklestein, S., Stoll, A.L., Yutzey, D.A., Denenberg, V.H. (1984) Neurochemical asymmetries in the albino rat's cortex, striatum and nucleus accumbens. Life Sci. 34:1143-1148.

Rosin, D.L., Clark, W.A., Goldstein, M., Roth, R.H., Deutch, A.Y. (1992) Effects of 6-hydroxydopamine lesions of the prefrontal cortex on tyrosine hydroxylase activity in mesolimbic and nigrostriatal dopamine systems. Neuroscience 48:831-839.

Ross, D.A. and Glick, S.D. (1981) Lateralized effects of bilateral frontal cortex lesions in rats. Brain Res. 210:379-382.

Ross, D.A., Glick, S.D., Meibach, R.C. (1981) Sexually dimorphic brain and behavioral asymmetries in the neonatal rat. Proc.Natl.Acad.Sci.U.S.A. 78:1958-1961.

Schaefer, G.J. and Michael, R.P. (1988) An analysis of the effects of amphetamine on brain self-stimulation behavior. Behavioural Brain Research 29:93-101.

Schenk, S., Horger, B.A., Peltier, R., Shelton, K. (1991) Supersensitivity to the reinforcing effects of cocaine following 6-hydroxydopamine lesions to the medial prefrontal cortex in rats. Brain Research 543:227-235.

Scott, P.A., Cierpial, M.A., Kilts, C.D., Weiss, J.M. (1996) Susceptibility and resistance of rats to stress-induced decreases in swim-test activity: A selective breeding study. Brain Research 725:217-230.

Shoemaker, W. J., Deckel, A. W., Hebert, D. M. (1996) Effects of a single dose of DMI on voluntary ethanol drinking and lateralized monoamine levels in rats. Soc.Neurosci.Abst. 22(Part 2), 1156.

Slopsema, J.S., Van der Gugten, J., De Bruin, J.P.C. (1982) Regional concentrations of noradrenaline and dopamine in the frontal cortex of the rat: dopaminergic innervation of the prefrontal subareas and lateralization of prefrontal dopamine. Brain Res. 250:197-200.

Soldo, B.L., Proctor, W.R., Dunwiddie, T.V. (1994) Ethanol differentially modulates GABAA receptor-mediated chloride currents in hippocampal, cortical, and septal neurons in rat brain slices. Synapse 18:94-103.

Sorg, B.A., Davidson, D.L., Kalivas, P.W., Prasad, B.M. (1997) Repeated daily cocaine alters subsequent cocaine-induced increase of extracellular dopamine in the medial prefrontal cortex. Journal of Pharmacology & Experimental Therapeutics 281:54-61.

Springer, S. and Deutsch, G. (1981) Left Brain, Right Brain. Freeman, San Francisco.

Starkstein, S.E., Moran, T.H., Bowersox, J.A., Robinson, R.G. (1988) Behavioral abnormalities induced by frontal cortical and nucleus accumbens lesions. Brain Research 473:74-80.

Suddath, R.L., Casanova, M.F., Goldberg, T.E., Daniel, D.G., Kelsoe, J.R Jr., Weinberger, D.R. (1989) Temporal lobe pathology in schizophrenia: a quantitative magnetic resonance imaging study. American Journal of Psychiatry 146:464-472.

Sullivan, R.M. and Szechtman, H. (1995) Asymmetrical influence of mesocortical dopamine depletion on stress ulcer development and subcortical dopamine systems in rats: implications for psychopathology. Neuroscience 65:757-766.

Tanda, G., Carboni, E., Frau, R., Di, C.G. (1994) Increase of extracellular dopamine in the prefrontal cortex: a trait of drugs with antidepressant potential?. Psychopharmacology (Berl) 115:285-288.

Tarter, R.E., Blackson, T., Brigham, J., Moss, H., Caprara, G.V. (1995) The association between childhood irritability and liability to substance use in early adolescence: a 2-year follow-up study of boys at risk for substance abuse. Drug & Alcohol Dependence 39:253-261.

Tarter, R.E. and Hegedus, A.M. (1985) Neurological mechanisms underlying inheritance of alcoholism vulnerability. International Journal of Neuroscience 28:1-10.

Tarter, R.E. and Ryan, C.M. (1983) Neuropsychology of alcoholism. Etiology, phenomenology, process, and outcome. [Review]. Recent Developments in Alcoholism 1:449-469.

Thierry, A.M., Tassin, J.P., Blanc, G., Glowinski, J. (1976) Selective activation of the mesocortical DA system by stress. Nature 263:242-244.

Ticku, M.K. (1989) Ethanol and the benzodiazepine-GABA receptor-ionophore complex. Experientia 45:413-418.

Tomarken, A.J., Davidson, R.J., Wheeler, R.W., Doss, R. (1992) Individual differences in anterior brain asymmetry and fundamental dimensions of emotion. Journ of Personality and Social Psychology 62:676-687.

Toomim, C. S., Greengard, P., Goldman Rakic, P. S. (1992) Hemispheric asymmetry of DARPP-32 in rat cingulate cortex. Soc.Neurosci.Abst. 18, 1419-1419. Ref Type: Abstract

Ungerstedt, U. (1971) Striatal dopamine release after amphetamine or nerve degeneration revealed by rotational behavior. Acta Physiol.Scand. 367:49-68.

van Wolfswinkel, L. and van Ree, J.M. (1985) Effects of morphine and naloxone on thresholds of ventral tegmental electrical self-stimulation. Naunyn Schmiedebergs Arch.Pharmacol. 330:84-92.

Varlinskaya, E.I., Petrov, E.S., Robinson, S.R., Smotherman, W.P. (1995) Asymmetrical development of the dopamine system in the fetal rat as indicated by lateralized administration of SKF-28393 and SCH-23390. Pharmacology, Biochemistry & Behavior 50:359-367.

Volkow, N.D., Wang, G.J., Fowler, J.S., Hitzemann, R., Angrist, B., Gatley, S.J., Logan, J., Ding, Y.S., Pappas, N. (1999) Association of methylphenidate-induced craving with changes in right striato-orbitofrontal metabolism in cocaine abusers: implications in addiction. American Journal of Psychiatry 156:19-26.

Westerink, B.H., Enrico, P., Feimann, J., De Vries, J.B. (1998) The pharmacology of mesocortical dopamine neurons: a dual-probe microdialysis study in the ventral tegmental area and prefrontal cortex of the rat brain. Journal of Pharmacology & Experimental Therapeutics 285:143-154.

Wieland, S., Boren, J.L., Consroe, P.F., Martin, A. (1986) Stock differences in the susceptibility of rats to learned helplessness training. Life Sci. 39:937-944.

Williams-Hemby, L. and Porrino, L.J. (1994) Low and moderate doses of ethanol produce distinct patterns of cerebral metabolic changes in rats. Alcoholism, Clinical & Experimental Research 18:982-988.

Willner, P. (1983c) Dopamine and depression: a review of recent evidence. Brain.Res. 287:211-224.

Willner, P. (1983b) Dopamine and depression: a review of recent evidence. II Theoretical approaches. Brain.Res. 287:225-236.

Willner, P. (1983a) Dopamine and depression: a review of recent evidence. III. The effects of antidepressant treatments. Brain.Res. 287:237-246.

Wise, R.A. (1978) Catecholamine theories of reward: a critical review. [Review]. Brain Research 152:215-247.

Yokel, R.A. and Wise, R.A. (1975) Increased lever pressing for amphetamine after pimozide in rats: implications for a dopamine theory of reward. Science 187:547-549.

Zimmerberg, B., Glick, S.D., Jerussi, T.P. (1974) Neurochemical correlate of a spatial preference in rats. Science 185:623-625.

10 ANIMAL MODELS OF BIPOLAR DISORDER: FROM A SINGLE EPISODE TO PROGRESSIVE CYCLING MODELS

Haim Einat, Ora Kofman and Robert H. Belmaker

INTRODUCTION - ANIMAL MODELS IN PSYCHOPHARMACOLOGY

Animal models of psychopathology are divided into three major groups: heuristic models that assume a common underlying mechanism between a superficially different animal behavior and a particular human pathology; theory-based evidential models, which place emphasis on a common feature (etiological or behavioral) of both the model and the pathology; representative models involving generalization of a well-validated behavior to model the pathology (Overmier and Patterson, 1988; Ursin and Murison, 1986). The choice of a particular model for research will depend ultimately on the extent to which the etiology of the disorder is known, the specificity and efficacy of the pharmacological treatments available, and the facility with which the pathological behaviors can be mimicked in laboratory animals.

Validation of animal models for psychopharmacology is a complex matter usually referring to three aspects of validity: face validity, predictive validity and construct validity (e.g., Willner, 1986; Willner, 1991). Face validity represents the commonalties in overt behavioral features between the model and the modeled disorder. Predictive validity represents the degree to which the specific drugs that are effective in treating the disorder will have a corresponding "therapeutic" effect on the behavioral model. Since the behavioral models are only gross approximations of psychiatric disorders, it is also critical to determine that non-therapeutic drugs do not also reverse the behavior in question. Construct validity represents a possible common mechanistic theory that can explain both the model and the modeled disorder (for review see Willner, 1991).

Most animal models of psychopathology are induced by pharmacological, behavioral or genetic manipulations. Reserpine, which induces depletion of presynaptic stores of monoamines, is a classic pharamcological model of depression. At appropriate doses, reserpine induces hypoactivity that can be reversed by antidepressant drugs (e.g., Einat et al., 1999). Behavioral models can include either analysis of spontaneous behaviors, or alterations in the behavioral repertoire of the animal induced by experimental manipulation. For example, chronic mild stress in rats was suggested to induce a depressive-like state used to model depression (e.g., Willner et al., 1987). A genetically-induced model can be developed by breeding animals for a specific trait that characterizes a psychiatric disorder. For example, rats were bred for alcohol preference in order to model alcohol addiction (e.g., Overstreet et al., 1992).

Hardly any of the frequently-used animal models in psychopharmacology meets all three types of validation criteria. The choice of an appropriate model may depend on the task facing the researcher. If one attempts to screen a new drug for the modeled disorder he may prefer to use a model with a strong and well-established predictive validity. If one tries to explore the mechanism of a disorder he may choose to utilize a model that emphasizes construct validity (e.g., Willner, 1995; Dixon and Fisch, 1998). For example, attempts to screen new antidepressant drugs may prefer to utilize predictive models that respond to acute treatment whereas attempts to study the mechanisms of depression may prefer to rely on models that respond only to chronic treatment (in a similar way to the pattern of responding in depressed patients).

Some animal models for psychiatric disorders have had significant value in the search for new treatments and in the study of mechanisms. For example, the Porsolt forced swim test model of depression is frequently used in both these contexts (e.g., Kirby and Lucki, 1997; Rossetti et al., 1993). The Porsolt swim test is composed of either two exposures (in rats) spaced one day apart, or one lengthy exposure (in mice) to a water tank that does not permit escape (Borsini and Meli, 1988; Porsolt et al., 1978; Redrobe et al., 1996; Sanchez and Meier, 1997). The attempts to escape and activity levels during the second exposure (in rats) or the later part of the exposure (in mice) are monitored and serve to represent the level of "despair" of the animal that is suggested to represent its depressive state (Porsolt et al., 1978). The forced swim test has some face validity (reduced activity and motivation are similar to frequently observed symptoms of depression), good predictive validity since treatment with antidepressant drugs but not other psychiatric drugs increase test activity levels, and some construct validity since the test was reported to influence brain monoaminergic systems (for review see Willner, 1991).

Recently, the Porsolt forced swim test was successfully used to evaluate the therapeutic potential of inositol as an antidepressant drug (Einat et al., 1999; Einat et al., in press). The study demonstrated that chronic inositol treatment at a 1.2 g/kg/day dose reduces immobility time and increases struggle time in the test. These results corroborated the results of controlled double-blind trials of inositol in humans (for review see Levine, 1997). The model was used to explore the mechanisms of the therapeutic action of inositol. Inhibition of the 5-HT system, specifically $5-HT_2$ receptors, but not other 5-HT or noradrenergic receptors can reverse the effects of inositol in the model, suggesting that the mechanism of action of inositol is related to $5-HT_2$ receptors (Einat et al., submitted).

ANIMAL MODELS OF BIPOLAR DISORDER

Bipolar affective disorder (BPD) is unique in that it is characterized by progressive and spontaneously alternating episodes of depression and mania. The need to model two behaviorally opposite states presents a particular challenge for neuroscientists. These two states can be viewed as extremes on a continuum, where depression includes behavioral symptoms such as psychomotor retardation, loss of appetite, sleep disturbances and anhedonia, and mania includes behavioral symptoms such as hyperactivity, pressured speech, hypophagia and hypersexuality (DSM IV). The oscillatory and progressive course of the disorder has been particularly difficult to mimic as an animal model. This dilemma is often resolved by either studying each aspect of the disorder in separate experiments or by seeking other examples of oscillatory physiological or behavioral phenomena, even if they bear little superficial resemblance to the symptomatology of BPD. Ideally, a model would manifest spontaneous and perhaps progressively escalating alterations in behavior between episodes of hyper- and hypo-activity that would respond to chronic, but not acute, treatment with lithium and several anticonvulsants that are effective in BPD.

Modeling a Single Manic Episode

Since models for unipolar depression are readily available, first attempts were made to develop valid animal models for the manic state that is a unique feature of BPD.

A number of models for mania focused on the hyperactivity aspect of the disorder and utilized a number of possibilities to create hyperactive animals. Some of these models were reviewed by Kofman and Belmaker (1991) and are briefly described here.

Baseline Locomotor Activity

Baseline locomotor activity and exploration of a novel environment vary greatly across time of day and across situation. Studies testing the effects of lithium (Li) on baseline activity had equivocal results. Acute or chronic injections did not affect open field or Y maze activity (Ushijama et al. 1986), while chronic dietary Li did attenuate locomotor activity (Berggren, 1985; Lerer et al., 1984). Interestingly, a clearer reduction in basal activity following Li treatment was observed during the dark phase (when rodents are more active) suggesting that Li may only suppress high levels of activity (similar to manic state) without affecting low baseline activity levels (Lerer et al., 1984; Kofman and Belmaker, 1991).

Psychostimulant-induced Hyperactivity

Psychostimulant treatment can produce a range of behaviors similar to that of mania including hyperactivity, heightened sensory awareness, alertness and changes in sleep patterns (for review see Gessa et al., 1995). Psychostimulant-induced hyperactivity is easily detectable (for an in depth analysis see Antoniou et al., 1998) and was demonstrated to be Li sensitive (e.g., Berggren, 1985; Lerer et al., 1984; Robbins and Sahakian, 1980; Smith, 1982; Ushijama et al., 1986) adding a predictive validity component to the apparent face validity. The validity of this frequently-used model received further support from studies indicating its sensitivity to antimanic anticonvulsant drugs, for example, carbamazepine reduction of amphetamine-induced hyperactivity (Maj et al., 1985) and valproate reduction of intracerebral dopamine-induced (Kuruvilla and Uretsky, 1981) or amphetamine-induced (Maitre et al., 1984) hyperactivity. However, at the same time, studies demonstrated that the sensitivity of the model to antibipolar drugs may be dependent on the mode of administration or the specific type of activity measured. For example, oral or peripheral intraperitoneal administration of Li did not reduce amphetamine-induced hyperactivity in rats (Ebstein et al., 1980; Smith, 1981) but there was a report indicating that central (ICV) Li did have an effect in the model (Smith, 1981). Li had no effect on the amphetamine-induced increase of the number of entries into the arms of a Y-maze (Aylmer et al., 1987; Cox et al., 1971), on amphetamine-induced hyperlocomotion in a familiar open field (Cappeliez and Moore, 1990). In addtion, neither valproate nor carbamazepine treatment altered apomorphine-induced locomotion (Green et al., 1985). One explanation for these inconsistencies, and a criticism of the construct validity of the model, is that high doses of amphetamine induce stereotypes, which are actually enhanced by lithium (Lerer et al., 1984). Thus, the "mania" induced by psychostimulants may refer to a narrow dose range which elicits increased locomotion and rearing. Beyond that range, psychostimulant-induced behaviors may be enhanced or unaffected by lithium.

The inconsistencies in the responses of psychostimulant-induced hyperactivity models to antibipolar drugs led to the suggestion that the hyperactivity induced by the combination of chlordiazepoxide and amphetamine may provide a better model. Although some studies did report good responsiveness of this combined drug model to antibipolar drugs including Li (Okada et al., 1990; Davies et al., 1974), valproate (Cao and Peng, 1993) and carbamazepine (Okada et al., 1990), the effectiveness of the drugs was limited to specific behavioral conditions (i.e., head-dipping, but not other forms of activity in novel, but not familiar environments) (for review see Kofman and Belmaker, 1991).

An attempt to construct a model of mania with both construct and face validity was based on the G protein hypothesis of BPD (Young et al., 1993). The latter group found enhanced levels and activity of stimulatory G proteins (Gs) in post-mortem cortex of bipolar patients, compared with controls and schizophrenics. Using the model developed by Kelley et al. (1993), cholera toxin (CTX) was micro-injected bilaterally into the nucleus accumbens, eliciting a short lasting depression of activity, followed by hyperactivity that lasted 3-5 days. Since the nucleus accumbens is critical for reward, this model furnished both a hypothesis-driven behavior (over-stimulation of Gs/olf proteins) with some face validity. However, the model did not provide pharmacological validity, as lithium actually enhanced the hyperactive effect, whereas carbamazepine appeared to attenuate the initial depressive response and had no significant effect on the hyperactivity (Kofman et al. 1998).

Motivation and Reward

Since a major component of manic behavior involves reward-seeking behavior (e.g., squandering money, hypersexuality), Kofman and Belmaker (1991) suggested that drugs that increase reward-seeking behavior or enhance the rewarding effects of brain-stimulation reward, or natural rewards, such as sweet solutions, might provide more a more valid model of mania. A variety of methods are frequently used to evaluate the reward properties of stimuli such as stimulus discrimination (e.g., Colpaert et al., 1978), self administration (e.g., Bozarth and

Wise, 1981), conditioned place preference (e.g., Mucha et al., 1982; Shippenberg and Heidreder, 1995) and intracranial self-stimulation. The possibility that studying reward systems in animals may be important for the understanding of bipolar disorder was already raised in the 70s (Kumar, 1979).

Although increased reward and motivation essentially provide an appropriate face validity component for models of mania, little work was done in an attempt to further validate such possible models and the results obtained from these studies are inconsistent. Lithium abolished morphine-induced but not amphetamine-induced (Shippenberg and Herz, 1991) or cocaine-induced (Shippenberg and Heidbreder, 1995; Suzuki et al., 1992) place preference. Li significantly reduced intracranial self-stimulation of the medial forebrain bundle in one study (Edlson et al., 1976) but had only minimal effects in another study (Takigawa et al., 1994), reversed amphetamine-induced depression of self stimulation to the substantia nigra (Predy and Kokkinidis, 1981) and reversed haloperidol-induced increase in self-stimulation of the A10 dopaminergic nucleus (Seeger et al., 1981). Valproate treatment did not alter self-stimulation of the nigral-ventral tegmental area (Ramana and Desiraju, 1989) and did not influence diazepam-induced place preference (Spyraki et al., 1985). Additionally, a problem that may influence the effects of li in motivation and reward experiments is its known aversive properties (for review, see Ossenkopp and Eckel, 1995). Accordingly, stimuli that are paired with li may become less rewarding through a classical conditioning mechanism and this pairing may detract from attempts to study pharmacological interactions and to infer from such studies to bipolar disorder.

Sleep Deprivation

A completely different approach to the development of an animal model for mania was taken recently with the proposal of the sleep deprivation model in the rat (Gessa et al., 1995). Sleep deprivation has a rapid (although transient) therapeutic effect in unipolar depressed patients (e.g., Post et al., 1987; Szuba et al., 1994) and this effect can be maintained with Li or antidepressant drugs treatment (Szuba et al., 1994). Sleep deprivation in depressed BPD patients is even more potent as a treatment compared to unipolar depressed patients (Barbini et al., 1998) but was also demonstrated to induce manic episodes and was suggested to be a final common pathway in the genesis of mania (Wehr et al., 1987). With these effects in mind, Gessa and his colleagues (1995) studied the effects of sleep deprivation in the rat and demonstrated the induction of behaviors that are similar to those characterizing manic episodes. After a 72 hour period of sleep deprivation, rats demonstrate a period of insomnia lasting about 30 minutes (Albert et al., 1970; Fratta et al., 1987; 1988). During this period, rats are hyperactive, irritable, aggressive (Hicks et al., 1979) and hypersexual (Morden et al., 1968). Furthermore, Gessa et al. (1994, cited in Gessa et al., 1995) demonstrated that the insomnia and hyperactivity components of this behavioral syndrome are reduced by Li treatment adding a predictive/ pharmacological validity component to the face validity component of the proposed model (for review see Gessa et al., 1995).

Using the sleep deprivation model, Gessa and his colleagues attempted to study the brain mechanisms underlying these manic-like behaviors. Their findings indicate that treatment with the dopaminergic D2 antagonist haloperidol or with the dopamine D1 receptor antagonist SCH 23390 significantly reduced the sleep latency (time to the onset of sleep after sleep deprivation) in the model (Fratta et al., 1987) whereas treatment with the dopamine D1 agonist SKF 38393 prolonged the period of insomnia (Gessa et al., 1995). Interestingly, the dopamine D2/D3 agonist quinpirole produced a biphasic effect with small doses, possibly acting pre-synaptically (Eilam and Szechtman, 1990) reducing sleep latency while higher doses, acting post-synaptically, prolonged sleep latency (Gessa et al., 1995). Furthermore, naloxone (opioid antagonist) reduced sleep latency whereas morphine, beta-endorphin and [D-Ala2, D-Leu5]enkephalin prolonged the period of insomnia (Fratta et al., 1987). Neurochemical studies of the model demonstrated that sleep deprivation induced only small effects related to adrenergic or serotonergic receptors (Siegel and Rogawski, 1988) but had stronger effects on the dopaminergic (DeMontis et al., 1990) and opioid (Fadda et al., 1991; 1992) systems in the brain (for review, see Gessa et al., 1995). Gessa et al. (1995) suggest that sleep deprivation in the rat may be a valid model for mania and that this model can offer new directions for the study of the pathological mechanism of the disorder.

Na, K-ATPase Modification - ouabain Treatment

Another recently proposed model for mania is based on manipulation of the sodium- and potassium-activated adenosine triphosphate pump (Na, K-ATPase) activity. A number of studies demonstrated that Li alters cation transport in bipolar patients (Wood et al., 1989), that Na, K-ATPase activity is altered in bipolar patients (el-Mallakh and Wyatt, 1995; Looney and el-Mallakh, 1997) and in postmortem brains of bipolar but not schizophrenic individuals (Rose et al., 1998). These findings led to the development of the Na, K-ATPase hypothesis for bipolar disorder (el-Mallakh and Wyatt, 1995; el-Mallakh et al., 1993a) and the suggestion that ouabain-like compounds may be related to the pathology of bipolar illness (Christo and el-Mallakh, 1993). Following this hypothesis, el-Mallakh et al. (1995) tested the effects of intracerebroventricular (ICV) injections of subconvulsive doses of ouabain on the behavior of rats and reported that with specific doses the rats demonstrated increased locomotion following treatment. Since hyperlocomotion provides at least one aspect of face validity and the Na, K-ATPase hypothesis for bipolar disorder provides plausible construct validity, ouabain treatment was suggested as a possible model of mania (el-Mallakh et al., 1995). The validity of the model was later supported by the report that seven days Li treatment prior to the ouabain injection completely abolished the ouabain-induced hyperactivity effect (Li et al., 1997).

The findings described above appear to support the use of ouabain treatment as a valid model for mania but this model also has a variety of problems. At the technical level, the model requires ICV injections, a time consuming procedure (demanding pre-treatment operations) that diminishes the practical value of the model at least for the purpose of drug screening. Moreover, the range of doses of ouabain that can be used in the induction of behavior is very narrow (to avoid convulsions and lethality) and the responses of animals are extremely variable (el-Mallakh et al., 1995). At a more conceptual level, the proposed model suggests that similar doses of ouabain may induce hyperactivity or hypoactivity (el-Mallakh et al., 1995; el-Mallakh et al., 1993b). Although such inverse responses are in line with the Na, K-ATPase hypothesis for bipolar disorder (el-Mallakh and Wyatt, 1995), the inability to dissociate between the two possible inverse responses combined with the individual variability in responses reduces the possible value of the model. Additionally, ouabain treatment was reported to increase horizontal locomotion while decreasing vertical (rearing) behavior and there is no clear explanation for this discrepancy within the framework of manic behaviors (el-Mallakh et al., 1995).

Modeling the Progressive and Cycling Nature of BPD

The models described to this point all have at least some components of validity and some of them were used as for the screening of new drugs or the study of new theories regarding the mechanism of bipolar disorder. One common flaw of the above-mentioned models is their focus on a single manic episode. However, important and intriguing features of bipolar disorder are its progressive and cyclical characteristics. Bipolar patients alternate between three conditions: a depressed state, a euthymic state and a manic state and the episodes of the disease tend to appear with increasing severity (e.g., Maj et al., 1992) and/or frequency (e.g., Post et al., 1984a). The development of animal models for a single manic episode was based on the notion that the uniqueness of bipolar disorder (compared with unipolar depression) is the manic state and therefore modeling this state may represent the entire disorder. Not ignoring the importance of modeling a manic episode, these models inherently fail to represent the full scope of the disorder and therefore efforts were invested in attempts to develop models that will reflect the progressive and the cycling nature of the disease. This requires inducing a long-term change in behavior that manifests itself in cycling episodes of depression and mania, with a progressive course.

Behavioral Sensitization to Psychostimulants

One clearly progressive phenomenon that was proposed as a possible model for the development of bipolar illness is behavioral sensitization. The repeated administration of many psychostimulant drugs leads to a gradual increase or sensitization of the drug-induced behavioral response (e.g., Einat et al., 1996; Robinson and Becker, 1986; Stewart and Badiani, 1993). Although behavioral sensitization was traditionally used to model psychosis (for review see Robinson and Becker, 1986), the development and expression of sensitized behavior may also resemble the progression of manic episodes in bipolar disorder, with gradual enhancement in severity and progressively faster onset (Post and Contel, 1981). Considering this face validity and possible shared mechanisms related to the involvement of the dopaminergic system in manic psychosis (e.g., Carli et al., 1997; Jimerson and Post, 1982), the phenomenon of behavioral sensitization was proposed to model the progressive nature of BPD (Post and Contel, 1981; 1983). Moreover, cocaine mimics several of the pharmacological effects of stress. Post's group proposed a model whereby psychosocial stressors can interact with immediate early genes and effector genes to exacerbate the clinical course of bipolar cycling (Post and Weiss, 1995), lending a strong element of construct validity to the sensitization model.

However, attempts to examine predictive (pharmacological) validity of the psychostimulant-sensitization proposed model were mostly unsuccessful. Li was first reported to inhibit the development of behavioral sensitization (Post et al.,

1984c) but later studies did not find similar effects (Cappeliez and Moore, 1990; Poncelet et al., 1987), and carbamazepine treatment had no effect on sensitization (Post et al., 1984c; Weiss et al., 1990). A different problem regarding the proposed sensitization model is the involvement of more than one behavior in the progression of response to most psychostimulants. The motor response usually involves the transition from hyperlocomotion to stereotyped, locally oriented movements, as mentioned above (e.g., Eilam and Szechtman, 1990; Ellinwood et al., 1972; Kilbey and Ellinwood, 1977). This transition in behaviors diminishes the face validity component of the model and introduces a practical difficulty in the measuring of behavior.

Amygdala Kindling

A major effort to develop a progressive model is based on the amygdala kindling phenomenon. Amygdala kindling includes repeated, initially sub-convulsive, stimulation (usually electric but also chemical) of the amygdala that results in an intensifying response culminating in the appearance of seizures either following stimulation or spontaneously (e.g., Racine, 1978; for review see Post and Weiss, 1997). Kindling serves as a model for epileptogenesis (e.g., Racine, 1978) and for learning and memory (e.g., Goddard and Douglas, 1975) and was suggested as a model for the progressing nature of bipolar disorder (Post and Ballenger, 1981; Post et al., 1984b). As in the progression of bipolar disorder, the response to amygdala stimulation shows an intensifying progression and a gradual transition from stressor vulnerability or dependence to autonomous episodes (Post and Weiss, 1997). Although the nature of the response is dissimilar from the nature of manic episodes and therefore behaviorally nonhomologous (Weiss and Post 1995), the pattern of responding across stimuli and time provides a component of face validity to the model.

The amygdala kindling model also has predictive (pharmaceutical) validity because the threshold for the appearance of seizures is elevated by pretreatment with Li (e.g., Minabe et al., 1987; 1988) or anticonvulsants such as carbamazepine, phenytoin and valproic acid (Albright and Burnham, 1980; Azorin and Tramoni, 1987; Babington, 1977; Leviel and Naquet, 1977; Post et al., 1984c; Post et al., 1998; Wada et al., 1976; Weiss et al., 1990) and by ECT (Post et al., 1984b). A number of physiological and molecular changes that are common to both bipolar disorder and kindling, such as the involvement of immediate early genes, alteration in gene expression and changes in synaptic structure (for review see Post and Weiss, 1997) provide a significant construct validity to the model. In fact, the development and use of the amygdala kindling model was a key factor in the introduction and validation of carbamazepine as an effective anti-bipolar drug (Post et al., 1984b; Post and Weiss, 1997) and in attempts to study the common mechanisms of action of mood stabilizers (Stoll and Severus, 1996).

Recently, patterns of drug tolerance in amygdala kindling were suggested to model the cyclic nature of bipolar illness (Post and Weiss, 1996). These authors found that in the course of treatment of amygdala kindled animals with anticonvulsant drugs the effects of the drugs show tolerance episodically with breakthroughs of seizures, and that the appearance of seizures during treatment may be similar to the periodic outbursts of bipolar episodes (Post and Weiss, 1996). The periodic appearance of seizures is related to the intensity and rate of stimulation and to the doses of anticonvulsants and is postulated to be the consequence of failure in the emergence of endogenous molecular compensatory mechanisms and the progression of pathological mechanisms (Post and Weiss, 1996). The finding regarding the periodic eruptions of seizures in anticonvulsant-treated amygdala kindled animals led to speculations regarding the role of endogenous and environmental factors involved in the progression of bipolar disorder and to postulations of better therapeutic approaches (Post and Weiss, 1996).

Extreme Sensitization-induced Oscillations

Recently a new model with possible cycling properties was proposed, based on the older notion (discussed above) of cocaine sensitization (Antelman and Caggiula, 1996). The idea behind the model was that when animals reach a level of extreme sensitization, their responses begin to oscillate (Antelman and Caggiula, 1996). In fact, this does not happen with frequently-measured behaviors such as hyperactivity or locally oriented movements (see above regarding the behavioral sensitization model) but oscillation does occur when other measures are used. A number of studies demonstrated a variety of biochemical measures that oscillate during chronic cocaine treatment such as the efflux of striatal and nucleus accumbens dopamine, hippocampal serotonin, and plasma levels of corticosterone and glucose (Antelman et al., 1995; Antelman and Caggiula, 1996; Caggiula et al., 1996). A behavioral measure, shock-induced hypoalgesia, was also reported to oscillate with repeated cocaine (Cagguila et al., 1998) or morphine (Kucinski et al., 1998) treatment. The oscillations in both biochemical (dopamine efflux from the striatum and the nucleus accumbens) and behavioral (hypoalgesia) measures were completely prevented by chronic lithium pre-treatment (Antelman et al., 1998).

This model may be of special interest because it is the first attempt to propose a specific manipulation that is both progressive (sensitization), that directly induces cyclicity, and that is responsive to Li. However, the model is clearly non-homologous since both the biochemical and the behavioral measures are dissimilar from the human disorder, whereas the cocaine-induced behaviors that do have face validity for mania, such as hyperactivity and reward-related behaviors, do not show cyclicity and are not clearly normalized by antibipolar treatment (see above). Also, whereas Li treatment was reported to eliminate the cyclicity (Antelman et al., 1998), the effects of other antibipolar drugs such as carbamazepine and valproate has not yet been evaluated. Still, the notion of a cycling phenomenon is important and additional study of this proposed model may be useful.

Biphasic Response to Quinpirole

A different derivative of the psychostimulant-induced model is now under study in our laboratory, examining the biphasic locomotor response to the D2/D3 agonist quinpirole. Unlike most dopamine agonists, quinpirole (in appropriate doses) induces a biphasic response over time starting with hypolocomotion and developing into a hyperlocomotion state (Eilam and Szechtman, 1989). It is our hypothesis that the biphasic profile of the response may provide some face validity for the two states of BPD. We are currently testing the effects of antibipolar drugs on quinpirole-induced hypoactivity and hyperactivity. Preliminary results are are that chronic treatment with oral carbamazepine or valproate seems to attenuate the late hyperlocomotion response to quinpirole.

CONCLUSION

Bipolar affective disorder is unique among the psychiatric illnesses in its cyclicity and this special property presents a major difficulty in attempts to develop an appropriate animal model for the disease. The traditional animal models for bipolar disorder focussed on a particular manic trait, such as elevated locomotor activity or responsivity to reinforcing stimuli. Models based on changes in locomotor activity are often confounded by the narrow range of increased activity that can be attenuated by lithium, whereas models based on reinforcement are confounded by the malaise caused by lithium treatment.

Other attempts to develop models for the disorder attempted to reflect its progressive nature and include psychostimulant-induced sensitization and amygdala kindling. Kindling and sensitization both reflect the progressive nature of some types of bipolar disorder and the fact that episodes which may have once been triggered by external events evolve into spontaneously occurring episodes. These models paved the way for systematic testing of the effects of anti-convulsants in bipolar disorder, but they did not always respond to lithium.

The cyclic nature of bipolar disorder was the focus of studies showing that chronic cocaine- and morphine-induced biochemical and behavioral changes were reported to have a cyclic nature that is abolished by antibipolar treatment. The quinpirole model may be able to combine both superficial behavioral similarities, i.e., a biphasic locomotor response with the element of progression and cycling. Another approach to drug development and research on the pathogenesis of bipolar disorder may require abandoning the unitary disease approach in favor of a more flexible approach to both research and treatment. Possibly the kindling/sensitization-based behaviors may be more representative of a subset of rapidly cycling patients and/or patients who respond better to anticonvulsant-like drugs than to lithium, but may not represent other patterns of the disorder. Insight into the changes in signal transduction that are purported to be involved in the pathogenesis of BPD may provide new pharmacological means of manipulating behavior to provide novel models for BPD.

REFERENCES

Albert, I., Cicala, G.A., Siegel, J. (1970) The behavioral effects of REM sleep deprivation in rats. Psychophysiol. 7: 552-60.

Albright, P.S. and Burnham, W.M. (1980) Development of a new pharmacological seizure model: effects of anticonvulsants on cortical- and amygdala-kindled seizures in the rat. Epilepsia 21: 681-89.

Antelman, S.M., Caggiula, A.R., Kucinski, B.J., Fowler, H., Gershon, S., Edwards, D.J., Austin, M.C., Stiller, R., Kiss, S., Kocan, D. (1998) The effects of lithium on a potential cycling model of bipolar disorder. Prog Neuropsychopharmacol Biol Psychiat. 22: 495-510.

Antelman, S.M., Caggiula, A.R. (1996) Oscillation follows drug sensitization: implications. Critic Rev Neurobiol. 10: 101-17.

Antelman, S.M., Caggiula, A.R., Kiss, S., Edwards, D.J., Kocan, D., Stiller, R. (1995) Neurochemical and physiological effects of cocaine oscillate with sequential drug treatment: possibly a major factor in drug variability. Neuropsychopharmacol. 12: 297-306.

Antoniou, K., Kafetzopoulos, E., Papadopoulou-Daifoti, Z., Hyphantis, T., Marselos, M. (1998) d-Amphetamine, cocaine and caffeine: a comperative study of acute effects on locomotor activity and behavioral patterns in rats. Neurosci Biobehav Rev 23: 189-96.

Aylmer, C.G.G., Steinberg, H., Webster, R.A. (1987) Hyperactivity induced by dexamphetamine/chlorodiazepoxide mixures in rats and its attenuation by lithium pretreatment: a role for dopamine? Psychopharmacol. 91: 198-206.

Azorin, J.M. and Tramoni, V. (1987) Kindling models and antikindling effects of mood normalizers. Pharmacopsychiatr. 20: 189-91.

Babington, R.G. (1977) The pharmacology of kindling. In: I. Hanin, E. Usdin, eds. Animal Models of Psychiatry and Neurology, NY: Pergamon Press. pp 141-149.

Barbini, B., Colombo, C., Bendetti, F., Campori, E., Bellodi, L., Smeraldi, E. (1998) The unipolar-bipolar dichotomy and the response to sleep deprivation. Psychiatr Res. 79: 43-50.

Berggren, U. (1985) Effects of chronic lithium treatment on brain monoamine metabolism and amphetamine-induced locomotor stimulation in rats. J Neural Trans. 64: 239-50.

Borsini, F. and Meli, A. (1988) Is the forced swimming test a suitable model for revealing antidepressant activity? Psychopharmacol. 94: 147-60.

Bozarth, M.A. and Wise, R.A. (1981) Localization of the reward relevant opiate receptors. In: L.S. Harris, ed. Problems of Drug Dependence, Washington, D.C.:National Institute of Drug Abuse.

Caggiula, A.R., Antelman, S.M., Palmer, A.M., Kiss, S., Edwards, D.J., Kocan, D. (1996) The effects of ethanol on striatal dopamine and cortical D-[3H] aspartate efflux oscillate with repeated treatment: relevance to individual differences in drug responsiveness. Neuropsychopharmacol. 15: 125-32.

Caggiula, A.R., Antelman, S.M., Kucinski, B.J., Fowler, H., Edwards, D.J., Austin, M.C., Gershon, S., Stiller, R. (1998) Oscillatory-sensitization model of repeated drug exposure: cocaine's effects on shock-induced hypoalgesia. Prog Neuropsychopharmacol Biol Psychiatr. 22: 511-21.

Cao, B.J. and Peng, N.A. (1993) Magnesium valproate attenuates hyperactivity induced by dexamphetamine-chlordiazepoxide mixure in rodents. Eur J Pharmacol. 237: 177-81.

Caggiula, A.R. and Hoebel, B.G. (1966) 'Copulation reward site' in the posterior hypothalamus. Science 153:1284-1285.

Cappeliez, P. and Moore, E. (1990) Effects of lithium on an amphetamine animal model of bipolar disorder. Prog Neuropsychopharmacol Biol Psychiatr. 14: 347-58.

Carli, M., Morissette, M., Hebert, C., Di Paolo, T., Reader, T.A. (1997) Effects of a chronic lithium treatment on central dopamine neurotransporters. Biochem Pharmacol 54: 391-97.

Christo, P.J. and el-Mallakh, R.S. (1993) Possible role of endogenous ouabain-like compounds in the pathophysiology of bipolar illness. Med Hypoth. 41: 378-83.

Colpaert, F.C., Niemeegers, C.J.E., Janssen, P.A. (1978) Discriminative stimulus properties of cocaine and d-amphetamine, and antagonism by haloperidol: A comparative study. Neuropharmacology 17: 937-942.

Cox, C., Harrison-Read, P.E., Steinberg, H., Tomkiewicz, M. (1971) Lithium attenuates drug-induced 'manic' activity in rats. Nature 232: 336-38.

Davies, C., Sanger, D.J., Steinberg, H., Tomkiewicz, M., U'Prichard, D.C. (1974) Lithium and alpha-methyl-p-tyrosine prevent 'manic' activity in rodents. Psychopharmacol 36: 263-74.

DeMontis, M.G., Fadda, P., Devoto, P., Martellotta, M.C., Fratta, W. (1990) Sleep deprivation increases dopamine D1 receptor antagonist [3H]SCH 23390 binding and dopamine-stimulated adenylate cyclase in the rat limbic system. Neurosci Let. 117: 224-27.

Dixon, A.K. and Fisch, H.U. (1998) Animal models and ethological strategies for early drug-testing in humans. Neurosci Biobehav Rev. 23: 345-58.

Ebstein, R.P., Eliashar, S., Belmaker, R.H., Ben-Uriah, Y., Yehuda, S. (1980) Chronic lithium treatment and dopamine-mediated behavior. Biol Psychiatr. 15: 459-67.

Edelson, A., Gottesfeld, Z., Samuel, D., Yuwiler, A. (1976) Effects of lithium and other alkali metals on brain-stimulation behavior. Psychopharmacol. 45: 233-37.

Eilam, D. and Szechtman, H. (1990) Dosing regime differentiates sensitization of locomotion and mouthing to D2 agonist quinpirole. Pharmacol Biochem and Behav. 36: 989-91.

Eilam, D. and Szechtman, H. (1989) Biphasic effect of D-2 agonist quinpirole on locomotion and movements. Eur J Pharmacol. 161: 151-57.

Einat, H., Karbovski, H., Korik, J., Tsalah, D., Belmaker, R.H. (1999) Inositol reduces depressive-like behaviors in two different animal models of depression. Psychopharmacol. 144: 158-62.

Einat, H., Einat, D., Allan, M., Talangbayan, H., Tsafnat, T., Szechtman, H. (1996) Associational and nonassociational mechanisms in locomotor sensitization to the dopamine agonist quinpirole. Psychopharmacol. 127: 95-101.

Einat, H. and Belmaker, R.H. (in press) The effects of inositol treatment in animal models of psychiatric disorders. J Affect Disord.

176

Einat, H., Clenet, F., Shaldevin, A., Belmaker, R.H., Bourin, M. (submitted) The antidepressant activity of inositol in the forced swim test involves 5-HT2 receptors.

Ellinwood, E.H., Sudilovski, A., Nelson, L. (1972) Behavioral analysis of chronic amphetamine intoxication. Biol Psychiatr. 4: 215-30.

el-Mallakh, R.S., Barrett, J.L., Wyatt, R.J. (1993a) The Na, K-ATPase hypothesis for bipolar disorder: implications of normal development. J Child Adolesc Psychopharmacol 3: 37-52.

el-Mallakh, R.S., Harrison, L.T., Changaris, D.G., Levy, R.S. (1993b) An animal model for bipolar illness. Society for Neuroscience Abstracts 19: 140 (abs. number 340.18).

el-Mallakh, R.S., Harrison, L.T., Li, R., Changaris, D.G., Levy, R.S. (1995) An animal model for mania: perliminary results. Prog Neuropsychopharmacol Biol Psychiatr. 19: 955-62.

el-Mallakh, R.S. and Wyatt, R.J. (1995) The Na, K-ATPase hypothesis for bipolar illness. Biol Psychiatr. 37: 235-44.

Fadda, P., Martellota, M.C., DeMontis, M.G., Gessa, G.L., Fratta, W. (1992) Dopamine D1 and opioid receptor binding changes in the limbic system of sleep deprived rats. Neurochem Int. 20 (supp): 153S-56S.

Fadda, P., Tortorella, A., Fratta, W. (1991) Sleep deprivation decreases mu and delta opioid receptor binding in the rat limbic system. Neurosci Let. 129: 315-17.

Fratta, W., Collu, M., Martellotta, M.C., Pichiri, M., Gessa, G.L. (1988) Opioid dopamine interactions in stress induced insomnia. In: P.F. Spano, G. Biggio, G. Toffano, G.L. Gessa, eds. Central and Peripheral Dopamine Receptors: Biochemistry and Pharmacology. Berlin: Springer Verlag. pp 197-204.

Fratta, W., Collu, M., Martellotta, M.C., Pichiri, M., Muntoni, F., Gessa, G.L. (1987) Stress-induced insomnia: opioid-dopamine interactions. Eur J Pharmacolog. 142: 437-40.

Gessa, G.L., Fadda, P., Serra, G., Fratta, W. (1994) Modelli animali di patologia psichiatrica e loro utilita nella sperimentazione del nuovi psicofarmaci. In: M. Maj, G. Racagni, eds. La Sperimentazione dei Nuovi Farmaci in Psichiatria. Milan: Masson. pp 17-28.

Gessa, G.L., Pani, L., Fadda, P., Fratta, W. (1995) Sleep deprivation in the rat: an animal model of mania. Eur Neuropsychopharmacol Supp.: 89-93.

Gessa, G.L., Pani, L., Serra, G., Fratta, W. (1995) Animal models of mania. In: G.L. Gessa, W. Fratta, I. Pani, G. Serra, eds. Depression and Mania: From Neurobiology to Treatment. NY: Raven Press. pp 43-66.

Goddard, G.V. and Douglas, R.M. (1975) Does the engram of kindling model the engram of normal long term memory? Can J Neurolog Sci. 2: 385-94.

Green, A.R., Johnson, P., Mountford, J.A., Nimgaonkar, V.L. (1985) Some anticonvulsant drugs alter monoamine-mediated behavior in mice in ways similar to electroconvulsive shock: implications for antidepressant therapy. Br J Pharmacol. 84: 337-46.

Hicks, R.A., Moore, J.D., Hayes, C., Phillips, N., Hawkins, J. (1979) REM sleep deprivation increases aggressiveness in male rats. Physiol Behav. 22: 1097-100.

Jimerson, D.C. and Post, R.M. (1982) Dopaminergic mechanisms in affective illness. In: R.M. Post, J.C. Ballenger, eds. The Neurobiology of Mood Disorders. Baltimore: Williams and Wilkins.

Kelley A.E., Finn, M., Cunnignham S.T., Renshaw, P., Sachs, G. (1993) Lithium diet enhances the behavioral response to cholera toxin infusion into the nucleus accumbens. Soc. Neurosci. Abstr. 19, 130, 15.

Kilbey, M.M. and Ellinwood, E.H. (1977) Reverse tolerance to stimulant-induced abnormal behavior. Life Sci. 20: 1063-76.

Kirby, L.G. and Lucki, I. (1997) Interaction between the forced swimming test and fluoxetine treatment on extracellular 5-hydroxytryptamine and 5-hydroxyindoleacetic acid in the rat. J Pharmacol Exp Therapeut. 282: 967-76.

Kofman, O. and Belmaker, R.H. (1991) Animal models of mania and bipolar affective illness. In: P. Soubrie, ed. Anxiety, Depression and Mania. Animal Models of Psychiatric Disorders. Basel: Karger. Vol. 3 pp 103-121.

Kofman, P., Li, P.P., Warsh, J.J (1998) Lithium, but not carbamazepine, potentiates hyperactivity induced by intra-accumbens cholera toxin. Pharmacol. Biochem. Behav. 59 (1), 191-200.

Kucinski, B.J., Antelman, S.M., Caggiula, A.R., Fowler, H., Gershon, S., Edwards, D.J., Austin, M.C. (1998) Oscillatory effects of repeated morphine on shock-induced hypoalgesia and beta-endorphin. Synapse 30: 30-37.

Kumar, R. (1979) Animal models of psychiatric disorders. In: Van Praag, H., Lader, Rafaelsen, Sachar, eds. Handbook of Biological Psychiatry. Disciplines Relevant to Biologcial Psychiatry, New York:Marcel Dekker.

Kuruvilla, A. and Uretsky, N.J. (1981) Effects of sodium valproate on motor function regulated by the activation of GABA receptors. Psychopharmacol. 72: 167-72.

Lerer, B., Globus, M., Brik, E., Hamburger, R., Belmaker, R.H. (1984) Effect of treatment and withdrawal from chronic lithium in rats on stimulant-induced responses. Neuropsychobiol. 11: 28-32.

Leviel, V. and Naquet, R. (1977) A study of the action of valproic acid on the kindling effect. Epilepsia 18: 229-34.

Levine, J. (1997) Controlled trials of inositol in psychiatry. Eur. Neuropsychopharmacol. 7:145-155.

Li, R., el-Mallakh, R.S., Harrison, L., Changaris, D.G., Levy, R.S. (1997) Lithium prevents ouabain-induced behavioral changes. Toward an animal model for manic depression. Mol Chem Neuropathol. 31: 65-72.

Looney, S.W. and el-Mallakh, R.S. (1997) Meta-analysis of erythrocyte Na, K-ATPase activity in bipolar illness. Depres Anxiet. 5: 53-65.

Maitre, L., Baltzer, V., Mondadori, C., Olpe, H.R., Baumann, P.A., Waldmeier, P.C. (1984) Psychopharmacological and behavioral effects of anti-epileptic drugs in animals. In: H.M. Emrich, T, Okuma, A.A. Muller, eds. Anticonvulsants in affective disorders. Amsterdam: Elsevier. pp 3-13.

Maj, J., Chojnacka-Wojcik, E., Lewandowska, A., Tatarczynska, E., Wiczynska, B. (1985) The central action of carbamazepine as a potential antidepressant drug. Pol J Pharmacol Pharmac. 37: 47-56.

Maj, M., Veltro, F., Piozzi, R., Lobrace, S., Magliano, L. (1992) Pattern of recurrence of illness after recovery from an episode of major depression: a prospective study. Am J Psychiatr. 149: 795-800.

Minabe, Y., Emori, K., Kurachi, M. (1988) Effects of chronic lithium treatment on limbic seizure generation in the cat. Psychopharmacol. 96: 391-94.

Minabe, Y., Tanii, Y., Tsunoda, M., Kurachi, M. (1987) Acute effect of TRH, flunarizine, lithium and zotepine on amygdaloid kindled seizures induced with low-frequency stimulation. Japan J Psychiatr Neurol. 41: 685-91.

Morden, B., Mullins, R., Levine, S. (1968) Effects of REM deprivation on the mating behavior of male rats. Psychophysiol. 5: 241-42.

Mucha, R.F., van der Kooy, D., O'Shaughnessy, M., Bucenieks, P. (1982) Drug reinforcement studied by the use of place conditioning in rat. Brain Res. 243:91-105.

Okada, K., Oishi, R., Saeki, K. (1990) Inhibition by antimanic drugs of hyperactivity induced by methamphetamine-chlordiazepoxide mixure in mice. Pharmacol Biochem Behav. 35: 897-901.

Ossenkopp, K.P. and Eckel, L.A. (1995) Toxin-induced conditioned changes in taste reactivity and the role of chemosensitive area postrema. Neurosci Biobehav Rev. 19: 99-108.

Overmier, J.B. and Patterson, J. (1988) Animal models of human psychopathology. In: P. Simon, P. Soubrie, D. Wildlocher, eds. Animal Models of Psychiatric Disorders, Volume 1. Basel: Karger. pp. 1-35.

Overstreet, D.H., Rezvani, A.H., Janowsky, D.S. (1992) Genetic animal models of depression and ethanol preference provide support for cholinergic and serotonergic involvement in depression and alcoholism. Biol Psychiatr. 31: 919-36.

Porsolt, R.D., Anton, G., Blavet, N., Jalfre, M. (1978) Behavioral despair in rats, a new model sensitive to antidepressant treatment. Eur J Pharmacol 47: 379-91.

Poncelet, M., Dangoumau, L., Sourbrie, P., Simon, P. (1987) Effects of neuroleptic drugs, clonidine and lithium on the expression of conditioned behavioral excitation in rats. Psychopharmacol. 92: 393-97.

Post, R.M. and Ballenger, J.C. (1981) Kindling models for the progressive development of behavioral psychopathology: sensitization to electrical, pharmacological , and psychological stimuli. In: H.M. van Praag, M.H. Lader, O.J. Rafaelsen, E.J. Shachar, eds. Handbook of Biological Psychiatry Part IV. NY: Marcel Dekker. pp 609-651.

Post, R.M. and Contel, N.R. (1981) Cocaine induced behavioral sensitization: a model for recurrent manic illness. In: C. Perris, G. Struwe, B. Jansson, eds. Biological Psychiatry. Amsterdam: Elsevier. pp 746-749.

Post, R.M. and Contel, N.R. (1983) Human and animal studies of cocaine: implications for development of behavioral pathology. In: I. Creese, ed. Stimulants: Neurochemical, Behavioral and Clinical Perspectives. NY: Raven Press.

Post, R.M., Denicoff, K.D., Frye, M.A., Dunn, R.T., Leverich, G.S., Osuch, E., Speer, A. (1998) A history of the use of anticonvulsants as mood stabilizers in the last two decades of the 20th century. Neuropsychobiol. 38: 152-66.

Post, R.M., Putnam, F., Contel, N.R., Goldman, B. (1984b) Electroconvulsive seizures inhibit amygdala kindling: implications for mechanisms of action in affective illness. Epilepsia 25: 234-39.

Post, R.M., Rubinow, D.R., Ballenger, J.C. (1984a) Conditioning, sensitization, and kindling: implications for the course of affective illness. In: R.M. Post, J.C. Ballenger, eds. Neurobiology of Mood Disorders. Baltimore, MD: Williams & Wilkins. pp 432-66.

Post, R.M., Weiss, S.R.B, Pert, A. (1984c) Differential effects of carbamazepine and lithium on sensitization and kindling. Prog Neuropsychopharmacol Biol Psychiatr. 8: 425-34.

178

Post, R.M., Unde, T.W., Rubinow, D.R., Huggins, T. (1987) Differential time course of antidepressant effects after sleep deprivation, ECT, and carbamazepine: clinical and theoretical implications. Psychiatr Res. 22: 11-9.

Post, R.M. and Weiss, S.R.B. (1997) Kindling and stress sensitization. In: L.T. Young, R.T. Joffe, eds. Bipolar disorders: biological models and their clinical application. NY: Marcel Dekker,. pp 93-126.

Post, R.M. and Weiss, S.R.B. (1995) The neurobiology of treatment-resistant mood disorders. In Bloom FE and Kupfer DJ Psychopharmacology: The Fourth Generation of Progress. Raven Press Ltd. N.Y. pp 1155-1170.

Post, R.M. and Weiss, S.R.B. (1996) A speculative model of affective illness cyclicity based on patterns of drug tolerance observed in amygdala-kindled seizures. Mol Neurobiol. 13: 33-60.

Predy, P.A. and Kokkinidis, L. (1981) Post-amphetamine depression of self-stimulation behavior in rats: prophylactic effects of lithium. Neurosci Let. 29: 343-47.

Racine, R.J. (1978) Kindling: the first decade. Neurosurger. 3: 234-52.

Ramana, S.V. and Desiraju, T. (1989) Investigation of influence of diazepam, valproate, cyproheptadine and cortisol on the rewarding ventral tegmental self-stimulation behavior. Indian J Physiol Pharmacol. 33: 179-85.

Redrobe, J.P., MacSweeney, C.P., Bourin, M. (1996) The role of 5-HT1A and 5-HT1B receptors in antidepressant drug actions in the mouse forced swimming test. Eur J Pharmacol. 318: 213-20.

Robbins, T.W. and Sahakian, B.J. (1980) Animal models of mania. In: H.M. Van Praag, R.H. Belmaker, eds. Mania, an Evolving Concept. Jamaica: MTP Press/ Spectrum Publication. pp 143-216.

Robinson, T.E. and Becker, J.B. (1986) Enduring changes in brain and behavior produced by chronic amphetamine administration: a review and evaluation of animal models of amphetamine psychosis. Brain Res Rev. 11: 157-98.

Rose, A.M., Mellett, B.J., Valdes, R. Jr., Kleinman, J.E., Herman, M.M., Li, R., el-Mallakh. R.S. (1998) Alpha 2 isoform of the Na, K-adenosine triphosphatase is reduced in temporal cortex of bipolar individuals. Biol Psychiatr. 44: 892-97.

Rossetti, Z.L., Lai, M., Hmaidan, Y., Gessa, G.L. (1993) Depletion of mesolimbic dopamine during behavioral despair: partial reversal by chronic imipramine. Eur J Pharmacol. 242: 313-15.

Sanchez, C. and Meier, E. (1997) Behavioral profiles of SSRIs in animal models of depression, anxiety and aggression. Are they all alike? Psychopharmacol 129: 197-205.

Seeger, T.F., Gardner, E.L., Bridger, W.F. (1981) Increase in mesolimbic electrical self-stimulation after chronic haloperidol: reversal by L-DOPA or lithium. Brain Res. 215: 404-09.

Shippenberg, T.S. and Heidbreder, C. (1995) The delta-opioid receptor antagonist naltrindole prevents sensitization to the conditioned rewarding effects of cocaine. Eur J Pharmacol. 280: 55-61.

Shippenberg, T.S. and Herz, A. (1991) Influence of chronic lithium treatment upon the motivational effects of opioids: alteration in the effects of mu- but not kappa-opioid receptor ligands. J Pharmacol Experiment Therapeut. 256: 1101-06.

Siegel, J.M. and Rogawski, M.A. (1988) A function for REM sleep: regulation of noradrenergic receptor sensitivity. Brain Res Rev. 13: 213-33.

Smith, D.F. (1981) Central and peripheral effects of lithium on amphetamine-induced hyperactivity in rats. Pharmacol Biochem Behav. 14: 439-42.

Smith, D.F., (1982) Central effects of acute lithium treatment on catecholaminergic behavior in rats. In: H.M. Emrich, Aldenhoff, H.D. Lux, eds. Basic Mechanisms in the Action of Lithium. Amsterdam: Excerpta Medica. pp 167-174.

Spyraki, C., Kazandjian, A., Varonos, D. (1985) Diazepam-induced place preference conditioning: appetitive and antiversive properties. Psychopharmacol. 87: 225-32.

Stewart, J. and Badiani, A. (1993) Tolerance and sensitization to the behavioral effects of drugs. Behav Pharmacol. 4: 289-312.

Stoll, A.L. and Severus, W.E. (1996) Mood stabilizers: shared mechanisms of action at postsynaptic signal-transduction and kindling processes. Harv Rev Psychiatr. 4: 77-89.

Suzuki, T., Shiozaki, Y., Masukawa, Y., Misawa, M., Nagase, H. (1992) The role of mu- and kappa-opioid receptors in cocaine-induced conditioned place preference. Japan J Pharmacol. 58: 435-42.

Szuba, M.P., Baxter, L.R., Altshuler, L.L., Allen, E.M., Guze, B.H., Schwartz, J.M., Liston, E.H. (1994) Lithium sustains the acute antidepressant effects of sleep deprivation: preliminary findings from a controlled study. Psychiatr Res. 51: 283-95.

Takigawa, M., Fukuzako, H., Ueyama, K., Tominaga, H. (1994) Intracranial self-stimulation and locomotor traces as indicators for evaluating and developing antipsychotic drugs. Japan J Psychiatr Neurol. 48: 127-32.

Ursin, H. and Murison, R. (1986) Ethical issues in stress research. Acta Physiolog Scan. 128 (supp): 242-43.

Ushijama, I., Yamada, K., Furukawa, T. (1986) Behavioral effects of lithium on presynaptic sites of catecholaminergic neurons in the mouse. Archs int Pharmachodyn 282:58-67.

Wada, J.A., Sato, M., Wake, A., Green, J.R., Troupin, A.S. (1976) Prophylactic effects of phenytoin, phenobarbital and carbamazepine examined in kindled cat preparations. Arch Neurol. 33: 426-34.

Wehr, T.A., Sack, D.A., Rosenthal, N.E. (1987) Sleep reduction as a final common pathway in the genesis of mania. Am J Psychiat. 144: 201-04.

Weiss. S.R.B. and Post, R.M. (1995) Caveats in the use of the kindling model of affective disorders.J. Toxicol. Indust. Hlth. 10:421-447.

Weiss, S.R.B., Post, R.M., Costello, M., Nutt, D.J., Tandeciarz, S. (1990) Carbamazepine retards the development of cocaine kindled seizures but not sensitization to cocaine-induced hyperactivity. Neuropsychopharmacol. 3: 273-281.

Willner, P. (1995) Animal models of depression: validity and applications. In: G. Gessa, W. Fratta, L. Pani, G. Serra, eds. Depression and Mania: From Neurobiology to Treatment. NY: Raven Press. pp 19-41.

Willner, P. (1991) Animal models of depression. In: P. Willner, ed. Behavioral Models in Psychopharmacology Theoretical, Industrial and Clinical Perspectives. Cambridge: Cambridge University Press. pp. 91-125.

Willner, P. (1986) Validation criteria for animal models of human mental disorders: learned helplessness as a paradigm case. Prog Neuropsychopharmacol Biol Psychiatr. 10: 677-90.

Willner, P., Towell, A., Sampson, D., Sophokleous, S., Muskat, R. (1987) Reduction of sucrose preference by chronic mild unpredictable stress, and its restoration by tricyclic antidepressant. Psychopharmacol. 93: 358-64.

Wood, A.J., Elphick, M., Aronson, J.K., Grahame-Smith, D.G. (1989) The effect of lithium on cation transport measured in vivo in patients suffering from bipolar affective illness. Br J Psychiatr. 155: 504-10.

Young, L.T., Li, P.P.,Kish, S.J., Siu, K.P., Kamble, A.,Hornykiewicz, O., Warsh, J.J. (1993) Cerebral cortex Gs protein levels and forskolin-stimulated cyclic AMP formation are increased in bipolar affective disorder. J. Neurochem. 61;890-898.

11 EMERGENCE OF PTSD-TYPE REACTIVITY IN SPRAGUE-DAWLEY RATS FOLLOWING PRENATAL GAMMA IRRADIATION

Matti Mintz and Michael Myslobodsky

INTRODUCTION

Posttraumatic Stress Disorder (PTSD) is believed to be precipitated by stressors which are markedly distressing to almost anyone (DSM-III), so that the major experimental paradigms relevant for modeling PTSD have emphasized the necessity of traumatic history for development of conditioned fear. By contrast, the necessity of an innate (unconditioned) fear as a prerequisite for PTSD has not received a proper hearing. The potential of the traumatic precipitant is somewhat reduced by the fact that not everyone will have gone to pieces in conditions of severe stress whereas others are expected to develop PTSD following relatively 'mild' psychological trauma (Foy et al., 1987). Lord Taylor (1978) noticed that during WWII, only a fraction of the civil population (about 10%) were afflicted in the bombed cities in England. Somewhat apologetically he called them "the psychopathic tenth." This variation in response to stress is in keeping with an old conviction that the syndrome "depends not only upon the kind of injury, but upon the kind of brain" (Symonds, 1937, p. 464).

The allusion to "the kind of brain" de-emphasizes the role of traumatic history, association, and learning. It posits that similar to schizophrenia, the premorbid innate readiness to respond to environmental stimuli with lingering fear may be a product of genetic liability (Foy et al., 1987; McFarlane, 1988, 1989) and/or neurodevelopmental abnormality. The possibility that such intrinsic vulnerability could be created by neurodevelopmental abnormalities was suggested elsewhere on the basis of anatomical brain findings using magnetic resonance imaging (Myslobodsky et al., 1995). Also, the presence of PTSD is significantly predicted by the pattern of psychopathology in the families (Reich et al., 1996), and premilitary school performance (Watson et al., 1998). These findings did not rule out an alternative possibility, there may be more than a single disorder behind the facade of PTSD. A good way to draw attention to the conundrum of PTSD is to show that it consists of overlapping but dissimilar disorders. This study attempts to achieve this goal by disrupting prenatal (intrauterine) development in a rat so as to reproduce an untoward psychopathological response to novel environmental stimuli and/or conditions later in life (i.e., to reproduce the state of unconditioned fear).

Prenatal stressor is a term commonly used as a synonym for any harmful developmental event. It can cause disruptions of embryonic/fetal development due to either direct effects or indirect effects. In the latter case, the stressor acts through maternal organisms by creating a state when adjustment is difficult or impossible but motivation is very strong, as Scott defined psychological stress in 1949. Put differently, maternal stress is made to be perceived and thus is dependent upon whether or not the afflicted dam adapts to it (Weinstock et al., 1992). It may be said to operate via 'harassment variables,' that is, via the features of the paradigm which inflict pain or require the mother to keep up a struggle throughout pregnancy (e.g., to cope with drug experience, excessive illumination, loud noise, electrical shock, unusual position, complete immobilization, etc.). But prenatal factors may be deleterious without being noticed. It seems preferable to avoid or minimize "harassment variables" when mother-infant relations are not at issue. For example, by exposing an animal to ionizing radiation in utero (when a dose is kept under 1.5 Gy), a spectrum of congenital abnormalities, growth retardation, and functional deficits, depending upon the dose and the specific gestational phase of irradiation, could be inflicted with neither excessive harassment, nor with significant maternal effects (Schull et al., 1990; Kimler, 1998).

The reference to 'specific gestational phase' is relevant vis-a-vis paradigms which tend to administer potentially harmful drugs from conception to birth while others are limited to exposures of a single day or a number of days of development. Both are useful. Prolonged exposures are justifiable etiologically, but have limited pathophysiological advantage. Early studies have shown that neuronal cells may have rather narrow time periods of radiosensitivity which creates an impression that malformations caused by prenatal injury are rather deterministic in character. In general, prior to the blastocyst stage, ionizing radiation acts in the threshold 'all-or-none' fashion, producing lethal effects, but no teratogenicity or growth retardation. Likewise, in the fetal stage, the radiosensitivity is greatly reduced and gross central and somatic malformations are absent (Brent and Bolden, 1961; Rugh, 1962; for review see Brent et al., 1987). Early organogenesis opens the major window of radiosensitivity when the embryo appears to be highly sensitive to growth-stunting, local teratogenic, and carcinogenic effects of ionizing radiation (Hicks, 1958; Hicks and D'Amato, 1978). The term 'window' implies that the effect has been claimed to occur at some periods of development and not at others. We thus opted for using ionizing radiation as a damaging agent given in specific periods of prenatal development. Our choice was dictated by previous experience and the recognized advantages of ionizing radiation in its application and dosing, as well as in the relative absence of 'harassment variables.'

The utility of using ionizing radiation applied at precise times has been explored elsewhere for reproducing the congenital form of epilepsy (Myslobodsky, 1976). The fitness of this approach can be supported by three founding assumptions:

(1) The process of prenatal development could be approximated by a series of categorical time-periods when vulnerability of different brain systems is maximal. Thus, a narrowly timed prenatal trauma could create a relatively discrete deficiency in the central nervous system (Rugh, 1962; Wilson et al., 1953).

(2) Prenatal injury could contribute to a variety of dissimilar states and responses, collectively designated as behavioral teratogenesis (Bruses et al., 1991; Elsner, 1992).

(3) A number of effects of developmental trauma become noticeable only in adulthood; their magnitude is partly accounted for by additional exogenous factors (see Lipska and Weinberger, this volume).

CREATING A MODEL

Model transfer profile (MTP). To our knowledge, a neurodevelopmental model of PTSD has yet to be created. We thus had to make a credible proposition and judge our product on the basis of features which fit clinical reality. Any phenomenological (naturalistic, clinical) model should be comprised of features, which conceive of either clinically-relevant elements of animal's behavior, or specific pathophysiological mechanisms. Such features may be said to be 'transferred' into the model domain. For example, a tendency of withdrawal could be modeled by rats becoming motionless in a novel environment, and/or reduced time spent in social interactions. The ratio of adequately transferred features (ΔS) to all diagnostically relevant features (ΣS) will be designated as MTP. To assess the present model, we placed such feature of PTSD as the enhanced startle reactivity in the numerator of MTP. The enhancement of the startle response magnitude as well as reduced startle habituation throughout the session are commonly encountered in PTSD (Butler et al., 1990; Morgan et al., 1995, 1997; Ornitz and Pynoos, 1989; Orr et al., 1995; Ross et al., 1989 ; Shalev et al, 1992). They have been recommended as useful markers of the disorder in DSM-IV.

The acoustic startle reflex is a short-latency response of the skeletal musculature elicited by a novel and/or strong auditory stimulus (Davis, 1984). The Collaborative Behavioral Teratology Study indicated that the startle response is a reliable measure of developmental deficits (Buelke-Sam et al., 1985). It provides information for which no training of animals is required, and can be elicited in rat pups as young as 12 days of age. As an example, there are indications of profound anomalies of startle in rodents exposed prenatally to ionizing radiation (Myslobodsky, 1976) or methylmercury (Geyer et al., 1985). Occasionally, they reach the magnitude of myoclonic responses (Myslobodsky, 1976). Another desirable feature of PTSD-prone rat is an excessive fear which could be operationally defined as a tendency to freeze in a novel environment.

In the present study, Sprague-Dawley rats were exposed to a single dose of γ radiation (1.5 Gy at 0.15 Gy/min for 10 min). The dose was delivered on one of embryonic days (E15, E17, or E19) through the whole body of pregnant rats. Day 15 is the crucial period as it is the time of heightened vulnerability to ionizing radiation for numerous postnatal behavioral end points (Kimler and Norton, 1988; Norton and Kimler, 1988). Sham prenatal exposure of controls consisted of placing pregnant rats in the same environment for 10 min without irradiation. To explore whether aberrant behaviors will emerge prepubertally or appear in adulthood, rats were examined behaviorally prepubertally (at day 25-27, P25) or postpubertally (at day 55-57, P55). These stages were based on the timing of development of rats (King, 1958). The details of methodology have been communicated elsewhere (Mintz et. al., 1998).

DEVELOPMENTAL LANDMARKS OF EXPOSED PROGENY

If prenatal manipulations were found to alter postnatal development, their effects could be seen in the disordered pattern of acquisition of developmental milestones ("pandysmaturation" of Fish, 1977, 1992), such as axial (postural) asymmetry and the rate of eye opening in rats.

Neonatal Axial Asymmetry (NAA)

NAA was assessed by the deviation of the pup's tail (Ross et al., 1981). It is presumably the first postnatal marker of laterality associated with imbalanced dopaminergic system. On the assumption that dopamine (DA) is as imbalanced in embryogeny as in neonates, the findings of Ross et al. may imply that the principle of spatial and temporal gradients of proliferation of the neuroepithelial germinal zone might be extended to the lateral maturational gradient of DAergic system. This gradient was expected to change following prenatal exposure to γ radiation. On the second postnatal day, Gigi et al. (1997) examined more than six hundred offspring of the Sprague-Dawley strain (368/233 exposed and sham-irradiated, respectively). Overall, 70% of pups in the exposed group showed tail asymmetry compared to 66% among sham-irradiated controls with no gender effect.

Exposed pups showed a small (16%), but statistically significant weight reduction. Given that low birth weight is a classical measure of embryotoxicity (Norton and Donoso, 1985; Jensh et al., 1986) we explored whether NAA was affected by reduced birth weight. Among the E15 group, NAA was more consistently manifested by low weight pups. Only females with left-biased posture showed significant weight reduction. No such association was obtained for the biased males. Neither among control pups, nor among irradiated E17 and E19 pups, was there a statistically significant difference in asymmetry as a function of weight.

Eye Opening Asymmetry

Rodents are born with closed eyes, and eye opening is a harbinger of an important leap in brain maturity which heralds an increment in exploratory activity and adult patterns of locomotion (Altman and Sudarshan, 1975). Bilateral (synchronous) eye opening is considered a standard event. The progeny of the Sprague-Dawley rats exposed prenatally to γ radiation manifested biased eye opening (Gigi et al., 1996). In exposed pups, the left eye was the leader in 62% (50 of 81) compared to 40% (31 of 78) in sham controls. The exposed vs. sham frequencies were statistically significant ($\chi 2 = 7.7$; $p < 0.01$). Exposed females showed left-biased eye opening in 59% (26 of 44) compared to 33% (12 of 36) in sham-exposed females ($\chi 2 = 5.3$; $p < 0.02$). No differences were obtained among the male pups.

Auditory Startle Response

Auditory startle response (ASR) was measured at one of the prepubertal days 27-29 (P27) in 216 rats (with 111/105 of male/female ratio) and the testing was repeated at one of the postpubertal days 57-59 (P57) (Mintz et al., 1998). This study showed normal ASR in exposed pups prepubertally. Enhanced startle in exposed rats was observed postpubertally due to significant hyperresponding in E15 exposed rats. A single injection of amphetamine, applied two days before the ASR test, unmasked the hyperresponding of the E15 exposed rats prepubertally and further enhanced their hyperresponding postpubertally. On these occasions E15 exposed rats showed delayed habituation of ASR across 16 tone-alone trials.

To further emphasize the loss of within-session habituation in the exposed E15 group we analyzed the amplitude of ASR on the last pulse-alone trial. On day P27 the analysis in the amphetamine sample resulted in a significant exposure effect, with E15 showing maximal ASR. In drug-naive conditions, there were no statistically significant differences of ASR. By P57 there was a significant exposure effect in amphetamine condition, but not in drug-naive rats. Again, E15 rats contributed the maximal ASR values.

Prepulse Inhibition (PPI) of Startle

There were no signs of PPI blunting in exposed and sham rats tested either at P27 or P57 (Mintz et al., 1998). This result, although negative, is instructive. For years, deficient sensory and cognitive gating was explored in the context of a search of the pathophysiology of schizophrenia (McGhie and Chapman, 1961; Braff and Geyer, 1990). A variety of techniques were designed and analyzed in experimental models of psychopathology and in the clinical setting. Lately, a triad of tests, comprised of (a) auditory startle response; (b) habituation of the startle response; and (c) prepulse inhibition of startle, has proved itself to be an inexpensive, reliable and replicable diagnostic battery. On these tests patients with schizophrenia exhibit a profile of virtually normal basal startle response (Braff et al., 1992), deficient habituation of startle (Geyer and Braff, 1982; 1987; Bolino et al., 1992) and consistent blunting of PPI (Braff et al., 1978; Braff and Geyer, 1990). By contrast, in combat-related PTSD patients, startle was enhanced, but showed normal PPI of the startle response (Butler et al., 1990). Thus, the dissociation between the magnitude of startle and PPI could be used as a certain marker with which to differentiate a model of PTSD from that of schizophrenia.

DISCUSSION

The major objective signs of PTSD are hypervigilance along with enhanced startle reactivity throughout the testing session (Butler et al., 1990; Shalev et al, 1992; Orr et al., 1995). This state is said to develop following excessively strong environmental stressors. We were able to reproduce a robust and lasting enhancement of startle in pups and adult rats exposed at E15 that were not subjected to excessive traumatic stress.

Initially, we pictured novel/strong stimuli to be intrinsically anxiogenic for E15 because of the activation of neuroendocrine axes. The reason for this attribution was the fact that infusion of corticotropin-releasing hormone (CRH) was shown to cause an increase in the ASR (Swerdlow et al., 1986; Liang et al., 1992). Lee and Davis (1997a,b) reported that intracerebroventricular CRH caused a robust startle-enhancing effect. However, *all* exposed rats showed higher basal CORT levels (Ben-Elyahu et al., 1996) whereas only E15 showed abnormal ASR values. Thus, there must be some other reasons for selective enhancement of ASR in E15.

A search for the system(s) responsible for enhanced intrinsic fear is not an easy one inasmuch as more than a single neuronal target must be lost after exposure at Day E15. Young neurons labeled at E14 - E18 migrate in a spatial synchrony and reach the cortical plate and other distant targets in about two days. By contrast, cells labeled at E19 - E21 may need 3 to 10 days to arrive at the destined location of the cortex (Hicks and D'Amato, 1968). As the synchrony of neuronal tides decreases, the resistance of the brain pool to damaging agents goes up.

Table 1. Distinction between Periamygdaloid and Lateral Temporal Phenomena with Electrical Stimulation (after Feindel, 1961; p. 528; with permission).

Reactions	Periamygdaloid	Lateral Temporal
Sensory	Abdominal; somatic; olfactory	Auditory; vertiginous
Motor	Complex automatism with mastication; tonic contralateral movement; tonic unconscious bilateral movement	Nil
Autonomic	Great variety of responses	Nil
Emotional	Fear , loneliness, detachment	Complex psychical
Perceptual	Behavior automatism	Hallucinations, illusions
Memory	Blocking of memory-recording with amnesia	Vivid recall
Consciousness	Confusion; unresponsiveness; drowsiness	No consistent effect
Electrical activity	Diffuse low-voltage "blanketing" and afterdischarge	Usually local afterdischarge; occasional "blanketing"
Spikes	Obliteration	Variable
Duration of response	Prolonged beyond stimulus	Brief, on-and-off

There is still another reason for uncertainty. More than four decades ago it was noticed that electrical stimulation of the limbic system in the course of neurosurgery can elicit distinctly dissimilar profiles of sensory, autonomic, emotional and mnemonic effects. Table 1, borrowed from Feindel (1961), shows that after stimulation periamygdaloid sites manifest lasting, rich and diverse autonomic, emotional, and sensory-motor responses along with alterations of consciousness. By contrast, lateral temporal sites chiefly cause brief hallucinatory effects with vivid recall. The former is more reminiscent of a state of intrinsic fear, whereas the latter looks like a brief retrieval from the repository of fragments of posttraumatic events. Although stimulation of the cerebral cortex of patients whose brains had been exposed for surgery is not a physiological method, the contrast between these effects suggests the presence of two dissimilar systems activated in PTSD. The amygdaloid network may be speculated to create undifferentiated fear, a sense of loneliness and detachment whereas lateral temporal sites may have secured the reexperience of rich perceptual material. These clinical studies are of interest for the understanding of the posttraumatic syndromes. They create an impression of the duality of the system of fear, operating in the complex and intertwined nuclei of the anterior limbic system.

The neuronal system controlling the startle response was worked out by the elegant studies of Davis and his associates (Davis et al., 1982; Davis, 1984; Rosen and Davis, 1988; Davis, 1992; Davis et al., 1993; Lee et al., 1996; Davis et al., this volume). Among the first sites of a 'defense network' we considered the contribution of the septum. The choice was explained by our previous observations of the unusually high incidence of the cavum of the septum pellucidum in PTSD patients (Myslobodsky et al., 1995) and army veterans who are HIV positive and have some cognitive deficits (Lalonde et al., 1996). There are indications (reviewed extensively by Lee and Davis, 1997a) that the septum controls amygdaloid activity such that a deficient septum could result in a disinhibition of the amygdala thereby precipitating fear and anxiety. Using a model of the intracerebroventricular CRH-enhanced startle, Lee and Davis (1997a) showed that electrolytic lesions of the medial septum, but not the lateral septum, blocked CRH-enhanced startle. Yet CRH microinfusions into the medial septum were ineffective in enhancing startle thereby suggesting that the effect could not have been contributed by the neurons of the 'septum gangliosum.' Rather the effects were associated with the fimbria fibers traversing through the medial septum. Indeed, fimbria transection blocked the startle almost completely. This experiment has narrowed the number of sites for CRH-enhanced startle to either the dorsal hippocampus, ventral hippocampus, and/or the bed nucleus of the stria terminalis (BNST), the target of projections of the ventral hippocampus through the fimbria/fornix.

BNST is a part of the "extended amygdala," comprised of the centro-medial amygdaloid (CA) nucleus and substantia innominata, along with their projections to the caudal lateral tegmental field, ventral part of the medullary medial reticular formation and the spinal cord. It is believed to set the gain of neuronal functioning and thus the output of the brain defense system (Holstege, 1990a). However, although CA-BNST neurons do carry identical neuropeptides and project to the same caudal brainstem structures (Holstege, 1990a; de Olmos, 1990), their role in coordinating defensive behaviors appears to be dissimilar. Davis and associates were able to demonstrate experimentally that the system controlling unconditioned fear overlaps only partially with that implicated in conditioned fear in these nuclei. They obtained a double dissociation between the effects of the CA and the BNST with respect to fear-potentiated startle, and CRH-enhanced startle (Lee and Davis, 1997b) and fear-potentiated and light-enhanced startle (Walker and Davis, 1997).

By juxtaposition, these studies suggest that innate fear is more dependent upon the BNST. By contrast, the expression of conditioned fear is initiated by the CA. It would be important to explore whether the CA/BNST imbalance contributed to the excessive vulnerability of E15 rats to mild stress. The BNST stretches rostrally from the CA which occupies the caudal part of the amygdaloid body. Given the rostro-caudal gradient of maturation of the limbic system, the BNST neurons must have settled in their places prior to Day 15 of embryogeny and thus could have been less sensitive to ionizing radiation inflicted at that period. By contrast, the peak of neuron production in CA falls around E15 (Bayer, 1981) so that exposure at that time could possibly produce a relatively more deficient central amygdala thereby producing a permanent imbalance of CA/BNST activity with a lasting predominance of unconditioned fear.

Two other signs of PTSD are the tendency of withdrawal and the disposition to reexperience traumatic events. In E15, withdrawal tendency from the potentially traumatic environment could be gleaned from freezing behavior in a novel environment. Prenatally, the major difference in activity between the groups of exposed rats was observed during the very first minutes of pups' encounter with the novel environment. At this initial period, E19 pups were visibly hyperactive whereas E15 pups, initially quiet, required an extra 2-4 min to regain normal level of motility. Postnatally, E15 and to a degree, E17 rats showed a familiar biphasic profile in the novel environment: a phase of inhibition during initial 2 min period followed by a phase of hyperactivity (Mintz et al., 1999). Clearly, the rather specific finding at E15 cannot be attributed to the differences between irradiated and control dames in building the nest, as well as cleaning and nursing the young. Unhealthy and sluggish mothers could have contributed to the 'separation syndrome' thereby hampering the proper development of the neuronal cells, destined to take control over behavioral and endocrine responses to stress. A possible answer to the suspicion of maternal failure is that it was not reflected in pregnancy outcome, offspring's mortality or development of exposed pups. Although we have no records on the nest building and mother-pup interactions these variables could be relevant at exposures close to the day of delivery. For example, E19 pups would be expected to suffer from maternal neglect. But that was not the case.

Model Transfer Profile (MTP)

We did not intend to model the disposition to "reexperience" traumatic events which may be tested by examining extinction of conditioned fear response in exposed progeny. Thus, given the ability of the paradigm to model enhanced startle and tendency to withdrawal, the MTP criteria of the model may be accepted as reaching 0.66.

Intrinsic Conformity Index (C_I)

Modeling of psychopathology is as successful as the proximity of laboratory phenomena to the emulated clinical reality. The presence of the desired effect should not obscure the possibility that applied maneuvers have produced a multitude of features which were not predicted. Dividing the number of planned (relevant) aberrant features (n) by all encountered behavioral aberrations in the model (Δn) will provide a quantitative expression of this disparity. We designated this ratio as the intrinsic conformity index (C_i) of the model ($C_i = n/\Delta n$).

The C_i is a post-hoc test of the model. It is concerned with the degree to which the model may spill over the target it was destined to emulate, whereas when discussing MTP one is concerned with the prospective feasibility and/or success of 'transfer' of clinical signs to their experimental analogues. It should be mentioned that some statisticians do not approve of the analysis of data that were not planned at the start of the experiment. They consider them at best, as fit for "hypothesis generation." There are, however, authoritative voices arguing that an honest body of data should not be rejected simply because it does not conform to "some favored theoretical scheme" (Cutler et al., 1966). We thus believe that C_i is useful as a descriptor of the number of potential confounds and unplanned features the model contains. If such a list is excessively long, the injury may be said to be nonspecific rather than reasonably selective. Understandably, the number of planned features may be high since most models are hypothesis-driven. Commonly, models are low on the number of unplanned features which require an exhaustive battery to be revealed. The higher the C_i, the better the model. Nonetheless, the advantage of 'unplanned' or spillover features is that they provide an important insight into some aspects of pathophysiology.

The 'Spillover' Features

As mentioned, any model may have more features than planned. In the present model we encountered such unplanned spillover items in the form of early signs of accelerated development and imbalanced infantile posture. Formally, this reduces the C_i value to 0.5 (50%). However, both items may be pathophysiologically relevant to PTSD; both may have important methodological ramifications for examining anomalies of brain laterality and their modulation by a multiplicity of systems, such as gonadal, hormonal, neurotransmitter, and lesion-related.

The disordered pattern of acquisition of developmental milestones is a typical feature of prenatal injury, and is rather common for E15 (Kimler and Norton, 1988; Norton and Kimler, 1988). The left-biased eye opening may be one of the disrupted postnatal end points. We have no explanation for the phenomenon which is hardly 'hormetic' (Wolff, 1989) for it does not seem to be of any developmental benefit. Also, it was not a specific feature, as it prevailed among females regardless of embryonic stage of exposure. Unlike other measures, it presumably implicates some systems with a long period of vulnerability. In fact, Smart et al. (1986) observed a reliable left-biased eye opening in male rats of a black and white-hooded Lister stock, following postnatal stress (an isolation and artificial feeding of newborn pups through a gastric cannula). Artificial feeding employed by Smart et al., much as other neonatal or early postnatal stressors, are more liable to affect structures characterized by an extensive mitotic activity in the early postnatal period (e.g., the cerebellum or hippocampus) (Angevine, 1974; Bayer, 1981). The late-generated hippocampal dentate granule cells and their synaptic connections are particularly responsive to this kind of stress during the first days of neonatal development (Cameron and Gould, 1996). By contrast, acute prenatal γ irradiation is associated with cell depletion as well as disturbances of migration of cells that are maximally vulnerable at a stage of exposure (Hicks, 1958; Hicks and D'Amato, 1978).*

The heuristic advantage of monitoring spillover variables can be demonstrated by pretending that we actually target a model of low birth weight following prenatal stress. That is precisely what E15 progeny permits us to do. We may then see some surprising forms of neurological and behavioral aberrations. One such unpredicted finding, in fact, appeared as the sharpened postural asymmetry in only one group with maximal signs of neurotoxicity (E15 pups with low body weight). The association of imbalanced posture with reduced weight may be juxtaposed with similar findings in humans, such as in twins discordant for schizophrenia when only the schizophrenic twin shows reduced weight along with 'soft' neurological signs (Mosher et al., 1971). Also, low birth weight is known to be associated with non-right-handedness (Ross et al., 1987; Powls et al., 1996) and increased risk of ocular and visual defects (Stayte et al., 1990).**

Finally, these data suggest the necessity to consider the possibility of imbalanced modulation of startle response in PTSD. Earlier findings suggesting the presence of imbalanced control of orienting-electrodermal activity in man were summarized elsewhere (Mintz and Myslobodsky, 1983). More recently, Morgan et al. (1997) showed a significant asymmetry of startle, albeit only in women with PTSD.

CONCLUDING REMARKS

By disrupting the normal course of embryogeny it proved possible to enhance vulnerability of a rat to environmental stressors. The effect was prenatally-induced and period-selective; it was almost exclusively noticeable in rats exposed at E15. The neurodevelopmental disorder created in E15 is a state of heightened intrinsic or unconditioned fear. Based on these findings it would not be a stretch of biological plausibility to suggest that at least in a certain category of individuals, a PTSD disorder develops on a background of neurodevelopmental deficit when a traumatic scenario sharpens rather than causes premorbid affective and autonomic deficit.

Although our findings do not allow us to make specific anatomical and or neurochemical hypotheses concerning the mechanism(s) responsible for these effects, departing from the duality of the systems controlling fear (Lee and Davis, 1997a,b; Walker and Davis, 1997; Davis, this volume) we speculated that exposure at E15 may have disrupted the CA/BNST balance. The question of whether baseline enhanced startle hyperresponding in E15 facilitates conditioned fear responses has yet to be explored.

The study of the startle response and its habituation in the rodent was dictated by psychophysiological findings in patients. However, PTSD patients are overwhelmingly tested using the eye-blink response, rather than somatic startle response. The unconditioned and conditioned eyelid closure responses are mediated by dissimilar neuronal circuits that converge on the same neuronal output (Holstege, 1990b). Yet these are different from those controlling the somatic startle response. In rodents, as well as in primates the orbicular oculi motoneurons cluster in the dorsal part of the facial nucleus. No direct projections are known from the CA and BNST to the facial nucleus, or to the oculomotor, trigeminal, trochlear or abducens (Holstege, 1990a). However, the medullary lateral tegmental field, one of the recipients of CA and BNST fibers, project to the orbicularis oculi (Holstege, 1990b). Given the differences in the organization of orbicularis control in humans it is not certain how the ratio of CA/BNST activity is relevant for the orbicular startle reflex. Also, in some cases of PTSD the facilitated ocular startle is plainly absent which makes it an imperfect physiological marker of the disorder. To mitigate this problem the present paradigm was constructed so as to co-examine the state of prepulse inhibition of startle which by and large is not deficient in PTSD. It proved to be intact in exposed E15 rats, too.

In summary, the state of heightened unconditioned fear may be greatly enhanced by mild traumatic events (e.g., amphetamine administration). DSM-III-R suggests that abnormalities precipitated by such 'mild' causes (e.g., bereavement, bankruptcy, or divorce) belong to the category of 'adjustment disorders.' But perhaps, such disorders could be more accurately designated as trauma facilitated stress disorder. Such a definition emphasizes the presence of premorbid vulnerability of the afflicted individual.

ENDNOTES

*The earlier, even if imbalanced, eye opening could conceivably signal a higher stage of brain maturation. Indeed, Narang (1977) showed that in intact rabbits the right eye is opened first. This eye showed a greater number of myelinated fibers in the optic nerve.

Among numerous signs of asymmetry in behavior and brain organization in vertebrates, ocular imbalance is an infrequent component. There is a possibility that the earlier opened eye ('the pioneer eye') becomes a dominant eye. There are occasional reports of asymmetrical eye use in lizards (Deckel, 1995), birds (Dharmaretnam and Andrew, 1994), and dolphins (Sobel et al., 1994). It is of interest that whereas both left and right eyes were used with equal frequency during non-aggressive movements, the most aggressive behaviors, including aggressive movements and biting, were done under the guidance of left eye (Deckel, 1995). In rodents, as in lizards, the optic tract is almost completely crossed which makes it likely that the right hemisphere responds earlier to communication from the left eye.

Developmental correlates of sighting dominance in humans are meager. Given that the majority of humans are right-handers with right ocular dominance, the only developmental correlate one might recall is the slightly warmer ocular temperature in the right eye in neonates (Alio and Padron, 1982), including prematurely born incubated babies (Fielder et al., 1986). Kagan et al. (1995) reported that children who had cooler skin on the left side of the forehead had lower heart rates, thereby suggesting that some autonomic reactivity and ocular dominance may be mediated by a common set of processes.

** The early trunk-tail imbalance has been compared in the past (Geschwind and Galaburda, 1985) with lateral head turning in infants placed in the supine position (Gesell, 1938; Goodwin and Michel, 1979) and may thus be conceived of as an expression of the proximodistal gradient of maturation (Altman and Sudarshan, 1975). It should be mentioned that imbalanced postnatal posture has been related to the intrauterine orientation of the fetus before delivery (Goodwin and Michel, 1979). Likewise, the tail was noticed to be asymmetric in rodent embryos younger than 15 days of age (Wilson, 1953) when the majority of embryos in the early limb-bud stages are seen with the tail curved toward the right. Only a small fraction of embryos have leftward tail flexion (Wilson, 1953; Fujinaga et al., 1988). Thus, although axial asymmetry is said to be present at birth, its 'larval' signs may well appear during the initial stages of DA prenatal history. In neonates, there is a tendency toward more symmetric posture. If this embryonic tail asymmetry is a precursor of neonatal tail deviation it might be attributed to the earlier maturation of left hemisphere machinery. Perhaps, the right hemisphere is catching up around the time of birth, thereby contributing to a more consistent bilateral activation pattern in the neonates, hence reducing the prenatal populational unidirectionality in axial asymmetry.

ACKNOWLEDGEMENTS

Supported by Theodore and Vada Stanley Foundation Research Award (1995-1996).

REFERENCES

Alio, J. and Padron, M. (1982) Influence of age on the temperature of the anterior segment of the eye. Measurements by infrared thermometry. Ophthalmic Res. 14: 153-59.

Altman, J., Sudarshan, K. (1975) Postnatal development of locomotion in the laboratory rat. Animal Behav. 23: 896-920.

Angevine, Jr., J.B. (1974) Critical cellular events in the shaping of neural centers. In: F.O. Schmitt, ed. The 2nd Neurosciences Program, Cambridge, MA: The MIT Press, pp. 62-71.

Bayer, S.A. (1981) Neurogenesis of the rat amygdala. In: Y. Ben-Ari, ed. The amygdaloid complex, Amsterdam: Elsevier, pp. 19-31.

Ben-Elyahu, S., Gigi, A., Mintz, M., Rossen, E., Myslobodsky, M.S. (1996) Stress and immune measures in rats gamma-irradiated in utero. Soc. for Neurosci. 190.9.

Bolino, F., Manna, V., DiCicco, L. (1992) Startle reflex habituation in functional psychoses: a controlled study. Neuroscience Lett. 145: 126-28.

Braff, D.L., Stone, C., Callaway, E., Geyer, M.A., Glick, I.D., Bali, L. (1978) Prestimulus effects on human startle reflex in normals and schizophrenics. Psychophysiol. 15: 339-43.

Braff, D.L. and Geyer, M.A. (1990) Sensorimotor gating and schizophrenia. Arch Gen Psychiat. 47: 181-88.

Braff, D.L., Grillon, C., Geyer, M.A. (1992) Gating and habituation of the startle reflex in schizophrenic patients. Arch Gen Psychiat. 49: 206-15.

Brent, R.L. and Bolden, B.T. (1961) The long-term effects of low dosage embryonic irradiation. Radiation Res. 14: 453-58.

Brent, R.L., Beckman, D.A., Jensh, R.P. (1987) Relative radiosensitivity of fetal tissues. Adv Radiat Biol. 12: 239-56.

Bruses, J.L, Berninsone, P.M., Ojea, S.I., Azcurra, J.M. (1991) The circling training rat model as a behavioral teratology test. Pharmacol Biochem Behav. 38: 739-45.

Buelke-Sam, J., Kimmel, C.A., Adams, J., Nelson, C.J., Reiter, L.W., Sobotka, T.J., Tilson, H.A., Nelson, B.K. (1985) Collaborative behavioral teratology study: Results. Neurobehav Toxicol Teratol. 7: 591-624.

Butler, R.W, Braff, D.L., Rausch, J.L., Jenkins, M.A., Sprock, J., Geyer, M.A. (1990) Physiological evidence of exaggerated startle response in the subgroup of Vietnam veterans with combat-related PTSD. Am J Psychiat. 147: 1308-12.

Cameron, H.A. and Gould, E. (1996) Distinct populations of cells in the adult dentate gyrus undergo mitosis or apoptosis in response to adrenalectomy. J Comp Neurol. 369: 56-63.

Cutler, S.J., Greenhouse, S.W., Cornfield, J., Schneiderman, M.A. (1966) The role of hypothesis testing in clinical trials. National Institute of Health biometrics seminar. J Chronic Dis. 19: 857-82.

Davis, M. (1984) The mammalian startle response. In: R.C. Eaton, ed. Neural mechanisms of startle behavior, New York: Plenum, pp. 287-351.

Davis, M. (1992) The role of the amygdala in fear and anxiety. Annu Rev Neurosci. 15: 353-75.

Davis, M., Gendelman, D.S., Tischler, M.D., Gendelman, P.M. (1982) A primary acoustic startle circuit: Lesion and stimulation studies. J Neurosci. 6: 791-805.

Davis, M., Falls, W.A., Campeau, S., Kim, M. (1993) Fear-potentiated startle: a neural and pharmacological analysis. Behav Brain Res. 58: 175-98.

Deckel, A.W. (1995) Laterality of aggressive responses in anolis. J Exp Zool. 272: 194-200.

de Olmos, J. (1990) Amygdala. In: G. Paxinos, ed. The human nervous system, San Diego: Academic Press, pp. 583-710.

Dharmaretnam, M. and Andrew, R.J. (1994) Age and stimulus-specific use of right and left eyes by the domestic chick. Animal Behav. 48: 1395-406.

Elsner, J. (1992) Animal-models for human behavioral deficiencies during development. Neurotoxicol. 13: 65-76.

Feindel, W. (1961) Response patterns elicited from the amygdala and deep temporo-insular cortex. In: D.E. Sheer, ed. Electrical stimulation of the brain, Austin: Texas University Press, pp. 519-532.

Fielder, A.R., Levene, M.I., Russell-Eggitt, I.M., Weale, R.A. (1986) Temperature: a factor in ocular development? Dev Med Child Neurol. 28: 279-84.

Fish, B. (1977) Neurobiologic antecedents of schizophrenia in children. Arch Gen Psychiat. 34: 1297-313.

Fish, B., Marcus, J., Hans, S.L., Auerbach, J.G., Perdue, S. (1992) Infants at risk for schizophrenia: sequel of a genetic neurointegrative defect. A review and replication analysis of pandysmaturation in the Jerusalem Infant Development Study. Arch Gen Psychiat. 49: 221-35.

Foy, D.W., Resnick, H.S., Sipprelle, R.C., Carroll, E.M. (1987) Premilitary, military, and postmilitary factors in the development of combat-related stress disorder. Behav Therapist 19: 3-9.

Fujinaga, M., Mazze, R.I., Baden, J.M., Shepard, T.H. (1988) Rat whole embryo culture: An in vitro model for testing nitrous oxide teratogenicity. Anesthesiol. 69: 401-04.

Geschwind, N. and Galaburda, A.M. (1985) Cerebral lateralization. Biological mechanisms, associations and pathology: I. A hypothesis and program for research. Arch Neurol. 42: 428-59.

Gesell, A. (1938) The tonic neck reflex in the human infant. J Pediatr. 13: 455-64.

Geyer, M.A. and Braff, D.L. (1982) Habituation of the blink reflex in normals and schizophrenic patients. Psychophysiol. 19: 1-6.

Geyer, M.A., Butcher, R.E., Fite, K. (1985) A study of startle and locomotor activity in rats exposed prenatally to methylmercury. Neurobehav Toxicol Teratol. 7: 483-88.

Geyer, M.A. and Braff, D.L. (1987) Startle habituation and sensorimotor gating in schizophrenia and related animal models. Schizophr Bull. 13: 643-68.

Gigi, A., Mintz, M., Ben-Elyahu, S., Myslobodsky, M. (1996) Left-biased eye opening in prenatally gamma irradiated rat pups. Soc Behav Neurosci Abstracts.

Gigi, A., Mintz, M., Ben-Elyahu, S., Myslobodsky, M. (1997) Prenatal gamma irradiation alters axial asymmetry in low birth weight pups. Behav Brain Res. 86: 205-07.

Goodwin, R.S. and Michel, G.F. (1981) Head Orientation position during birth and in infant neonatal period, and hand preference at nineteen weeks. Child Dev. 52: 819-26.

Hicks, S.P. (1958) Radiation as an experimental tool in mammalian developmental neurology. Physiol Rev. 38: 337-58.

Hicks, S.P. and D'Amato, C.J. (1968) Cell migrations to the isocortex in the rat. Anat Record. 160: 619-34.

Hicks, S.P. and D'Amato, C.J. (1978) Effects of ionizing radiation on developing brain and behavior. In: G. Gottlieb, ed. Studies on the development of behavior and the nervous system. Early influences, London: Academic Press, V. 4, pp. 35-72.

Holstege, G. (1990a) Subcortical limbic system projections to the ventral part of the caudal brainstem and spinal cord. In: G. Paxinos, ed. The human nervous system, San Diego: Academic Press, pp. 261-286.

Holstege, G. (1990b) Neuronal organization of the blink reflex. In: G. Paxinos, ed. The human nervous system, San Diego: Academic Press, pp. 287-296.

Kagan, J., Snidman, N., Arcus, D. (1995) The role of temperament in social development. Ann. N.Y. Acad. Sci. 771: 485-90.

Kimler, B.F. (1998) Prenatal irradiation: a major concern for the developing brain. Int J Radiat Biol. 73: 423-34.

Kimler, B.F. and Norton, S. (1988) Behavioral changes and structural defects in rats irradiated in utero. Inter J Radiat Oncol Biol Phys. 15: 1171-77.

King, J.A. (1958) Parameters relevant to determining the effect of early experience upon the adult behavior of animals. Psychol Bull. 55: 46-58.

Jensh, R.P., Brent, R.L., Vogel, W.H. (1986) Studies concerning the effects of low level prenatal X-irradiation on postnatal growth and adult behaviour in the Wistar rat. Int J Radiat Biol Relat Stud Phys Chem Med. 50: 1069-1081.

Lalonde, F.M., Martin, A., Myslobodsky, M.S. (1996) Increased prevalence of septal cavitation in a nonschizophrenic sample: An MRI study of HIV-infected individuals. J Neuropsychiat Clin Neurosci. 8: 47-53.

Lee, Y., Lopez, D.E., Meloni, E.G., Davis, M. (1996) A primary acoustic startle pathway: obligatory role of cochlear root neuron and the nucleus reticularis pontis caudalis. J Neurosci. 16: 3775-89.

Lee, Y. and Davis, M. (1997a) Role of the septum in the excitatory effect of corticotropin releasing hormone on the acoustic startle reflex. J Neurosci.17: 6424-33.

Lee, Y. and Davis, M. (1997b) Role of the hippocampus, the bed nucleus of the stria terminalis, and the amygdala in the excitatory effect of corticotropin-releasing hormone on the acoustic startle reflex. J Neurosci. 17: 6434-46.

Liang, K.C., Melia, K.R., Miserendino,.M.J., Falls, W.A., Campeau, S., Davis, M. (1992) Corticotropin-releasing factor: long-lasting facilitation of the acoustic startle reflex. J Neurosci. 12: 2303-12.

McFarlane, D.W. (1988) The aetiology of posttraunatic stress disorders following a natural disaster. Br J Psychiat. 152: 116-21.

McFarlane, D.W. (1989) The aetiology of posttraumatic morbidity: Predisposing, precipitating and perpetuating factors. Br J Psychiat. 154: 221-28.

McGhie, A. and Chapman, J. (1961) Disorders of attention and perception in early schizophrenia. Br J Med Psychol. 34: 103-16.

Mintz, M. and Myslobodsky, M.S. (1983) Two types of hemisphere imbalance in hemi-Parkinsonism coded by brain electrical activity and electrodermal activity. In: Myslobodsky, M. ed. Hemisyndromes: Psychobiology, Neurology, Psychiatry. New York: Academic Press, pp. 213-238.

Mintz, M., Yovel, G., Gigi, A., Myslobodsky, M.S. (1998) Dissociation between startle and prepulse inhibition in rats exposed to gamma radiation at day 15 of embryogeny. Brain Res Bull. 45: 289-96.

Mintz, M., Gigi, A., Shohami, D., Myslobodsky, M.S. (1999) Effects of prenatal exposure to gamma rays on circling and activity behavior in prepubertal and postpubertal rats. Behav Brain Res. 98: 45-51.

Morgan, C.A., Grillon, C., Southwick, S.M., Davis, M., Charney, D.S. (1995) Fear potentiated startle in posttraumatic stress disorder. Biol Psychiat. 38: 378-85.

Morgan, C.A., Grillon, C., Lubin, H., Southwick, S.M. (1997) Startle reflex abnormalities in women with sexual assault-related posttraumatic stress disorder. Am J Psychiat. 154: 1076-80.

Mosher, L.R., Pollin, W., Stabenau, J.R. (1971) Identical twins discordant for schizophrenia: Neurological findings. Arch Gen Psychiat. 24: 422-30.

Myslobodsky, M. (1976) Petit Mal Epilepsy. A search for precursors of petit mal activity. New York: Academic Press.

Myslobodsky, M. S., Glicksohn, J., Singer, J., Stern, M., Bar-Ziv, J., Friedland, N., Bleich, A. (1995) Changes of brain anatomy in patients with posttraumatic stress disorder: A pilot magnetic resonance imaging study. Psychiat Res Neuroimag. 58: 259-64.

Narang, H.K. (1977) Right-left asymmetry of myelin development in epiretinal portion of rabbit optic nerve. Nature 266: 855-66.

Norton, S. and Donoso, J.A. (1985) Forebrain damage following prenatal exposure to low-dose x-irradiation. Exp Neurol. 87: 185-97.

Norton, S. and Kimler, B.F. (1988) Comparison of functional and morphological deficits in the rat after gestational exposure to ionizing radiation. Neurotoxicol Teratol. 10: 363-71.

Ornitz, E.M. and Pynoos, R.S. (1989) Startle modulation in children with posttraumatic stress disorder. Am J Psychiat. 146: 866-71.

Orr, S.P., Lasko, N.B., Shalev, A.Y., Pitman, R.K. (1995) Physiologic responses to loud tones in Vietnam veterans with posttraumatic stress disorder. J Abnorm Psychol. 104: 75-82.

Powls, A., Botting, N., Cooke, R.W.I., Marlow, N. (1996) Handedness in very low-birthweight (VLBW) children at 12 years of age: relation to perinatal and outcome variables. Dev Med Child Neurol 38: 594-602.

Reich, J., Lyons, M., Cai, B. (1996) Familial vulnerability factors to post-traumatic stress disorder in male military veterans. Acta Psychiat Scand 93: 105-112.

Rosen, J.B. and Davis, M. (1988) Enhancement of acoustic startle by electrical stimulation of the amygdala. Behav Neurosci. 102: 195-202.

Ross, G.F., Glick, S.D., Meibach, R.C. (1981) Sexually dimorphic brain and behavioral asymmetries in the neonatal rat. Proc Natl Acad Sci USA 78: 1958-61.

Ross, G., Lipper, E.G., Gauld, P.A. (1987) Hand preference of four-year-old children: its relationship to premature birth and neurodevelopmental outcome. Devel Med Child Neurol. 29: 615-22.

Ross, R.J., Ball, W.A., Cohen, M.E., Silver, S.M., Morrison, A.R., Dinges, D.F. (1989) Habituation of the startle reflex in posttraumatic stress disorder. J Neuropsychiat. 1: 305-07.

Rugh, R. (1962) Low level of X-irradiation and the early mammalian embryo. Amer J Rentgenol. 87: 559-66.

Schull, W.J., Norton, S., Jensh, R.P. (1990) Ionizing radiation and the developing brain. Neurotoxicol Teratol. 12: 249-60.

Scott, cited by Janis, I.L., Leventhal, H. (1968) Human reaction to stress. In: E.F. Bogratta, W.W. Lambert, eds. Handbook of personality. Theory and Research, Chicago: Rand McNally and Co, pp. 1041-85.

Shalev, A.Y., Orr, S.P., Peri, T., Schreiber, S., Pitman, R.K. (1992) Physiologic responses to loud tones in Israeli patients with posttraumatic stress disorder. Arch Gen Psychiat. 49: 870-74.

Smart, J.L., Tonkiss, J., Massey, R.F. (1986) A phenomenon: Left-biased asymmetrical eye-opening in artificially reared rat pups. Develop. Brain Res. 28: 134-136.

Sobel, N., Supin, A.Y., Myslobodsky, M.S. (1994) Rotational swimming tendencies in the dolphin (Tursiops truncatus). Behav Brain Res. 65: 41-45.

Stayte, M., Johnson, A., Wortham, C. (1990) Ocular audio visual defects in a geographically defined population of 2-year-old children. Br J Ophthalmol. 74: 465-68.

Symonds, C.P. (1937) The assessment of symptoms following head injury. Guys Hosp Gazette 51: 461-68.

Swerdlow, N.R., Geyer, M.A., Vale, W.W., Koob, G.F. (1986) Corticotropin-releasing factor potentiates acoustic startle in rats: blockade by chlordiazepoxide. Psychopharmacol. 88: 147-52.

Taylor, S. (1978) Psychiatry and natural history. Brit Medic J. 2: 1754-58.

Walker, D.L. and Davis, M. (1997) Double dissociation between the involvement of the bed nucleus of the stria terminalis and the central nucleus of the amygdala in startle increases produced by conditioned versus unconditioned fear. J Neurosci. 17: 9375-83.

Watson, C.G., Davenport, E., Anderson, P.E.D., Mendez, C.M., Gearhart, L.P. (1998) The relationships between premilitary school record data and risk for posttraumatic stress disorder among Vietnam war veterans. J Nerv Ment Disease 186: 338-44.

Weinstock, M., Matlina, E., Maor, G.I., Rosen, H., McEwen, B.S. (1992) Postnatal stress selectively alters the reactivity of the hypothalamic-pituitary adrenal system in the female rat. Brain Res. 595: 195-200.

Wilson, J.G., Jordan, H.C., Brent, R.L. (1953) Effects of irradiation on embryonic development. Am J Anat. 92: 153-87.

Wolff, S. (1989) Are radiation-induced effects hormetic? Science 245: 575.

12 THE LATENT INHIBITION MODEL OF SCHIZOPHRENIA

Ina Weiner

INTRODUCTION

As detailed by McKinney (1988) and Willner (1991), there are several ways of going about building an animal model of psychopathology. The LI model of schizophrenia begun its way with mimicking a widely documented behavioral manifestation of the disorder, an inability to ignore irrelevant stimuli (face validity) coupled with a central neurotransmitter dysfunction postulated to occur in schizophrenia, i.e., dopaminergic (construct validity). The development of the model included its extension to normal humans and schizophrenia patients on the one hand, and an analysis of the underlying neural and cognitive mechanisms in the rat model on the other hand. I believe that the results of these lines of LI research have now converged to provide interesting leads on the neuropsychology and pathophysiology of schizophrenia, at present largely speculative, but ripe to be tested in the clinic.

LATENT INHIBITION (LI)

While a variety of behavioral tasks and conditioning procedures is used to demonstrate LI, all of them share the basic procedure: Subjects are repeatedly exposed in the first stage (preexposure) to a stimulus which has no consequences, and this stimulus is then used as a signal of a target event (e.g., reinforcement) in the second stage (conditioning). LI consists of the fact that the preexposed subjects show slower learning that the stimulus predicts the target event in the second stage compared to subjects that were not preexposed. LI can be demonstrated in many different behavioral procedures, and in many mammalian species, including humans (Lubow, 1973, 1989; Lubow et al., 1981). An extensive review of human LI data has concluded that LI is similar (i.e., sensitive to the same manipulations) in humans and animals, and can be viewed as reflecting the operation of analogous processes across species (Lubow and Gewirtz, 1995).

Based on findings that nonreinforced stimulus preexposure decreases the attention to, or the associability of, that stimulus, without affecting its associative strength, the construct of attention has been adopted by most major theorists who have attempted to explain the LI effect (e.g., Lubow, 1989; Lubow et al., 1981;

Mackintosh, 1975; Pearce and Hall, 1980; Schmajuk and Moore, 1985, 1988; Wagner and Rescorla, 1972). In short, the retarded conditioning to the preexposed stimulus is considered to index the capacity not to attend to, or to ignore, stimuli that predict no significant consequences.

DISORDER OF ATTENTION IN SCHIZOPHRENIA AND LATENT INHIBITION

Beginning with Kraepelin's (1919) observation that a "disorder of attention" is "conspicuously developed" in patients with dementia praecox, and Bleuler's (1911) analogous description of schizophrenia as the loss of "selectivity which normal attention ordinarily exercises among the sensory impressions," attentional deficit in schizophrenia has retained its centrality in numerous theoretical formulations (e.g., Anscombe, 1987; Cornblatt et al., 1985; Frith, 1979; Gjerde, 1983; Hemsley, 1993, 1994; Maher, 1983; McGhie and Chapman, 1961; Nuechterlein and Dawson, 1984; Oades, 1982; Venables, 1984). Most often, this deficit has been described as an inability to filter out, or ignore, irrelevant or unimportant stimuli, and it has been argued that the major abnormalities of schizophrenia can be derived from this single underlying deficit. Studies of high risk individuals (e.g., children of schizophrenic parents) indicate that attentional deficits may constitute a biological marker for the liability to schizophrenia (Cornblatt and Erlenmeyer-Kimling, 1984; Cornblatt et al., 1989), and there is evidence that the amelioration of schizophrenic symptoms with neuroleptic treatment is related to the normalization of attentional processes (Asarnow et al., 1988; Braff and Sacuzzo, 1982; Kornetzky, 1972; Rappaport et al., 1971).

The LI model of schizophrenia was launched by Solomon et al., (1981) and Weiner et al., (1981, 1984, 1988), who proposed that disrupted LI may provide an animal model of the widely described failure of schizophrenic patients to ignore irrelevant stimuli. Given that the predominant hypothesis regarding the pathophysiology of schizophrenia stated that excessive dopamine (DA) neurotransmission in the forebrain contributes to schizophrenia (Snyder, 1976; Meltzer and Stahl, 1976), these authors showed that rats treated with the DA releaser amphetamine, which produces and exacerbates psychotic symptoms in humans, learn about the preexposed stimulus as if it were novel. This finding established an animal model which combined the most prominent neurochemical dysfunction implied in schizophrenia, and a widely described cognitive dysfunction of this disorder, i.e., inability to ignore irrelevant stimuli.

The original demonstration of amphetamine-induced LI disruption has been often replicated (e.g., Bakshi et al., 1995; Gosselin et al., 1996; Killcross et al., 1994b; Killcross and Robbins, 1993; Moran et al., 1996; Ruob et al., 1997; Weiner et al., 1996b, 1997a,c). Importantly, LI disruption is restricted to DA enhancement produced by low doses of amphetamine: high doses of this drug as well as direct DA agonists such as apomorphine, leave LI intact (Weiner et al., 1987c; Feldon et al., 1991). A mirror effect is obtained following blockade of DA transmission by haloperidol, namely, LI potentiation (Christison et al., 1988; Dunn et al., 1993; Feldon and Weiner, 1991; Peters and Joseph, 1993; Shadach et al., in press; Weiner and Feldon, 1987; Weiner et al., 1987a, 1997b), and this effect has been shown with a wide range of antipsychotic drugs (APDs, see below). In other words, the effects of preexposure are inflated in rats treated with APDs.

Two further empirical observations have contributed to the establishment and the validity of the LI model. First, the extension of the LI model to the clinic has shown that LI is disrupted in acutely psychotic schizophrenic patients tested within the first weeks of the current episode of illness or being in an acute phase of an otherwise chronic disorder (Baruch et al., 1988a; Gray et al., 1992a, 1995b). The initial study has also shown, using repeated testing in the same patients, that LI is absent in the first 2 weeks of a schizophrenic episode and is restored to more or less normal levels after 7-8 weeks of neuroleptic treatment. Second, it was shown that amphetamine-treated normal humans, like amphetamine-treated rats, are incapable of ignoring the preexposed stimulus (Gray et al., 1992b; Thornton et al., 1996). Moreover, as in the rat, this effect shows an inverse dose-dependency, with low but not high dose abolishing LI. In addition, it was shown that normal humans scoring high on questionnaires measuring schizotypy show reduced LI relatively to subjects with low schizotypy scores (Baruch et al., 1998b; Braunstein-Bercovitz and Lubow, 1998; De la Casa et al., 1993b; De la Casa and Lubow, 1994; Della Casa et al., 1999; Lipp and Vaitl, 1992; Lubow et al., 1992). Finally, normal humans treated with haloperidol, like the haloperidol-treated rats, showed excessive LI (Williams et al., 1996; 1997). These results strengthened the likelihood that the LI effect observed in the two species is indeed functionally and pharmacologically the same phenomenon.

THE SWITCHING MODEL OF LI

While most theoretical accounts of the LI phenomenon have stressed its attentional nature, and focused primarily on processes occurring during the nonreinforced stimulus preexposure, I had argued (Weiner, 1990) that the LI paradigm could be more profitably analyzed if viewed as involving the acquisition of two independent and conflicting contingencies in preexposure (stimulus-no event) and conditioning (stimulus-reinforcement), which compete for expression during conditioning, when mismatch arises between conflicting predictions signaled by the CS. In other words, LI is a selection problem. In order to show LI, the organism must remain under the control of the information acquired in preexposure (stimulus-no event); in contrast, absence of LI indicates that the organism switches to respond according to the new stimulus-reinforcement contingency.

It should be pointed out that the switching model distinguished between the acquisition and the expression of stimulus irrelevance: while in preexposure, the organism learns that a stimulus is irrelevant, it is in the conditioning stage that the "irrelevance" of the stimulus is manifested in the fact that the organism continues to treat it as irrelevant in spite of the fact that it signals a significant outcome. In this manner, the model allowed the shift of the critical locus of "ability to ignore" from preexposure, where it had been exclusively located, to conditioning The same applies to an "inability to ignore": the deficit may lie not in the ability to ignore the inconsequential stimulus in preexposure but in the failure to continue to ignore it under changed reinforcement contingencies in conditioning; in other words, there is an excessive yielding to the immediate situational demands, and enhanced cognitive switching between conflicting associations.

In addition, the switching model emphasized that LI is a "window" phenomenon, whereby the effects of preexposure are expressed under a very specific balance between the behavioral impact of preexposure and conditioning.

Thus, LI is obtained only with a certain combination of preexposure and conditioning parameters, and changes in these parameters, such as reduction in the number of preexposures, an increase in the number of conditioning trials, or a context shift between preexposure and conditioning, cause the organism to switch responding according to the stimulus-reinforcement contingency and thus not to show LI. Moreover, manipulations which affect switching, will shift this window, so that manipulations which lead to excessive switching, will disrupt LI under conditions in which normal rats exhibit LI, and manipulations which retard switching will promote the expression of LI under conditions in which normal rats fail to show it. As will be seen below, the concept of switching has guided our research as well as the interpretation of the LI results, and has led to some predictions and consequent experimental data which would not be possible without it (see also Weiner and Feldon, 1997).

THE NEURAL SUBSTRATES OF LI

The investigation of the neural substrates of LI has naturally focused on the dopaminergic system, and on brain regions presumed to play a role in the pathophysiology of schizophrenia, namely, the limbic system (the hippocampus, the entorhinal cortex, the amygdala), the frontal cortex, and the nucleus accumbens, the target of the mesolimbic dopaminergic system which receives afferents from all of the above regions.

Dopamine, Switching and LI

Weiner and colleagues showed that both amphetamine-induced disruption and haloperidol-induced potentiation of LI do not occur in the preexposure stage. Thus, rats preexposed under amphetamine (given acutely or following repeated treatment) but conditioned without the drug, showed intact LI (Weiner et al., 1981, 1984, 1988). Similarly, rats preexposed under haloperidol but conditioned without it, showed a normal, non-potentiated LI effect (Weiner et al., 1987a). This was interpreted by the switching model to imply that both drugs do not affect the acquisition of the stimulus-no event association, but affect its expression in conditioning, so that amphetamine promotes a rapid switch of responding according to the stimulus-reinforcement association, whereas haloperidol retards such switching.

Consistent with the position that DA manipulations affect LI via conditioning, it was shown that after low number of preexposures which was insufficient to produce LI in controls, administration of haloperidol confined to conditioning, led to LI (Peters and Joseph, 1993). Later, Weiner et al., (1997b) showed that rats treated with haloperidol or clozapine only in conditioning, persisted in showing LI when the number of conditioning trials was increased to a level at which normal animals switch to respond according to the stimulus-reinforcement contingency and thus ceased to display LI. We have recently confirmed (Shadach et al., 1999) that the site of APD-induced "super-LI" is the conditioning stage, using clozapine administration in either the preexposure stage, the conditioning stage, or in both, and two sets of parameters which do not yield LI in control rats (low number of stimulus preexposures, and high number of conditioning trials). As expected, no LI was evident in vehicle-treated rats under both sets of conditions. Likewise, no LI was evident in rats which received clozapine only in the preexposure stage. In contrast, clozapine administered in the conditioning stage, irrespective of drug condition in preexposure, led to the emergence of LI. These results demonstrated conclusively that APDs do not facilitate the acquisition of the stimulus-no event contingency in the preexposure stage, but promote the expression of this learning in conditioning. Thus, when the parameters of the LI procedure are manipulated so as to either decrease the impact of the stimulus-no event contingency (low number of preexposures), or to increase the impact of the stimulus-reinforcement contingency (increased number of conditioning trials), normal rats switch to respond according to the changed contingency of reinforcement in the conditioning stage. In contrast, APD-treated animals persist in responding to the stimulus according to the information acquired in preexposure.

Compared to systemic injection of DA blockers, a demonstration of conditioning-based amphetamine effect has encountered difficulties. Weiner et al., (1988) found that amphetamine did not disrupt LI when given once only in conditioning but needed to be administered twice, at the time of both preexposure and conditioning. This double-injection regime was itself not effective if preexposure and conditioning were separated by 30 min and the injections given before each stage, whereas LI was abolished when the two stages were given 24 h apart. Thus, the requirement for amphetamine to disrupt LI is not simply that it must be present at the time of preexposure and conditioning. Weiner et al (1988) suggested that disruption of LI requires behavioral sensitization, with the injection in preexposure only serving to sensitize the animal to the second injection in conditioning. In line with this suggestion, they found that under certain conditions, LI is disrupted by two amphetamine injections when the first one is given after and not before preexposure (Gray et al., 1995a). Later, other studies showed that LI can be disrupted by one amphetamine injection given prior to a one-session preexposure and conditioning procedure (McAllister, 1997), or given once only before the conditioning session (Gray et al., 1997), provided that the injection-test interval was long (30 min and longer, see below). It should be pointed out that only one amphetamine injection is sufficient to disrupt LI in Man.

Further evidence that DA manipulations exert only modulatory influence on the expression of the preexposure effect comes from findings that the effects of both amphetamine and APDs on LI can be modified by altering the preexposure and conditioning parameters. Thus, APD-induced potentiation of LI is much more pronounced when a low number of stimulus preexposures is used which does not lead to LI in control animals, as compared to conventional numbers of preexposures which yield LI in control animals. The results are less consistent for conditioning, but the overall picture is one in which the LI potentiating effect of APDs depends on the specific combinations of preexposure and conditioning parameters (Dunn et al., 1993; Killcross et al., 1994a; Ruob et al., 1998; Weiner et al., 1996b, 1997b; Schadach et al., in press). With regard to clozapine, we have found that whereas this drug potentiates LI with 10 preexposures and 2 conditioning trials (which do not produce LI in vehicle-treated rats), when the number of preexposures is increased to 20 or 40 while the number of conditioning trials remains 2 (leading to LI in vehicle-treated rats), clozapine looses its effectiveness to potentiate LI; further increase in the number of conditioning trials to a level leading to LI disruption in controls (40 preexposures and 5 conditioning trials) restores clozapine's effectiveness (Weiner et al., 1996b, 1997b; Schadach et al., 1997b, 1999, in press). A further increase in the number of conditioning trials (e.g., 40 preexposures and 10 conditioning trials) would most likely block the capacity of clozapine to potentiate LI, as was found by Killcross et al., (1994a) with a comparable set of parameters. As for amphetamine, it has been shown that the disruptive effects of this drug can be counteracted by either increasing the impact of preexposure (prolonging the duration of stimulus preexposure; De la Casa et al., 1993a) or by decreasing the impact of conditioning (decreasing the intensity of the reinforcer; Killcross et al., 1994b). In general, since dopaminergic manipulations apparently affect the balance between the impact of preexposure and conditioning on behavior, these manipulations can be expected to be highly sensitive to and to interact with parametric manipulations of the LI procedure. This should be born in mind when investigating and interpreting drug effects on LI.

In sum, studies with amphetamine and neuroleptics indicate that the DA system is not involved in the acquisition of the stimulus-no event contingency, but modulates its expression in conditioning. Enhancement of dopaminergic transmission disrupts the control of the stimulus-no event contingency by promoting rapid switch of responding according to the stimulus-reinforcement contingency, while blockade of dopaminergic transmission enhances this control by retarding such switching. Low doses of amphetamine are known to increase, while neuroleptics, as well as other means of DA blockade, are known to reduce, animals' capacity to switch ongoing behavior in response to changed environmental contingencies (Cools et al., 1984; Gelissen and Cools, 1988; Oades, 1985; Robbins and Everitt, 1982; Robbins and Koob, 1980; Robbins and Sahakian, 1983; Van den Bos and Cools, 1989), and such effects on switching apparently underlie also the LI-disrupting and LI-potentiating effects of these drugs.

Finally, consistent with the switching hypothesis albeit somewhat paradoxical, we showed that also high doses of amphetamine produce "persistent LI." We reasoned that since such doses produce behavioral perseveration, they should block the ability to switch responding in the conditioning stage, and thus act like APDs. Indeed, when the number of stimulus-reinforcement pairings is increased to a level at which normal animals switch to respond according to the new stimulus-reinforcement contingency, rats treated with high dose of amphetamine persevered in displaying LI. That this effect was DA-mediated was attested to by the fact that haloperidol (which produced persistent LI on its own) blocked high amphetamine-induced LI potentiation (unpublished observations; Feldon et al., 1995).

Nucleus Accumbens

Solomon and Staton (1982) showed that the locus of amphetamine-induced disruption of LI was the nucleus accumbens (NAC), the target of the mesolimbic DA system, since LI was disrupted by intra-accumbal but not by intra-caudate amphetamine infusion. This was consistent with the results of systemic administration (Weiner et al., 1987c) which showed that LI was disrupted by low doses of amphetamine which act primarily via the mesolimbic DA system but not by high dose of this drug, which act via the nigrostriatal DA system. Since switching is apparently mediated by the NAC, so that enhancement of dopaminergic activity in the NAC promotes switching, whereas dopaminergic blockade in this structure gives rise to perseveration (Koob et al., 1978; Le Moal and Simon, 1991; Oades, 1985; Robbins and Everitt, 1982; Swerdlow and Koob, 1987; Taghzouti et al., 1985a,b; Van den Bos and Cools, 1989), it was only a natural step for the switching model to attribute the NAC a key role in the expression of LI. In general, the switching model posited that enhanced activation of the NAC is the final common path via which all manipulations which abolish LI, act. Conversely, blockade of NAC DA activity or NAC lesion should prevent LI abolition by manipulations that do so, and have no effect on LI or produce LI potentiation on its own, because they block the ability to switch. Studies investigating NAC involvement in LI have been in general supportive of this proposition.

Measurement of extracellular DA in NAC with microdialysis showed changes in DA release that mirror LI: whereas a novel stimulus paired with shock subsequently potentiated DA release, such potentiation was prevented if conditioning was preceded by nonreinforced preexposure to that stimulus (Young et al., 1993). The differences between preexposed and nonpreexposed stimuli in their capacity to affect extracellular NAC DA was first seen in the conditioning stage; no changes in NAC DA release were seen during preexposure. Gray and his colleagues conducted an extensive series of experiments showing that manipulations of DA transmission within the NAC influence LI (summarized in Gray et al., 1997). First, these authors showed that the LI potentiating effect of haloperidol is mediated via the NAC: Following 10 nonreinforced stimulus preexposures, NAC vehicle-injected rats did not show LI, whereas an intra-accumbens injection of haloperidol led to the emergence of LI; importantly, the potentiating effect was obtained with haloperidol injection confined to the time of conditioning. The same LI potentiating effect was obtained following destruction of dopaminergic terminals in the NAC by means of 6-OHDA lesions. Gray et al., further showed that intra-accumbens injection of haloperidol reversed the disruption of LI caused by systemic amphetamine administration; also this effect was obtained when the intra-accumbens haloperidol injection was confined to the time of conditioning. Finally, they showed that after a single systemic injection of amphetamine, which by itself was insufficient to disrupt LI, a subsequent injection of amphetamine into the NAC at the time of conditioning, disrupted LI, supporting the hypothesis that amphetamine disrupts LI by virtue of an action in the NAC at the time of conditioning, and that this action may require sensitization, as suggested by Weiner et al., (1988). With regard to the conditions which enable LI disruption by one injection of low dose systemic amphetamine prior to conditioning, Gray et al., pointed out that the long time interval required for such an effect, parallels the time course of changes in extracellular NAC DA levels evoked by such an injection, and therefore suggested that systemic amphetamine-induced LI disruption requires impulse-dependent DA release in the NAC. This can also explain why LI is not disrupted by the direct agonist apomorhine as well as by a high amphetamine dose, because they do not release DA in an impulse-dependent manner, as was suggested by Weiner et al., (1987c). We have recently replicated Gray et al.,'s finding that 6-OHDA NAC lesion potentiated LI with low number of preexposures which did not yield LI in controls while having no effect on LI with parameters which led to LI in controls; In addition, such a lesion prevented LI disruption by systemic administration of amphetamine (Gal, 2000).

The above results indicate that NAC DA is involved in normal LI as well as in its disruption and potentiation. Moreover, the critical alterations of DA transmission occur at the time of conditioning. Finally, the fact that depletion or blockade of DA in this structure produces persistent LI and prevents the disruptive effects of systemic amphetamine administration is in line with the prediction of the switching model that animals with NAC DA blocked or depleted, are incapable of switching to respond according to the stimulus-reinforcement contingency in conditioning. However, the conclusion on the role of NAC DA in LI is limited by reports that LI was left intact following intra-accumbens injection of amphetamine (Ellenbroek et al., 1997; Killcross and Robbins, 1993). As noted by Gray et al., (1995a, 1997), it does not necessarily follow from the assumption that systemic amphetamine acts via NAC DA release that intra-accumbens amphetamine should mimic the effects of systemic injection, and our recent lesion studies suggest that it might be difficult to obtain LI disruption with intra-accumbal manipulations (see below). At present however, it can be concluded that the effects of direct injection of amphetamine into the NAC do not always mimic those of systemic low dose injection, and remain controversial.

The Hippocampus and the Entorhinal Cortex

With the exception of one study which found that LI was spared by aspiration lesion of the ventral hippocampal formation (Clark et al., 1992), studies using conventional hippocampal lesions have consistently shown LI disruption (Ackil et al., 1969; Kaye and Pearce, 1987a, b; Schmajuk et al., 1994; Solomon and Moore, 1975), suggesting that intact hippocampus is necessary for LI. However, excitotoxic lesions as well as muscimol inactivation of this structure have been shown to leave LI intact (Coutureau et al., 1999; Holt and Maren, 1999; Honey and Good, 1993; Reilley et al., 1993). Consistent with the latter findings, destruction of the fornix-fimbria was also found not to affect LI (Pouzet et al., 1999; Weiner et al., 1998a). Moreover, rats sustaining excitotoxic lesion or muscimol inactivation of the hippocampus were found to persist in showing LI under conditions which disrupted the phenomenon in controls, namely, context shift. Thus, whereas in normal rats, LI was disrupted by changing the context between preexposure and conditioning, in lesioned rats LI was resistant to such context change (Holt and Maren, 1999; Honey and Good, 1993). These results indicate that LI disruption following conventional hippocampal lesions is due to destruction of axons passing through this structure but not of cell bodies within it. Furthermore, they indicate that in the intact brain, the hippocampus is not necessary for the expression of the preexposure effect in the context of preexposure but rather for the prevention of its expression when conditioning takes place in a different context. In contrast to the hippocampus, an excitotoxic lesion of the entorhinal cortex and ventral subiculum was shown to disrupt LI (Yee et al., 1995), indicating that cells in one or both of these regions are essential for the expression of LI. Spared LI after fimbria-fornix transection has led us (Pouzet et al., 1999; Weiner et al., 1998a) to conclude that the critical pathway to the NAC is from the entorhinal cortex, because subicular projections reach the NAC via the fimbria-fornix, whereas a large portion of entorhinal projections to the NAC do not traverse the fimbria-fornix (Totterdell and Meredith, 1997). Recently, Coutureau et al., (1999) compared between the effects of excitotoxic lesions to the hippocampus proper, the subiculum, or the entorhinal cortex, and found that only the latter disrupted LI. It should be noted that the disruptive effect of both a conventional hippocampal lesion and an excitotoxic entorhinal cortex lesion was reversed by systemic treatment with haloperidol (Schmajuk et al., 1994; Yee et al., 1995), suggesting that they led to DA hyperactivity, presumably in the NAC.

Medial Prefrontal Cortex and Amygdala

Both the medial prefrontal cortex (mPFC) and the basolateral amygdala (BLA) provide extensive input to the NAC, and perturbations of both regions can modify ventral striatal DA function (Cador et al., 1991; Grace, 1991; Groenewegen et al., 1990, 1991, 1996, 1999; Louilot et al., 1985; Moore et al., 1999; O'Donnel and Grace, 1998; Zahm and Brog, 1992). Electrolytic lesions of the mPFC as well as smaller lesions confined to two of its subregions, the dorsal anterior cingulate area or the infralimbic cortex, spared LI (Joel et al., 1997). Intact LI was also shown following excitotoxic lesion of the mPFC (Lacroix et al., 1998) or direct injections of DA agonists or antagonists into the mPFC (Broersen et al., 1996, 1999; Ellenbroek et al., 1996; Lacroix et al., 2000). Finally, LI was also unaffected by electrolytic lesions of the BLA (Weiner et al., 1996c).

Switching, Nucleus Accumbens Shell and Core, Disrupted and Undisruptable LI

Consistent with the predictions of the switching model, Konstandi and Kafetzopoulus (1993) reported that excitotoxic NAC lesion left LI intact. However, Tai et al., (1995) reported that LI was disrupted by electrolytic and excitotoxic lesion of the medial NAC, and this was not easily accommodated by the switching model, which predicted that NAC lesion would either not affect or potentiate rather than disrupt LI. Since anatomical and immunohistochemical studies have indicated that the NAC can be divided into two subregions, a more caudomedially located "shell," and a more rostrolaterally located "core," which are cytoarchitecturally, physiologically, pharmacologically, and functionally distinct (Deutch and Cameron, 1992; Groenewegen et al., 1987, 1991, 1999; Maldonado-Irizarry and Kelley, 1994, 1995; Pennartz et al., 1994; Zahm and Brog, 1992), we have embarked on the investigation of the roles of the two accumbens subregions in LI (Gal, 2000; Weiner et al., 1996a).

In the first series of experiments we found that electrolytic shell and core lesions affected LI in different fashions. Confirming Tai et al's result, shell lesion disrupted LI, and this disruption could be prevented by systemic administration of the DA antagonist haloperidol. In contrast, core lesion left LI intact (Weiner et al., 1996a). While the straightforward interpretation of these results was that the shell is a critical substrate for LI while the core plays no role in this phenomenon, we raised an alternative possibility based on our assumption that the switching mechanism subserving LI disruption resides in the NAC. Thus, if disrupted LI stems from excessive switching to respond according to the CS-reinforcement contingency, then the fact that LI is disrupted by shell but not core lesion implies that shell lesion leads to rapid switching (disruption of LI), whereas core lesion spares the capacity not to switch (spared LI). From this it follows that: a. the switching mechanism of the NAC resides in the core subterritory; b. in the intact brain, the switching mechanism is inhibited (modulated) by the shell. On this account, it should be impossible to disrupt LI in rats with a core lesion, leading to two major predictions: 1.While shell lesion will abolish LI, a larger NAC lesion which includes a lesion to the core in addition to the same shell lesion, will restore LI; 2. Rats with a combined shell-core lesion or only core lesion will show LI under conditions in which normal rats cease to show LI, i.e., switch to respond according to the stimulus-reinforcement contingency.

We have completed a series of experiments that have shown just that: 1. With parameters of preexposure and conditioning which lead to LI in normal rats, an electrolytic shell lesion abolished LI, while a combined shell-core lesion restored the phenomenon (Gal, 2000; Weiner et al., 1999). 2. Next, we tested rats with a combined shell-core lesion using two conditions which disrupt LI in normal rats, namely, extended conditioning and a context shift. Sham-lesioned rats showed LI with low but not high number of conditioning trials, and when preexposure and conditioning were conducted in the same context but not when they were conducted in a different context. In marked contrast, NAC-lesioned rats showed LI under all of these conditions. 3. Finally, in order to ensure that our effects were not due to damage to fibers on passage, we tested the effects of excitotoxic (NMDA) shell and core lesions. Under conditions which led to LI in vehicle-injected rats, shell lesion disrupted LI, whereas core lesion left it intact. Moreover, core lesioned rats persisted in showing LI with high number of conditioning trials and a context shift (Gal, 2000).

Taken together, the results of the shell-core experiments supported our proposition that in the intact brain, the switching mechanism resides in the core, and the shell can inhibit the switching mechanism of the core. This proposition is consistent with the pattern of results we have obtained with different combinations of shell and core lesions. 1. When both subterritories are intact, shell inhibits the switching mechanism of the core, leading to LI. 2. Damage to the shell while the core remains intact leads to LI disruption due to the removal of shell's inhibition of the switching mechanism. 3. When the switching mechanism is damaged, the inhibitory function of the shell is redundant. Therefore, with core lesion, LI is present whether the shell is intact or damaged. 4. Moreover, with core lesion, LI persists under conditions which lead to LI disruption in intact animals.

Before continuing, it should be noted that the above results carry an important implication for investigations of NAC involvement in LI. More specifically, findings that NAC manipulations (amphetamine microinfusion, Ellenbroek et al., 1997; Killcross and Robbins, 1993, or 6-OHDA lesion, Hijzen et al., 1996) left the LI effect intact were interpreted as demonstrating that the NAC plays no role in LI. Our results suggest that presence of LI following NAC manipulations may reflect disrupted core function and thus be actually an "undisruptable," or persistent LI. To clarify this question, LI must be tested under conditions which do not yield LI in normal rats. The same applies to other lesions/manipulations which spare LI. Thus, the findings that mPFC and BLA lesions, similarly to core lesion, leave LI intact (Joel et al., 1997; Lacroix et al., 1998; Weiner et al., 1996c), raise the possibility that such lesions also produce persistent LI. Therefore, the effects of mPFC and BLA lesions on LI should be re-evaluated in conditions in which normal animals fail to show LI.

SO HOW IS IT DONE IN THE INTACT BRAIN?

The findings surveyed above can be summarized as follows: 1. It is clear that the NAC and its dopaminergic innervation forms a crucial component of the neural circuitry of LI; 2. The role of the NAC in LI is apparently more complex than previously thought in that there is a clear functional differentiation between the shell and the core subregions; 3. Moreover, the effects of shell and core lesions parallel those produced by lesions to the major sources of input to the NAC: entorhinal cortex lesion, like shell lesion, disrupts LI, whereas hippocampal, BLA and mPFC lesions, like core lesion, leave LI intact; in addition, hippocampal lesion, like core lesion, produces context-independent LI. 4. The differential effects of shell/entorhinal cortex and core/hippocampal lesions demonstrate that LI can exhibit two poles of abnormality, namely, to be disrupted under conditions in which normal animals show LI and to persist under conditions in which normal animals do not show LI, and that these abnormalities are subserved by damage to different brain circuitries. 5. Finally, our analysis of shell and core involvement in LI suggests that the site of all NAC DA alterations which were shown to be correlated with normal LI, as well as with its disruption and potentiation, is the core NAC, in which the switching mechanism resides.

What is, then, the function/s of the intact NAC and its inputs in "normal" LI, or how the two NAC subterritories interact in the intact brain to allow such LI? My answer to this question requires the reminder that LI involves the acquisition of conflicting contingencies in preexposure and conditioning, which compete for behavioral expression in conditioning, and that it is a "window" phenomenon, obtained under limited and specific environmental conditions.

I suggest that the function of the NAC is to determine which of the two contingencies, stimulus-no event or stimulus-reinforcement, gains control over behavior. More specifically, the switching mechanism which resides in the core, is activated at the time of conditioning, when the previously nonreinforced stimulus is followed by reinforcement. Under conditions which lead to LI (low mismatch between conditions of preexposure and conditioning), shell inhibits the switching mechanism of the core, so that the stimulus-no event contingency gains control over behavior. Under conditions which do not lead to LI (high mismatch between conditions of preexposure and conditioning), shell's inhibition is removed, allowing the expression of the stimulus-reinforcement contingency.

On the present view, then, the NAC is not necessary in order to exhibit LI; indeed, without the NAC, LI is "undisruptable." Instead, the NAC is necessary in order to ensure that LI is flexible and adapted to environmental demands; in other words, the role of the NAC is to enable disruption of LI when environmental contingencies demand so. The relevant information for such modulation is provided to the NAC from its major sources of input.

Since entorhinal cortex lesion disrupts LI, it follows that the critical input to the shell which subserves the inhibition of the switching mechanism, i.e., "stimulus-no event," arrives from the entorhinal cortex. This information subserves what may be called "stimulus-dependent LI," i.e., attribution of low associability to the stimulus under all circumstances.

This stimulus-dependent LI is modulated by the different types of information which are fed, during conditioning, into the switch circuitry, such as the similarity/dissimilarity of context and the number of times the stimulus is followed by a significant outcome, or US intensity, etc. Since hippocampal lesion, like core lesion, produces context shift-resistant LI, it can be concluded that the hippocampus provides the information about the context; Moreover, given that fornix-fimbria transection leaves LI intact (Pouzet et al., 1999; Weiner et al., 1998a) and disrupts contextual conditioning (Phillips and LeDoux, 1995), it is likely that information on context is carried by the projections from the hippocampus via the fornix-fimbria to the NAC. In addition, since lesions to the mPFC and the BLA, similarly to core lesion, leave LI intact (Joel et al., 1997; Lacroix et al., 1998; Weiner et a!., 1996c), I expect that these two regions provide input to the core which normally subserves switching. Since the amygdala in general, and the BLA in particular, is critical for the emotional and motivational aspects of behavior, including the formation of stimulus-reinforcement associations (Davis et al., this volume; Everitt and Robbins, 1992; Gallagher and Chiba, 1996; LeDoux, 1992), this region is likely to provide the information about the US, or associative strength. As for the mPFC, this region is known to be involved in switching and flexible behavior in general, but at present it remains unclear what specific function it may discharge in LI.

Low mismatch, under which the preexposure effect is expressed, occurs with the following combination of signals during conditioning: from the entorhinal cortex = same stimulus; from the hippocampus = same context; from the amygdala = low impact of US. In this case, comparison between past and present conditions results in assigning the CS a low associability value, and inhibition of the switching mechanism, enabling the continuation of responding according to past predictions. High mismatch occurs when the hippocampal and/or amygdalar (and/or mMPC?) inputs signal a change in context and/or high impact of US. In this case, comparison between present and past conditions results in assigning the CS a high associability value, and a removal of inhibition from the switching mechanism, leading to responding according to present predictions. Switching is subserved by increased DA release in the core, whereas a decrease in core DA results in inhibition of switching.

While it is clear that the results of the mismatch analysis are enacted in the core, where the switching mechanism resides, it is not yet clear how the different types of information reach the core, and where mismatch is calculated. It is clear that the input from the entorhinal cortex does not reach the core directly but is channeled via the shell. There are at least two pathways via which information from the shell can reach the core. The first is an "open pathway" originating in the shell and traversing the ventral pallidum, thalamus and cortex to reach the core (Zahm, 1999; Zahm and Brog, 1992). The second is the shell projections to the ventral tegmental area (VTA), and the latter's DA projections to the core (Berendse et al., 1992; Groenewegen, 1991, 1996; Zahm and Brog, 1992). While it is possible that the information from the shell reaches the core via both pathways, the second pathway is of particular importance since it is likely to provide the anatomical substrate for the here postulated shell-mediated control of the switching mechanism of the core. Thus, it is suggested that via its inhibitory projections to the VTA, the shell can attenuate DA input to the core, thus preventing the switch to the stimulus-reinforcement contingency and allowing the expression of the stimulus-no event contingency.

It is also not clear where the information from the entorhinal cortex is combined with information from the hippocampus/amygdala/mPFC. Since the latter regions project to both the VTA and the core, it is possible that the calculation of mismatch is performed at the level of either the VTA or core, or both. Given that DA cells are suggested to compute an "error signal" between predicted and actual events (Schultz, 1998), and that a phasic increase in accumbal DA has been suggested to facilitate behavioral switching (Pennartz et al., 1994; Redgrave et al., 1999), it is suggested that information favoring a switch (e.g., a context-shift or large associative strength), which is channeled from the hippocampus/amygdala/mPFC to both the core and the VTA, would act simultaneously to direct switching in the core and to facilitate such a switch via the projections to the VTA. The latter can be counteracted by switch-inhibiting information channeled from the entorhinal cortex, via the shell to the VTA.

In sum, it is suggested that: a. the mechanism responsible for switching to respond according to the new stimulus-reinforcement contingency in the conditioning stage resides in the NAC core; b. presence of LI, i.e., continuing to respond according to the previous stimulus-no event contingency, or it absence, i.e., switching to respond according to the stimulus-reinforcement contingency, is mediated by signals from the entorhinal cortex/hippocampus/amygdala/mPFC. If the sum of the converging signals signifies low mismatch, the switching mechanism is inhibited, and LI is present; if the sum of signals signifies high mismatch, inhibition is removed, and LI is absent; c. damage to the switch inhibiting mechanism (shell or its entorhinal input) disrupts LI; d. damage to the core switching mechanism produces LI which persists under all conditions which disrupt it in normal rats; damage to the sources of mismatch information (hippocampus, amygdala, mPFC?) produces LI which persists under some of the conditions which lead to its disruption in control rats (only context-independent LI, or only US impact-independent LI, etc.). e. switching is subserved by increased DA release in the core, which can be inhibited by the shell via its control of DA input to the core. This conceptualization resonates with the current emphasis on the functional differentiation between the shell and core subterritories, and the view of the NAC as the site of convergence and integration of cortical inputs (Groenewegen et al., 1999; O'Donnell and Grace, 1998; Moore et al., 1999; Pennartz et al., 1994; Zahm and Brog, 1992).

Finally, I would like to note that the pattern of results obtained with LI has more general implications for structure-function relationships. Conventionally, results of brain manipulations such as lesions or stimulation are expected either to disrupt a behavioral phenomenon or to be without an effect, because it is assumed that a given brain region either plays a role in the behavioral phenomenon or not. The results of lesion studies of LI show that different structures are responsible for the expression and for the disruption of the same behavioral phenomenon; consequently, a more complex pattern of effects should be expected following different manipulations of such structures. Damage (permanent lesion or reversible inactivation) to structures which normally subserve the expression of LI, will lead to its disruption, whereas stimulation of such structures will enhance it. Conversely, damage to structures normally subserving the disruption of LI, will leave it intact or enhance it, whereas stimulation of such structures will disrupt it. Therefore, stimulation of the entorhinal cortex will spare or enhance LI, whereas stimulation of the hippocampus or the amygdala will disrupt LI. Also it should be pointed out, that unlike the outcomes of lesions to the latter sites, which can unravel the type of specific information provided by the structure (e.g., context or US), the outcomes of stimulation will not be specific with regard to the function of the structure in LI.

THE LI MODEL OF ANTIPSYCHOTIC DRUG ACTION

An animal model of schizophrenia should by definition provide an animal model of antipsychotic drug action. This means that the behavior indexed by the model should be specifically and selectively sensitive to APD treatment, and this effect should in turn be able to shed light on the mechanisms of action of APDs.

Accordingly, typical APDs were shown to produce two effects in the LI model: to block amphetamine-induced disruption of LI, and to potentiate LI under conditions that are insufficient to produce LI in control animals, namely, low number of preexposures or high number of conditioning trials (Christison et al., 1988; Dunn et al., 1993; Gosselin et al., 1996; Feldon and Weiner, 1991; Killcross et al., 1994a; Peters and Joseph, 1993; Ruob et al., 1998; Solomon et al., 1981; Warburton et al., 1994; Weiner and Feldon, 1987; Weiner et al., 1987a, 1996b, 1997b). The predictive validity of the LI model has been further strengthened by the demonstrations of its sensitivity to atypical APDs such as clozapine, sertindole, olanzapine and remoxipride (Gosselin et al., 1996; Moran et al., 1996; Trimble et al., 1997, 1998; Weiner et al., 1994, 1996b, 1997b, Shadach et al., 1999, in press) and putative APDs (Gracey et al., 2000; Millan et al., 2000a,b; Weiner et al., 1992). As pointed out above, the potentiating effect is due to the action of APDs in the conditioning stage, and it is most likely subserved by their action within the NAC. In addition, the likely mechanism is blockade of DA2 receptors, because LI potentiation is obtained with typical APDs like haloperidol which are DA2 antagonists; importantly, clozapine produces lower DA2 blockade compared to typical APDs (Arnt and Skarsfeldt, 1998), indicating that low DA2 receptor occupancy suffices for LI enhancement, as it suffices for an antipsychotic action.

APDs-induced potentiation of LI is notable in several respects: 1. It predicts antipsychotic activity for both typical and atypical APDs; 2. It is specific and selective for APDs and is not produced by a wide range of non-antipsychotic agents (Dunn et al., 1993; these authors did not find LI potentiation with clozapine, but this was shown in later studies); 3. It is obtained also in normal humans (Williams et al., 1996, 1997); 4. Most importantly, it does not require previous administration of DA agonists or other drugs so that the model does not rely on pharmacological means to elicit the behavioral index of antipsychotic activity. While these features lend the LI model important advantages as a tool for screening both typical and atypical APDs, until recently the model has not been able to dissociate between these two classes of drugs. We have now demonstrated such a dissociation (Shadach et al., in press), based on the following rationale:

While atypical APDs are characterized by a broad receptor profile, their mixed DA2-5HT2 receptor antagonism has been the feature most often suggested to account for their greater antipsychotic efficacy in general, and their efficacy in improving negative symptoms in particular (e.g., Arnt and Skarsfeldt, 1998; Brunello et al., 1995; Leysen et al., 1993; Meltzer 1989; Meltzer and Nash 1991; Nordstrom et al., 1993; Schotte et al., 1996). The serotonergic component of atypicality is particularly relevant to LI, because LI is disrupted by brain serotonin depletion (Asin et al., 1980; Cassaday et al., 1993b; Lorden et al., 1983; Solomon et al., 1978, 1980), as well as by systemic administration of the 5-HT2 antagonist ritanserin (Cassaday et al., 1993a). In spite of this, there has been no evidence that atypical APDs disrupt LI. Since serotonergic antagonists disrupt LI when given in both the preexposure and conditioning stages (Cassaday et al., 1993a), and atypical APDs potentiate LI when given in conditioning but not when given in preexposure (Weiner et al., 1997c; Shadach et al., 1999), it follows that if atypical APDs disrupt LI via serotonergic antagonism, the site of such an effect must be the preexposure stage; in addition, the demonstration of LI disruption requires the use of parameters which yield LI in controls.

We therefore tested the effects of haloperidol and clozapine, as well as of the selective 5HT2 antagonist ritanserin, on LI, using two sets of conditions: 40 preexposures and 5 conditioning trials, which do not lead to LI in control rats and 40 preexposures and 2 conditioning trials, which produce LI in normal rats. We predicted and showed that: 1. With parameters which did not yield LI in controls, both haloperidol and clozapine were without an effect when administered in preexposure and potentiated LI when administered in conditioning and in both stages, whereas ritanserin was ineffective in all three administration conditions. 2. With parameters which led to LI in controls, haloperidol was without an effect in all three administration conditions; clozapine had no effect when administered in conditioning and in both stages but disrupted LI when administered in preexposure; ritanserin had no effect when administered in conditioning but disrupted LI when administered in preexposure and in both stages (Shadach et al., in press).

These results provide the first demonstration that clozapine disrupts LI when given in preexposure. As for the mechanism of this disruptive action, it cannot stem from DA blockade, because DA mechanisms are not involved in preexposure; since the preexposure-based disruptive effect was also exerted by the selective 5HT2 antagonist ritanserin, it is likely that clozapine-induced disruption is 5HT2-mediated. In addition, the fact that clozapine disrupted LI via preexposure but spared LI when administered in both stages indicates that clozapine's action in conditioning overrode its disruptive effect in preexposure, implying that the 5HT2 and DA2 antagonistic actions of clozapine compete in LI. While the possibility of such a competition has been raised previously (Dunn et al., 1993; Trimble et al., 1998), our results showed that: 1. the competing actions of clozapine are exerted at different stages of the LI procedure; and 2. the manifestation of such a competition is dependent on the parameters of the LI procedure. In addition, since the relative potency of the two actions are dose-dependent, with 5HT2 receptor occupancy predominating at lower doses and DA2 receptor occupancy occuring at higher doses (Schotte et al., 1996), the effects of clozapine and other atypical APDs on LI should be dose-dependent. Given the above, depending on the parametric conditions and doses of clozapine, the serotonergic component should be able to override the dopaminergic component, or vice versa, leading to either potentiated LI, intact LI or disrupted LI. This may explain why clozapine-induced potentiation of LI is obtained within a relatively narrow dose range (Moran et al., 1996; Trimble et al., 1998).

Taken together, our results showed that the LI model has the capacity to dissociate between typical and atypical APDs, so that 1. both classes of drugs potentiate LI via their action at the conditioning stage under conditions which do not lead to LI in controls and 2. atypical but not typical APDs disrupt LI via action at the preexposure stage under conditions which lead to LI in controls. In addition, the results suggest that the LI potentiating and disrupting effect of atypical APDs may be due to their DA2 and 5HT2 antagonism, respectively. We have now completed experiments with additional doses of clozapine and haloperidol and with additional atypical APDs, which support these conclusions (in preparation).

THE NEURODEVELOPMENTAL LI MODEL

In recent years, there has been a growing emphasis on the contribution of neurodevelopmental factors to the pathophysiology of schizophrenia. The fact that the course of schizophrenia is characterized by the onset of clinical symptoms after puberty, and the accumulating findings emerging from brain imaging and neuropathological studies on subtle brain abnormalities which are not progressive, have led to an increasing acceptance of the notion that schizophrenia is a neurodevelopmental disorder (e.g., Bogerts 1991; Harrison, 1995; Lipska and Weinberger, this volume; Mednick and Cannon, 1991; Murray and Lewis 1987; Torrey, 1991; Weinberger and Lipska 1995).

The central postulates of the neurodevelopmental hypothesis of schizophrenia include:
1. There is a vulnerable period of prenatal development during which an acquired or present "lesion" to critical limbic structures (most notably, the hippocampus and the entorhinal cortex) alters the normal course of development but does not fully manifest itself until later in life; 2. The typical course of schizophrenia, characterized by the onset of clinical symptoms after puberty, implicates age-related factors that lead to a functional breakdown of the vulnerable limbic substrates; 3. The greater vulnerability of the male brain to prenatal insults may underlie the observed sex differences in severity, age at onset (males having an earlier onset) and other aspects of schizophrenia.

There is evidence that LI is sensitive to environmental manipulations during the vulnerable period of neonatal development, and moreover, that such manipulations affect LI in an age- and gender-dependent manner. Thus, in a series of studies we showed that LI is present in adult male and female rats which underwent "early handling," namely, a brief daily removal from their mothers between birth and weaning, as well as in female rats which underwent "early nonhandling," i.e., were left completely undisturbed from birth to weaning. In marked contrast, LI was lost in nonhandled male rats. Importantly, LI loss in nonhandled males could be restored following antipsychotic treatment (Feldon et al., 1990; Feldon and Weiner, 1988, 1992; Weiner et al., 1987b; Weiner et al., 1985). These results showed that LI is susceptible to developmental manipulations, and moreover, that the abnormality in LI exhibits an 'in-built' gender difference which may provide an animal parallel to the susceptibility of young adult males to schizophrenia (Cowell et al., 1996; Gur et al., 1996; Hafner et al., 1993; Lewis, 1992; Torrey, 1991). Thus, the selective loss of LI in non-handled young male rats may tap an early onset, gender-dependent expression of an environmentally induced brain abnormality. Indeed, consistent with the observation that gender differences in schizophrenia lessen with age, we found that whereas only nonhandled male rats failed to show LI at 3 months, both nonhandled males and females failed to show LI at 16 months (Shalev et al., 1998). In line with the hypothesis that the detrimental effects of early developmental damage are mediated by hippocampal pathology, we found that nonhandling reduced the density of NADPH-diaphorase reactive hippocampal neurons in adulthood (Vaid et al., 1997), similarly to findings in schizophrenia (Akbarian 1993). In a more direct support, Grecksch et al., (1999) have recently shown that neonatal ventral hippocampal lesion led to disruption of LI at adulthood. Recently we also found that exposure to inescapable footshock or corticosterone administration during the last trimester of pregnancy led to LI loss in the adult male but not female offspring (Shalev, 1998). Finally, given the often stressed association of schizophrenia with exposure in utero to viral infections (Adams et al., 1993; Mednick et al., 1988; O'Callaghan et al., 1991; Pearce, this volume; Torrey, 1991) and the findings of distinct immune abnormalities in schizophrenic patients (Altamura et al., 1999; Ganguli et al., 1995; Maes et al., 1995), we tested the effects of prenatal administration of the synthetic double-stranded RNA Polyriboinosinic-Polyribocytidilic acid (Poly I:C), which simulates an in vivo viral response (produces cytokines and interferons in mammalian cells), on LI in the offspring. The male offspring of rats which were injected with Poly I:C on days 15 and 17 of pregnancy, failed to show LI at 3 months. While the early manipulations described above led to LI disruption at adulthood, other pre-weaning manipulations lead to LI persistence (Feldon et al., this volume).

ADDITIONAL DIRECTIONS

Some of the additional directions of research in LI include c-fos immunoreactivity studies, and tests of LI in different strains and lines. Sotty et al., (1996) showed that nonreinforced stimulus preexposure followed by conditioning produces a distinct pattern of c-fos immunolabelling in rats' brain as compared to conditioning alone. First, areas that showed increased activity (increased labeled cell density) following conditioning, showed a decrease in the preexposed groups. Second, and most relevant to the switching model, labeled cell density was higher exclusively in the preexposed animals in parts of the hippocampal formation, the subiculum, and the NAC. As for strain differences, we (Weiner et al., 1998b) found that the inbred Dark Agouti strain differed from the outbred Wistar strain both in the development of LI as a function of the nature of the stimulus and in their response to APDs. Thus, Wistar rats developed LI to a tone as well as to a flashing light stimulus, whereas the Dark Agouti rats developed LI to the flashing light but failed to show LI to tone. Increasing the number of preexposures or administration of haloperidol failed to produce LI to tone in the Dark Agouti rats. Finally, Kline et al., (1998) assessed LI in mice bidirectionally selected for response (NR line) or non-response (NNR line) to neuroleptic-induced catalepsy and showed that resistant NNR line had a deficit in LI.

OTHER SYSTEMS

This presentation omitted the involvement of the serotonergic system in LI, although this system undoubtedly plays an essential role in this phenomenon (Asin et al., 1980; Cassaday et al., 1993a,b; Hitchcock et al., 1997; Moser et al., 1996; Solomon et al., 1978, 1980), as it apparently does in schizophrenia (Meltzer, 1989; Meltzer and Nash, 1991). Recently, there has been a renewed interest in the serotonergic substrates of LI, mainly because of the atypical APDs. Also, Rochford (1996a,b) has recently began to unravel the cholinergic substrates of LI. Given that both systems, contrary to the DA system, are apparently involved in preexposure, their investigation may reveal the hitherto unknown neural system/s responsible for the stimulus-no event association. Lastly, since all of the critical inputs to the NAC are glutamatergic (GLU), and given the well documented GLU-DA interactions in the NAC (Burns et al., 1994; Freed, 1994), as well as the growing popularity of the glutamate hypothesis of schizophrenia (Carlsson and Carlsson, 1990; Tamminga, 1999), it is high time to investigate the role of GLU transmission in LI. To date, the few available results are inconsistent: In two studies, PCP and MK-801 were reported not to affect LI (Weiner and Feldon, 1992; Robinson et al., 1993), and in one, PCP was reported either not to affect or disrupt LI depending on the mode of administration (Schroeder et al., 1998). In line with Carlsson and Carlsson's (1989) report that MK-801 blocks switching, we have now found that this compound did not affect LI with low number of conditioning trials but produced persistent LI with high number of conditioning trials (in preparation).

BACK TO SCHIZOPHRENIA

The LI model of schizophrenia has originally focused on the disruption of this phenomenon, and research on the neural substrates of LI has accordingly concentrated on LI-disrupting manipulations as valid models. The dependence of LI upon the hippocampal and the entorhinal inputs to the NAC has been considered highly consistent with the central role attributed to hippocampal and mesolimbic DA pathology in schizophrenia (e.g., Beckmann and Jakob, 1991; Bogerts, 1993; Csernansky et al., 1991; Kovelman and Scheibel, 1984; Pearce, this volume; Swerdlow and Koob, 1987), and has been therefore taken to provide further support for the validity of the LI model. Finally, the focus on LI disruption has received support and a major impetus from demonstrations of disrupted LI in schizophrenic patients.

However, the picture is now more complicated both in the laboratory and in the clinic. Lesion and drug studies in the rat have shown that LI can exhibit two poles of abnormality: a failure to ignore irrelevant stimuli (as reflected in disrupted LI under conditions which yield LI in normal rats) and a failure to dis-ignore irrelevant stimuli when they become relevant (as reflected in persistent LI under conditions which normally lead to LI disruption). In terms of the switching model, these poles reflect two extremes of deficient cognitive switching: excessive switching between associations (disrupted LI) and retarded switching between associations (persistent LI), or in more conventional attentional terms, attentional overswitching and attentional perseveration. Second, the fact that LI is disrupted following damage to some mesolimbocortical structures, but not affected or potentiated following damage to others, shows that the relationship between mesolimbocortical pathology and LI is more complex than previously conceived. In parallel, inconsistent findings have emerged with regard to LI in different studies testing this phenomenon in schizophrenic patients.

The initial clinical reports were consistent in indicating that LI disruption was associated with acute schizophrenia (Baruch et al., 1988a; Gray et al., 1992a, 1995b). Since in the first and most cited report on LI loss in acute schizophrenics, this loss was positively related to positive but not negative symptoms (Baruch et al., 1988a) and since temporal lobe and ventral striatum changes may be particularly significant in the development of positive symptoms (Liddle et al., 1992), Gray et al., (1991) proposed that LI disruption provides an animal model of positive symptoms. Indeed, these authors presented a forceful argument that positive symptoms would arise from the kind of breakdown in normal information processing that disrupted LI represents, and attributed these symptoms to disrupted hippocampal (subicular) input to the NAC, as the latter was believed to subserve loss of LI in rats (Weiner, 1990). However, in the study of Gray et al., (1992a), the acute and chronic groups of medicated patients were matched for positive-symptom score, yet LI was absent in the former but present in the latter. Moreover, in a further study with never-medicated patients Gray et al., (1995b) found that LI was absent at the start of the illness, confirming earlier results, but was reinstated as a function of chronicity of the disorder. Taken together, these results may be interpreted as indicating that LI disruption in schizophrenia is associated with the acute, or very early stages of the disorder, and that by corollary, LI disruption in rats can serve only as a model of acute psychosis.

Recently, also the relationship between LI disruption and acute schizophrenia has been challenged, as Swerdlow et al., (1996) reported on intact LI in acute medicated schizophrenic patients, and Williams et al., (1998) reported on intact LI in acute unmedicated patients. It is difficult if not impossible to explain the reasons for the inconsistency between the earlier and later results (see Swerdlow et al., for such an attempt); the difficulties associated with the diagnosis of "acute" schizophrenia, as well as the elusiveness/obscurity of many additional variables potentially affecting such research, e.g., medication history and status or the determination of the beginning of the psychotic episode, are only few likely factors. Indeed, Vaitl and Lipp (1997) found disrupted LI in acute unmedicated and medicated patients, and Dunn and Scibilia (1996) reported on LI disruption in chronic schizophrenic patients. To complicate matters further, Lubow et al., (in press) found intact LI in chronic male schizophrenics, but disrupted LI in chronic female patients.

Clearly, such results seriously undermine the validity and attractiveness of the LI model, and maybe more critically, simply discourage investigators from using LI in schizophrenic patients. The LI data collected in rats are well-timed to shed light on the confusing clinical results. Thus, from the rat we learn that: 1. Abnormality of LI has two opposite behavioral manifestations: loss of LI and perseveration of LI. Importantly, the latter appears as normal LI unless an appropriate procedure is used to unravel its "excess." 2. Disrupted LI is associated with increased DA release in the core and a rather circumscribed neural dysfunction limited to entorhinal cortex and/or shell NAC. 3. Dysfunction of most regions considered critically involved in schizophrenia, namely, prefrontal cortex, amygdala, and hippocampus, as well as NAC core, should not be expected to disrupt LI; rather, dysfunction in these regions will lead to normal LI. Likewise, both decreased and massively enhanced DA transmission should not be expected to disrupt LI. 4. Normal or reinstated LI found in schizophrenic patients is most probably, a "persistent LI," but as shown for rats, this can be only disclosed under conditions which disrupt LI in normal humans. For example, it is known that processing of contextual information is deficient in schizophrenia (Shervan-Schreiber et al., 1996), and according to rat data, such deficient contextual information should lead to spared/potentiated rather than disrupted LI.

The above implies that the relationship between mesolimbic DA and mesolimbocortical pathology and LI is complex and that such pathology in schizophrenia can be reflected in disrupted, normal or persistent LI. Moreover, the different manifestations of LI abnormality should be expected to differ in their stability over time depending on the underlying dysfunction they reflect. Thus, since disrupted and persistent LI would result from increased and decreased mesolimbic DA transmission, respectively, and given that both DA hyperfunction and hypofunction may be present in schizophrenia (O'Donnel and Grace, 1998; Moore et al., 1999), LI abnormality should be expected to behave in a state-dependent manner; in other words, LI may be present or absent in a schizophrenic patient at any given time, correlating with the underlying level of DA. Consequently, LI can be used as a state-marker of DA fluctuations.

However, more permanent dysfunction of the regions implicated in schizophrenia, as the case may be in some subpopulations of schizophrenic patients, will also be manifested in either LI disruption (entorhinal cortex dysfunction) or persistence (hippocampal dysfunction); however, these kinds of LI aberration are expected to be permanent. While I prefer to refrain from equaling operational phenomena with clinical states, it should be evident that there is more chance to obtain normal or persistent LI in the chronic state of the disorder, and/or in patients with pronounced/predominant negative symptomatology, because these states: a. are characterized by increased perseveration in general and attentional perseveration in particular; b. may be more associated with structural abnormalities in the brain; c. may be characterized by lowered rather than increased DA levels. This is consistent with findings of spared or reinstated LI in chronic schizophrenia.

The above account has several important implications for clinical research with LI: First, what is needed is a development of LI procedures in humans which can pick up both its disruption and its perseveration. While this might be a tedious task, some procedures are already available; thus, Lubow and colleagues (Lubow et al., 1976; Zalstein-Orda and Lubow, 1995) developed LI procedures which are sensitive to context shift, so that in normal humans LI is obtained in the "same-context" but not in the "different context" condition. I predict that if such procedures are used in schizophrenic patients who show intact LI, they will show LI both in the same and different context conditions. Not less important is a need to employ LI procedures in humans which are closer to those used in infra-human species, namely, without the use of a masking task. Such procedures are available (Lipp and Vaitl, 1992; Vaitl and Lipp, 1997; Surwit and Posner, 1974), and some of them have been used to show disrupted LI in schizophrenia; they should be modified to detect super-LI.

Second, LI research with schizophrenic patients (and any other pathological groups) must use a within-subject design (i.e., one in which each subject serves as his own nonpreexposed control and thus provides an index of subject-specific LI) and not a between-subject design. The use of between-subject design is indeed counterproductive if we consider the fact that it is impossible to match patients with identical states in the nonpreexposed and preexposed conditions, whereas a within-subject design assures perfect matching (see Lubow, 1997).

Third, and relatedly, groups of schizophrenic patients categorized by any criteria (symptoms, stage of illness, etc.) are likely to contain individuals who do or do not have LI. Therefore, group statistics are not appropriate because they might mask the differential manifestations of LI and thus preclude appropriate interpretation of the results. Instead, individual LI scores should be calculated and used either as a continuous measure or for grouping subjects into those showing or not showing LI. These data can then be used for various purposes, such as simultaneous correlations with several aspects of patient characteristics such as specific symptoms, illness duration, drug response, performance on other tests, etc., thus delineating distinctive subsets of patients.

Forth, LI studies should use repeated testing because only with such testing, it is possible to determine whether LI abnormality is transient or permanent, and thus to relate it to the likely source of such dysfunction.

It is customary and indeed deemed desirable to relate behaviors produced in animal models to clinical symptomatology. Given that amphetamine, which disrupts LI, produces positive symptoms in humans, and that increased DA levels are considered to be involved in the expression of positive but not negative symptoms (Laruelle et al., 1999; O'Donnel and Grace, 1998), LI disruption can be seen as a model of positive symptoms, as was indeed argued by Gray et al., (1991). By the same token, persistent LI can be seen as a model of negative symptoms; indeed, as noted above, cognitive perseveration and inflexibility, e.g., as reflected in performance on the Wisconsin Card Sorting Test, have been related to negative symptoms. While attempts to relate LI disruption and perseveration to symptomatology may be valuable in that they could foster the understanding of the functional disorder of schizophrenia as well as the research into the relationship between experimental evidence and clinical assessment instruments, I believe that the relationship between schizophrenia symptoms and LI is too complex to benefit from such attempts.

If LI disruption and perseveration are to have greater relevance to schizophrenia, the question to be asked is not what "stage" (acute or chronic) or what class of symptoms (positive, negative) they model. Rather, there are two questions: One, what brain aberration they tap, and what are the behavioral, neurochemical and physiological variables that subserve/modulate/alleviate such aberration. Animal research indicates that LI disruption represents a phenomenon which taps a rapid transient DA release in the NAC core. Such DA release most probably plays a role in the pathogenesis of schizophrenia (Grace, 1991) but it is difficult to link this neural state to particular schizophrenic symptomatology as it appears in the clinical rating scales used. On the other hand, spared or reinstated LI can be obtained under a broad range of insults to the brain as well as with decreased dopaminergic transmission in the NAC.

The second question is what specific cognitive aberration they tap, and whether they can be used to characterize distinct subsets of schizophrenic patients. The question then becomes targeted at a specific cognitive deficit rather than a complex and heterogeneous pathology. The present account offers one answer to this question, namely, that LI measures switching capacity, and that it can be used to distinguish between "overswitchers" (disrupted LI) and "underswitchers" (spared or persistent LI). Beginning from Kraeplin's (1919) classical observation that schizophrenics are unable to focus on relevant stimuli on the one hand, and are irresistibly drawn to irrelevant stimuli on the other hand, disturbances in switching capacity have been repeatedly noted in schizophrenia. Thus, on the one hand, the schizophrenic deficit has been described as an inability to maintain a major response set or a dominant interpretation of a given situation, excessive yielding to the immediate situational demands, and enhanced switching from one associative content to another (e.g., Anscombe, 1987; Bleuler, 1911; Broen, 1968; Frith, 1979; Magaro, 1980; Payne, 1966; Shakow, 1962). On the other hand, schizophrenics are known to exhibit behavioral inflexibility and perseveration (e.g., Carpenter et al., 1985; Crider, 1997; Karnath and Wallesch, 1992; Robbins, 1991; Spitzer et al., 1993; Wolkin et al., 1992). Indeed, Lyon (1991) has persuasively argued that most of the schizophrenic symptoms can be subsumed under the categories of increased and decreased switching. The advantage of LI is that it can reveal both overswitching and perseveration, and that these behavioral manifestations can apparently be mapped onto underlying brain pathology of systems which are considered dysfunctional in schizophrenia.

LI AND APDs

It is commonly asserted that both typical and atypical APDs are effective against positive symptoms whereas atypical APDs have higher efficacy for negative symptoms/ treatment-resistant schizophrenia, and that therefore, an animal model which is sensitive to both classes of APDs, may have predictive validity for the former condition whereas a model which is sensitive to atypical but not typical APDs may have predictive validity for the latter condition/s (Arnt and Skarsfeldt 1998; Brunello et al., 1995; Kinon and Lieberman 1996). Viewed in this light, APD-induced LI potentiation may have predictive validity for the treatment of positive symptoms whereas APD-induced LI disruption may have predictive validity for the treatment of negative symptoms/treatment resistant schizophrenia

However, the conclusions with regard to the relationship between the differential effects of typical and atypical APDs in animal models and their differential clinical efficacy are circular. Thus, the differential efficacy of these drugs in the clinic against positive vs negative symptoms is taken as evidence that their differential effects in the animal model are analogous to their effects in the clinic, and visa versa. Furthermore, although the distinction between positive and negative symptoms is considered as a major tool for subtyping schizophrenia, there is a considerable debate over the validity and value of such subtyping (Breier et al., 1987; Carpenter et al., 1985, 1988, 1993; Kane, 1995; Kane et al., 1994; Kay and Singh, 1989; King, 1998; Rao and Moller, 1994; Serban et al., 1992; Tandon, 1995; Tandon et al., 1990, 1993). Consequently, it is difficult to envisage how animal models can be related to the complex and debatable symptomatology of schizophrenia and its improvement by APDs.

Extending the argument presented above, if an animal model is to have relevance to the treatment of schizophrenia, the question to be asked is not what class of symptoms it models, but what specific cognitive aberration it taps, and how APDs affect such an aberration. Re-phrased with regard to LI, the question is what do the LI potentiating versus disruptive actions of the APDs reflect in relation to the processes involved in LI and by extension, how can these actions be beneficial in terms of normalization of cognitive impairment in schizophrenia.

Our answer to this question is derived from the switching model. Thus, disruption of LI under conditions which lead to LI in normal rats (as found with atypical APDs in preexposure), and persistence of LI under conditions which disrupt it in normal rats (as found with both typical and atypical APDs in conditioning), stem from excessive and retarded switching, respectively, between the cognitive sets/associations acquired in preexposure and in conditioning (it must be emphasized that I refer here to excessive and retarded switching only in terms of the behavioral outcomes, without implying specific underlying neural mechanisms; e.g., it is clear that atypical APDs produce excessive switching via different mechanisms than amphetamine, because they act via preexposure, and probably via serotonergic mechanisms). Therefore, we suggest that APDs alter cognitive switching, and that they may alleviate some of the schizophrenic symptoms by normalizing disturbances in switching capacity characteristic of schizophrenia. It also follows that atypical APDs which can exert a bi-directional effect on switching, should be more effective than typical APDs, and that typical APDs which can only retard switching, can in fact be ineffective or even deleterious in schizophrenia states characterized by retarded switching capacity/perseveration. Indeed, the latter condition is associated to a greater extent with negative symptoms/chronic schizophrenia, consistent with our suggestion that atypical APDs, which are more effective against these symptoms, can increase switching.

Clearly, the translation of the above suggestion to clinical treatment is not simple. In the laboratory rat, we use parameters of preexposure and conditioning which produce different levels of switching and thus enable to tap separately the switch-retarding and the switch-enhancing action of APDs. In clinical use, both actions are exerted on the same level of switching of the patient, and therefore, the capacity of atypical APDs to modulate switching will be a function of a complex interaction with the underlying level of switching of the patient. Moreover, if D2 and 5HT2 antagonisms compete, the relative capacity of atypical APDs to retard/enhance switching should be a function of dose, which will determine the relative balance between 5HT2 and D2 antagonism. While the above is highly speculative, it should be pointed out that if we are correct, then one could use performance of schizophrenic patients on cognitive tests measuring switching/perseveration for the choice of drugs and dose. Clearly, absence or presence of LI may provide one test which can aid in determining the current state of switching of the patient, and thus determine the choice of treatment.

It is of interest to note here that we found that clozapine has lower efficacy to potentiate LI with high number of conditioning trials than haloperidol, suggesting that at least at some doses, this drug has an in-built mechanism, presumably its 5HT2 antagonism, which counteracts excessive retardation of switching by the DA antagonism. Therefore, if 5HT2 action and D2 action compete in their effects on switching, it follows that in comparison to typical APDs, atypical APDs will always produce a more balanced regulation of switching capacity, and are thus better suited to regulate switching relative to the current abnormal state of switching. This is reminiscent of Meltzer's (1989, 1991) suggestion that the dysfunction characterizing schizophrenia may result from imbalance between dopaminergic and serotonergic activity and that clozapine may exert its unique effects by correcting this imbalance.

To the best of my knowledge, APDs effects have not been related to normalization of switching capacity; but the latter might explain why atypical APDs may improve cognitive deficits, given that many such deficits have the form of perseveration (e.g., on the WCST), as well as their beneficial effects on depressive symptoms.

CONCLUSION

Not surprisingly, the more we investigate the LI model, the more complicated it becomes. At the time I formulated the switching model of LI in 1990, the story of switching was simple: mismatch analysis was performed by the hippocampus, which in turn inhibited directly the switching mechanism of the NAC via the subiculum-NAC projection. Indeed, the subiculo-accumbal projection has become a basis for a neuropsychology of schizophrenia (Gray et al., 1991). Today it is clear that the subiculum-NAC substrate is a gross oversimplification, and that the circuitry of a seemingly simple phenomenon like LI is exquisitely complex and sophisticated: from what we know (and most of it we do not know yet), the hippocampus is responsible for only one aspect of mismatch calculation (context), switching is determined by inputs from several sources to the NAC, the switching mechanism is in the core, and it is modulated by the shell.

Likewise, till recently, the APD story seemed orderly: amphetamine disrupts LI, APDs prevent such disruption and on their own, potentiate LI; the latter was considered as a congruent manifestation of antipsychotic action, and it was (conveniently) disregarded that presence of LI under conditions which disrupt it in normal rats is not normal. With the discovery that atypical APDs disrupt LI, the story becomes more complicated; indeed, it is rather remarkable, although at second thought, not surprising, that atypical APDs produce the same two alterations of switching which, if produced by other mechanisms, are considered as analogs of cognitive deficits in schizophrenia. The answer to this seeming paradox is trivial: while certain drug effects are abnormal when they occur in a normal system, they can be beneficial when they are exerted on an abnormal system. Thus, if the system overswitches, a drug which retards switching will be beneficial, and the opposite will be true for a system which perseverates.

In view of this increasing complexity, I would like to note two points: one, although the LI model has become more complex in the laboratory, its implications to the clinic have not lessened but have grown. Second, while the LI model can apparently be applied to the clinic, and such an application is viewed as the most impressive criterion of models' validity, I am not sure this is very important. I believe that animal models should not necessarily be judged by their direct application to the clinic, but rather by their success to provide a reasonably "closed" picture of a cognitive/behavioral deficit, its underlying brain substrates and its sensitivity to relevant treatment, which can demonstrate the plausibility of a certain conception of the modeled psychopathological condition and its treatment. In the case of LI, the model demonstrates the plausibility of the concept that dysfunction of various components of the limbic and the mesolimbic DA system, including one of a developmental origin, can indeed give rise to two behavioral/cognitive aberrations, attentional overswitching and attentional perseveration, which are thought to be core characteristics of schizophrenia from the very inception of the dementia praecox (Kraepelin, 1913), and that APDs may exert their beneficial effects by counteracting these aberrations.

I believe that further research into the involvement of brain systems implicated in schizophrenia (notably, serotonergic, glutamatergic and GABAergic), in LI, will continue to provide insights into the behavioral, pharmacological, and neural mechanisms underlying organisms' capacity to effectively ignore unimportant aspects of their environment. Indeed, I will not be surprised if various manipulations of all of these systems are shown to produce both disrupted and persistent LI, albeit via different mechanisms and sites of action.

Acknowledgements. I am indebted to Daphna Joel for her critical reading of the manuscript.

REFERENCES

Ackil, J., Mellgren, R.L., Halgren, C., Frommer, S.P. (1969) Effects of CS preexposure on avoidance learning in rats with hippocampal lesions. J Comp Physiol Psychol. 69: 739-747.

Adams, W., Kendell, R.E., Hare, E.H., Munk-Jorgensen, P. (1993) Epidemiological evidence that maternal influenza contributes to the aetiology of schizophrenia. An analysis of Scottish, English, and Danish data. Br J Psychiatry 163: 522-34.

Akbarian, S., Vinuela, A., Kim, J.J., Potkin, S.G., Bunney, W.E., Jr., Jones, E.G. (1993) Distorted distribution of nicotinamide-adenine dinucleotide phosphate- diaphorase neurons in temporal lobe of schizophrenics implies anomalous cortical development. Arch Gen Psychiatry 50: 178-87.

Altamura, A.C., Boin, F., Maes, M. (1999) HPA axis and cytokines dysregulation in schizophrenia: Potential implications for the antipsychotic treatment. Eur J Neuropsychopharmacol. 10: 1-4.

Anscombe, F. (1987) The disorder of consciousness in schizophrenia. Schiz Bull. 13: 241-260.

Arnt, J. and Skarsfeldt, T. (1998) Do novel antipsychotics have similar pharmacological characteristics? A review of the evidence. Neuropsychopharmacology 18: 63-101.

Asarnow, R.F., Marder, S.R., J., M., Van Putten, T., Zimmerman, K.E. (1988) Differential effect of low and conventional doses of fluphenazine on schizophrenic outpatients with good or poor information-processing abilities. Arch Gen Psychiatry 45: 822-826.

Asin, K.E., Wirtshafter, D., Kent, E.W. (1980) The effects of electrolytic median raphe lesions on two measures of latent inhibition. Behav Neur Biol. 28: 408-417.

Bakshi, V.P., Geyer, M.A., Taaid, N., Swerdlow, N.R. (1995) A comparison of the effects of amphetamine, strychnine and caffeine on prepulse inhibition and latent inhibition. Behav Pharmacol. 6: 801-809.

Baruch, I., Hemsley, D., Gray, J.A. (1988a) Differential performance of acute and chronic schizophrenics in a latent inhibition task. J Nerv Ment Dis. 176: 598-606.

Baruch, I., Hemsley, D.R., Gray, J.A. (1988b) Latent inhibition and 'psychotic pronness' in normal subjects. Pers Indiv Differ. 9: 777-783.

Beckmann, H. and Jakob, H. (1991) Prenatal disturbances of nerve cell migration in the entorhinal region: a common vulnerability factor in functional psychoses. J Neural Trans. 84: 155-164.

Berendse, H.W., Groenewegen, H.J., Lohman, A.H.M. (1992) Compartmental distribution of ventral striatal neurons projecting to the ventral mesencephalon in the rat. J Neurosci. 12: 2070-2103.

Bleuler, E. (1911) Dementia Praecox or the Group of Schizophrenias. New York: International Universities Press.

Bogerts, B. (1991) The neuropathology of schizophrenia: Pathophysiological and neurodevelopmental implications. In S.A. Mednick, T.D. Cannon, C.E. Barr and M. Lyon, ed. Fetal neural development and adult schizophrenia, Cambridge: Cambridge University Press.

Bogerts, B. (1993) Recent advances in the neuropathology of schizophrenia. Schizophr. Bull. 19: 431-445.

Braff, D.L. and Sacuzzo, D.P. (1982) Effect of antipsychotic medication on speed of information processing in schizophrenic patients. Am J Psychiatry 139: 1127-1130.

Braunstein-Bercovitz, H., Lubow, R.E. (1998) Are high schizotypal normal participants distractible or limited in attentional resources? A study of latent inhibition as a function of masking task load and schizotypy. J Abn Psychol. 107: 659-670.

Breier, A., Wolkowitz, O.M., Doran, A.R., Roy, A., Boronow, J., Hommer, D.W., Pickar, D. (1987) Neuroleptic responsivity of negative and positive symptoms in schizophrenia. Am J Psychiatry 144: 1549-1555.

Broen, W.E. (1968) Schizophrenia: research and theory. New York: Academic Press.

Broersen, L.M., Feldon, J., Weiner, I. (1999) Dissociative effects of apomorphine infusions into the medial prefrontal cortex of rats on latent inhibition, prepulse inhibition and amphetamine-induced locomotion. Neuroscience 94: 39-46.

Broersen, L.M., Heinsbroek, R.P., de Bruin, J.P., Olivier, B. (1996) Effects of local application of dopaminergic drugs into the medial prefrontal cortex of rats on latent inhibition. Biol Psychiatry 40: 1083-90.

Brunello, N., Masotto, C., Steardo, L., Markstein, R., Racagni, G. (1995) New insights into the biology of schizophrenia through the mechanism of action of clozapine. Neuropsychopharmacolog 13: 177-213.

Burns, L.H., Everitt, B.J., Kelley, A.E., Robbins, T.W. (1994) Glutamate-dopamine interactions in the ventral striatum: role in locomotor activity and responding with conditioned reinforcement. Psychopharmacology 115: 516-28.

Cador, M., Robbins, T.W., Everitt, B.J., Simon, H., LeMoal, M., Stinus, L. (1991) Limbic-striatal interactions in reward-related processes: modulation by the dopaminergic system. In P. Willner and J. Scheel-Kruger, ed. The mesolimbic dopamine system: from motivation to action, Chichester: John Wiley.

Carlsson, M. and Carlsson, A. (1989) The NMDA antagonist MK-801 causes marked locomotor stimulation in monoamine-depleted mice. J Neural Transm. 75: 221-6.

Carlsson, M. and Carlsson, A. (1990) Schizophrenia: a subcortical neurotransmitter imbalance syndrome? Schizophr Bull. 16: 425-32.

Carpenter, W.T., Buchanan, R.W., Kirkpatrick, B., Tamminga, C., Wood, F. (1993) Strong inference, theory testing, and the neuroanatomy of schizophrenia. Arch Gen Psychiatry 50: 825-831.

Carpenter, W.T., Heinrichs, D.W., Alphs, L.D. (1985) Treatment of negative symptoms. Schiz Bull. 11: 440-452.

Carpenter, W.T., Heinrichs, D.W., Wagman, A.M. (1988) Deficit and nondeficit forms of schizophrenia: The concept. Am J Psychiatry 145: 578-583.

Cassaday, H.F., Hodges, H., Gray, J.A. (1993a) The effects of ritanserin, RU 24969 and 8-OH-DPAT on latent inhibition in the rat. Psychopharmacology 7: 63-71.

Cassaday, H.J., Mitchell, S.N., Williams, J.H., Gray, J.A. (1993b) 5,7-Dihydroxytryptamine lesions in the fornix-fimbria attenuate latent inhibition. Behav Neural Biol. 59: 194-207.

Christison, G.W., Atwater, G.E., Dunn, L.A., Kilts, C.D. (1988) Haloperidol enhancement of latent inhibition: Relation to therapeutic action? Biol Psychiatry 23: 746-749.

Clark, A.J.M., Feldon, J., Rawlins, J.N.P. (1992) Aspiration lesions of rat ventral hippocampus disinhibit responding in conditioned suppression or extinction, but spare latent inhibition and the partial reinforcement extinction effect. Neuroscience 48: 821-829.

Cools, A., Jaspers, R., Schwartz, M., Sontag, K.H., Vrijmoed de Vries, M., Van den Bereken, J. (1984) Basal ganglia and switching motor programs. In J.S. McKenzie, R.E. Kemm and N. Wilcock, ed. The basal ganglia, New York: Plenum Press.

Cornblatt, B., Erlenmeyer- Kimling, L. (1984) Early attentional predictors of adolescent behavioral disturbances in children at risk for schizophrenia. In N.F. Watt, E.F. Anthony, L.C. Wynne and J.E. Rolf, ed. Children at risk for schizophrenia: A longitudinal perspective, New York: Cambridge University Press.

Cornblatt, B. and Winters, L., Erlenmeyer-Kimling, L. (1989) Attentional markers of schizophrenia: Evidence from the New York high-risk study. In S.C. Schulz and C.A. Tamminga, ed. Schizophrenia: Scientific Progress, New-York: Oxford University Press.

Cornblatt, B.A., Lezenweger, M.F., Dworkin, R.H., Erlenmeyer-Kimling, L. (1985) Positive and negative schizophrenic symptoms, attention, and information processing. Schiz Bull. 11: 397-408.

Coutureau, E., Galani, R., Gosselin, O., Majchrzak, M., Di Scala, G. (1999) Entorhinal but not hippocampal or subicular lesions disrupt latent inhibition in rats. Neurobiol Learn Mem. 72: 143-57.

Cowell, P.E., Kostianovsky, D.J., Gur, R.C., Turetsky, B.I., Gur, R.E. (1996) Sex differences in neuroanatomical and clinical correlations in schizophrenia. Am J Psychiatry 153: 799-805.

Crider, A. (1997) Perseveration in schizophrenia. Schiz Bull. 23: 63-74.

Csernansky, J.G., Murphy, G.M., Faustman, W.O. (1991) Limbic/mesolimbic connections and the pathogenesis of schizophrenia. Biol Psychiatry 30: 383-400.

De la Casa, G. and Lubow, R.E. (1994) Memory for attended and nominally unattended stimuli in low and high psychotic-prone normal subjects: the effects of test-anticipation. Pers Ind Diff. 17: 783-789.

De la Casa, L.G., Ruiz, G., Lubow, R.E. (1993a) Amphetamine-produced attenuation of latent inhibition is modulated by stimulus preexposure duration: implications for schizophrenia. Biol Psychiatry 33: 707-711.

De la Casa, L.G., Ruiz, G., Lubow, R.E. (1993b) Latent inhibition and recall/recognition of irrelevant stimuli as a function of preexposure duration in high and low psychotic-prone normals. Br J Psychol. 84: 119-132.

Della Casa, V., Hofer, I., Weiner, I., Feldon, J. (1999) Effects of smoking status and schizotypy on latent inhibition. J Psychopharmacol. 13: 45-57.

Deutch, A.Y. and Cameron, D.S. (1992) Pharmacological characterization of dopamine systems in the nucleus accumbens core and shell. Neuroscience 46: 49-56.

Dunn, L.A., Atwater, G.E., Kilts, C.D. (1993) Effects of antipsychotic drugs on latent inhibition: Sensitivity and specificity of an animal behavioral model of clinical drug action. Psychopharmacology 112: 315-23.

Dunn, L.A. and Scibilia, R.J. (1996) Reaction time and pupil response measures show reduced latent inhibition in chronic schizophrenia. Soc Neurosci. 22:

Ellenbroek, B.A., Budde, S., Cools, A.R. (1996) Prepulse inhibition and latent inhibition: The role of dopamine in the medial prefrontal cortex. Neuroscience 75: 535-542.

Ellenbroek, B.A., Knobbout, D.A., Cools, A.R. (1997) The role of mesolimbic and nigrostriatal dopamine in latent inhibition as measured with the conditioned taste aversion paradigm. Psychopharmacology 129: 112-120.

Everitt, B. and Robbins, T.W. (1992) Amygdala-ventral striatal interactions and reward-related processes. In J.P. Aggleton, ed. The Amygdala. Neurobiological Aspects of Emotion, Memory and Mental Dysfunction, Chichester: Wiley-Liss.

Feldon, J., Avnimelech-Gigus, N., Weiner, I. (1990) The effects of pre- and postweaning rearing conditions on latent inhibition and partial reinforcement extinction effect in male rats. Behav Neural Biol. 53: 189-204.

Feldon, J., Shalev, U., Weiner, I. (1995) "Super" latent inhibition (LI) with high dose of amphetamine. Soc Neurosci Abstracts. 21: 1230.

Feldon, J., Shofel, A., Weiner, I. (1991) Latent inhibition is unaffected by direct dopamine agonists. Pharmacol Biochem Behav. 38: 309-314.

Feldon, J. and Weiner, I. (1988) Long-term attentional deficit in nonhandled males: possible involvement of the dopaminergic system. Psychopharmacology 95: 231-236.

Feldon, J. and Weiner, I. (1991) The latent inhibition model of schizophrenic attention disorder: Haloperidol and sulpiride enhance rats' ability to ignore irrelevant stimuli. Biol Psychiatry 29: 635-646.

Feldon, J. and Weiner, I. (1992) From an animal model of an attentional deficit towards new insights into the pathophysiology of schizophrenia. J Psychiat Res. 26: 345-366.

Freed, W.J. (1994) Glutamatergic mechanisms mediating stimulant and antipsychotic drug effects. Neurosci Biobehav Rev. 18: 111-120.

Frith, C.D. (1979) Consciousness, information processing and schizophrenia. Br J Psychiatry 134: 225-235.

Gal, G. (2000) Disrupted and undisruptable latent inhibition following shell and core lesions: The dual role of the nucleus accumbens in latent inhibition. Dept Psychol, Tel Aviv University.

Gallagher, M. and Chiba, A.A. (1996) The amygdala and emotion. Curr Opin Neurobiol. 6: 221-7.

Ganguli, R., Brar, J.S., Chengappa, K.R., DeLeo, M., Yang, Z.W., Shurin, G., Rabin, B.S. (1995) Mitogen-stimulated interleukin-2 production in never-medicated, first-episode schizophrenic patients: The influence of age at onset and negative symptoms. Arch Gen Psychiatry 52: 668-72.

Gelissen, M. and Cools, A. (1988) Effect of intracaudate haloperidol and apomorphine on switching motor patterns upon current behavior of cats. Behav Brain Res. 29: 17-26.

Gjerde, P.F. (1983) Attentional capacity dysfunction and arousal in schizophrenia. Psychol Bull. 93: 57-72.

Gosselin, G., Oberling, P., Di Scala, G. (1996) Antagonism of amphetamine-induced disruption of latent inhibition by the atypical antipsychotic olanzapine in rats. Behav Pharmacol. 7: 820-826.

Grace, A.A. (1991) Phasic versus tonic dopamine release and the modulation of dopamine system responsivity: A hypothesis for the etiology of schizophrenia. Neuroscience 41: 1-24.

Gracey, D.J., Bell, R., King, D.J. (2000) PD-135,158, a cholecystokinin(B) antagonist, enhances latent inhibition. Pharmacol Biochem Behav. 65: 459-463.

Gray, J.A., Feldon, J., Rawlins, J.N.P., Hemsley, D.R., Smith, A.D. (1991) The neuropsychology of schizophrenia. Behav Brain Sci. 14: 1-84.

Gray, J.A., Joseph, M.H., Hemsley, D.R., Young, A.M.J., Warburton, E.C., Boulenguez, P., Grigoryan, G.A., Peters, S.L., Rawlins, J.N.P., Tai, C.T., Yee, B.K., Cassaday, H., Weiner, I., Gal, G., Gusak, O., Joel, D., Shadach, E., Shalev, U., Tarrasch, R., Feldon, J. (1995a) The role of mesolimbic dopaminergic and retrohippocampal afferents to the nucleus accumbens in latent inhibition: implications for schizophrenia. Behav Brain Res. 71: 19-31.

Gray, J.A., Moran, P.M., Grigoryan, G., Peters, S.L., Young, A.M.J., Joseph, M.H. (1997) Latent inhibition: the nucleus accumbens connection revisited. Behav Brain Res. 88: 27-34.

Gray, N.S., Hemsley, D.R., Gray, J.A. (1992a) Abolition of latent inhibition in acute, but not chronic, schizophrenics. Neurol Psychiatr Brain Res. 1: 83-89.

Gray, N.S., Pickering, A.D., Hemsley, D.R., Dawling, S., Gray, J.A. (1992b) Abolition of latent inhibition by a single 5 mg dose of d-amphetamine in Man. Psychopharmacology 107: 425-430.

Gray, N.S., Pilowsky, L.S., Gray, J.A., Kerwin, R.W. (1995b) Latent inhibition in drug naive schizophrenics: relationship to duration of illness and dopamine D2 binding using SPET. Schiz Res. 17: 95-107.

Grecksch, G., Bernstein, H.G., Becker, A., Hollt, V., Bogerts, B. (1999) Disruption of latent inhibition in rats with postnatal hippocampal lesions. Neuropsychopharmacology 20: 525-32.

Groenewegen, H.G., Wright, C.I., Beijer, V.J., Voorn, P. (1999) Convergence and segregation of ventral striatal inputs and outputs. In J.F. McGintry, ed. Advancing from the ventral striatum to the extended amygdala, New York: Annals of the New York Academy of Sciences.

Groenewegen, H.J., Berendse, H.W., Meredith, G.E., Haber, S.N., Voorn, P., Wolters, J.G., Lohman, A.H.M. (1991) Functional anatomy of the ventral, limbic system-innervated striatum. In P. Willner and J. Scheel-Kruger, ed. The mesolimbic dopamine system: from motivation to action, Chinchester: John Wiley.

Groenewegen, H.J., Berendse, H.W., Wolters, J.G., Lohman, A.H.M. (1990) The anatomical relationship of the prefrontal cortex with the striatopallidal system, the thalamus and the amygdala: evidence for a parallel organization. Prog Brain Res. 85: 95-118.

Groenewegen, H.J., Vermeulen-Van der Zee, E., te Kortschot, A., Witter, M.P. (1987) Organization of the projections from the subiculum to the ventral striatum in the rat. A study using anterograde transport of phaseolus vulgaris leucoagglutinin. Neuroscience 23: 103-120.

Groenewegen, H.J., Wright, C.I., Beijer, A.V.J. (1996) The nucleus accumbens: gateway for limbic structures to reach the motor system? Prog Brain Res. 107: 485-511.

Gur, R.E., Petty, R.G., Turetsky, B.I., Gur, R.C. (1996) Schizophrenia throughout life: Sex differences in severity and profile of symptoms. Schiz Res. 21: 1-12.

Hafner, H., Riecher-Rossler, A., An Der Heiden, W., Maurer, K., Fatkenheuer, B., Loffler, W. (1993) Generating and testing a causal explanation of the gender difference in age at first onset of schizophrenia. Psychol Med. 23: 925-40.

Harrison, P.J. (1995) On the neuropathology of schizophrenia and its dementia: neurodevelopmental, neurodegenerative, or both? Neurodegeneration 4: 1-12.

Hemsley, D.R. (1993) A simple (or simplistic?) cognitive model for schizophrenia. Behav Res Ther. 31: 633-645.

Hemsley, D.R. (1994) Cognitive disturbance as the link between schizophrenic symptoms and their biological bases. Neurol Psychiatry Brain Res. 2: 163-170.

Hijzen, T., Gommans, J., Poth, M., Wolterink, G. (1996) 6-OHDA lesion in the nucleus accumbens do not affect latent inhibition. Behav Pharmacol. 5 (Suppl1): 121.

Hitchcock, J.M., Lister, S., Fischer, T.R., Wettstein, J.G. (1997) Disruption of latent inhibition in the rat by the 5-HT2 agonist DOI: effects of MDL 100,907, clozapine, risperidon and haloperidol. Behav Brain Res. 88: 43-49.

Holt, W. and Maren, S. (1999) Muscimol inactivation of the dorsal hippocampus impairs contextual retrieval of fear memory. J Neurosci. 19: 9054-62.

Honey, R.C. and Good, M. (1993) Selective hippocampal lesions abolish the contextual specificity of latent inhibition and conditioning. Behav Neurosci. 107: 23-33.

Joel, D., Weiner, I., Feldon, J. (1997) Electrolytic lesions of the medial prefrontal cortex in rats disrupt performance on an analog of Wisconsin Card Sorting Test but do not disrupt latent inhibition: Implications for animal models of schizophrenia. Behav Brain Res. 85: 187-201.

Kane, J.M. (1995) Current problems with the pharmacotherapy of schizophrenia. Clin Neuropharmacol. 18: S154-S161.

Kane, J.M., Safferman, A.Z., Pollack, S., Johns, C. (1994) Clozapine, negative symptoms, and extrapyramidal side effects. J Clin Psychiatry 55: S74-S77.

Karnath, H.O. and Wallesch, C.W. (1992) Inflexibility of mental planning: a characteristic disorder with prefrontal lobe lesions? Neuropsychologia 30: 1011-6.

Kay, S.R. and Singh, M.M. (1989) The positive-negative distinction in drug-free schizophrenic patients. Arch Gen Psychiatry 46: 711-718.

Kaye, H. and Pearce, J.M. (1987a) Hippocampal lesions attenuate latent inhibition and the decline of the orienting response in rats. Quart J Exp Psychol. 39B: 107-125.

Kaye, H. and Pearce, J.M. (1987b) Hippocampal lesions attenuate latent inhibition of a CS and of a neutral stimulus. Psychobiology 15: 293-299.

Killcross, A.S., Dickinson, A., Robbins, T.W. (1994a) Effects of the neuroleptic alpha-flupenthixol on latent inhibition in aversively - and appetitively - motivated paradigms: Evidence for dopamine-reinforcer interactions. Psychopharmacology 115: 196-205.

Killcross, A.S., Dickinson, A., Robbins, T.W. (1994b) Amphetamine-induced disruptions of latent inhibition are reinforcer mediated: Implications for animal models of schizophrenic attentional dysfunction. Psychopharmacology 115: 185-195.

Killcross, A.S. and Robbins, T.W. (1993) Differential effects of intra-accumbens and systemic amphetamine on latent inhibition using an on-baseline, within-subject conditioned suppression paradigm. Psychopharmacology 110: 479-489.

King, D.J. (1998) Drug treatment of the negative symptoms of schizophrenia. Eur J Neuropsychopharmacol. 8: 33-42.

Kinon, B.J. and Lieberman, J.A. (1996) Mechanisms of action of atypical antipsychotic drugs: A critical analysis. Psychopharmacology 124: 2-34.

Kline, L., Decena, E., Hitzemann, R., McCaughran, J. (1998) Acoustic startle, prepulse inhibition, locomotion, and latent inhibition in the neuroleptic-responsive (NR) and neuroleptic-nonresponsive (NNR) lines of mice. Psychopharmacology 139: 322-331.

Konstandi, M. and Kafetzopoulos, E. (1993) Effects of striatal or accumbens lesions on the amphetamine-induced abolition of latent inhibitions. Pharmacol Biochem Behav. 44: 751-754.

Koob, G.F., Riley, S.J., Smith, S.C., Robbins, T.W. (1978) Effects of 6-hydroxydopamine lesions of the nucleus accumbens septi and olfactory tubercle on feeding, locomotor activity, and amphetamine anorexia in the rat. J Comp Physiol Psychol. 92: 917-27.

Kornetzky, C. (1972) The use of simple test of attention as a measure of drug effects in schizophrenic patients. Psychopharmacology 24: 99-106.

Kovelman, J.A. and Scheibel, A.B. (1984) A neurobiological correlate of schizophrenia. Biol Psychiatry 19: 601-621.

Kraepelin, E. (1919) Dementia praecox and paraphrenia. New York: Robert E. Kreiger Publishing Co.

Lacroix, L., Broersen, L.M., Feldon, J., Weiner, I. (2000) Effects of local infusions of dopaminergic drugs into the medial prefrontal cortex of rats on latent inhibition, prepulse inhibition and amphetamine induced activity. Behav Brain Res. 107: 111-21.

Lacroix, L., Broersen, L.M., Weiner, I., Feldon, J. (1998) The effects of excitotoxic lesion of the medial prefrontal cortex on latent inhibition, prepulse inhibition, food hoarding, elevated plus maze, active avoidance and locomotor activity in the rat. Neuroscience 84: 431-42.

Laruelle, M., Abi-Dargham, A., Gil, R., Kegeles, L., Innis, R. (1999) Increased dopamine transmission in schizophrenia: Relationship to illness phases. Biol Psychiatry 46: 56-72.

Le Moal, M. and Simon, H. (1991) Mesocorticolimbic dopaminergic network: Functional and regulatory roles. Physiol Rev. 71: 155-234.

LeDoux, J.E. (1992) Brain mechanisms of emotion and emotional learning. Curr Opin Neurobiol. 2: 191-7.

Lewis, S. (1992) Sex and schizophrenia: Vive la différence. Br J Psychiatry 161: 445-50.

Leysen, J.E., Janssen, P.M.F., Schotte, A., Luyten, W.H.M.L., Megens, A.A.H.P. (1993) Interaction of antipsychotic drugs with neurotransmitter receptor sites in vitro and in vivo in relation to pharmacological and clinical effects - role of 5HT(2) receptors. Psychopharmacology 112: S40-S54.

Liddle, P.F., Friston, K.J., Frith, C.D., Jones, T., Hirsh, S.R., Frackowiak, R.S.J. (1992) Patterns of cerebral blood flow in schizophrenia. Br J Psychiatry 160: 179-186.

Lipp, O.V. and Vaitl, D. (1992) Latent inhibition in human Pavlovian differential conditioning: Effect of additional stimulation after preexposure and relation to schizotypal traits. Pers Indiv Differ. 13: 1003-1012.

Lorden, J.F., Rickert, E.J., Berry, D.W. (1983) Forebrain monoamines and associative learning: I. Latent inhibition and conditioned inhibition. Behav Brain Res. 9: 181-199.

Louilot, A., Simon, H., Taghzouti, K., Le Moal, M. (1985) Modulation of dopaminergic activity in the nucleus accumbens following facilitation or blockade of the dopaminergic transmission in the amygdala: A study by in vivo differential pulse voltammetry. Brain Res. 346: 141-145.

Lubow, R.E. (1973) Latent inhibition. Psychol Bull. 79: 398-407.

Lubow, R.E. (1989) Latent inhibition and conditioned attention theory. Cambridge, England: Cambridge University Press.

Lubow, R.E. (1997) Latent inhibition as a measure of learned inattention: some problems and solutions. Behav Brain Res. 88: 75-83.

Lubow, R.E. and Gewirtz, J.C. (1995) Latent inhibition in humans: data, theory, and implications for schizophrenia. Psychol Bull. 117: 87-103.

Lubow, R.E., Ingberg-Sachs, Y., Zalstein-Orda, N., Gewirtz, J.C. (1992) Latent inhibition in low and high 'psychotic-prone' subjects. Pers Indiv Differ. 13: 563-572.

Lubow, R.E., Kaplan, O., Rudnick, A., Laor, N. (in press) Visual search in schizophrenics: latent inhibition and novel pop-out effects. Schiz Res.

Lubow, R.E., Rifkin, B., Alek, M. (1976) The context effect: the relationship between stimulus preexposure and environmental preexposure determines subsequent learning. J Exp Psychol: Animal Behav Proc. 2: 38-47.

Lubow, R.E., Weiner, I., Schnur, P. (1981) Conditioned attention theory. In G.H. Bower, ed. The psychology of learning and motivation, New York: Academic Press.

Lyon, M. (1991) Animal models of mania and schizophrenia. In P. Willner, ed. Behavioral models in psychopharmacology: Theoretical, industrial and clinical perspectives., Cambridge: Cambridge University Press.

Mackintosh, N.J. (1975) A theory of attention: Variations in the associability of stimuli with reinforcement. Psychol Rev. 82: 276-298.

Maes, M., Meltzer, H.Y., Buckley, P., Bosmans, E. (1995) Plasma-soluble interleukin-2 and transferrin receptor in schizophrenia and major depression. Eur Arch Psychiatry Clin Neurosci. 244: 325-9.

Magaro, P.A. (1980) Cognition in schizophrenia and paranoia: The integration of cognitive processes. Hillsdale: Lawrence Erlbaum.

Maher, B.A., Manschreck, T.C., Molino, M.A. (1983) Redundancy, pause distributions and thought disorder in schizophrenia. Lang Speech. 26: 191-9.

Maldonado-Irizarry, C.S., Kelley, A.E. (1994) Differential behavioral effects following microinjection of an NMDA antagonist into nucleus accumbens subregions. Psychopharmacology 116: 65-72.

Maldonado-Irizarry, C.S. and Kelley, A.E. (1995) Excitotoxic lesions of the core and shell subregions of the nucleus accumbens differentially disrupt body weight regulation and motor activity in rat. Brain Res Bull. 38: 551-9.

McAllister, K.H. (1997) A single administration of d-amphetamine prior to stimulus pre-exposure and conditioning attenuates latent inhibition. Psychopharmacology 130: 79-84.

McGhie, A. and Chapman, J. (1961) Disorders of attention and perception in early schizophrenia. Br J Med Psychol. 34: 103-116.

226

McKinney, W.T. (1988) Models of mental disorders: A new comparative psychiatry. New-York: Plenum Press.

Mednick, S.A. and Cannon, T.D. (1991) Fetal development, birth and the syndroms of adult schizophrenia. In S.A. Mednick, T.D. Cannon and C.E. Barr, ed. Fetal development and adult schizophrenia, Cambridge: Cambridge University press.

Mednick, S.A., Machon, R.A., Huttunen, M.O., Bonett, D. (1988) Adult schizophrenia following prenatal exposure to an influenza epidemic. Arch Gen Psychiatry 45: 189-92.

Meltzer, H.Y. (1989) Clinical studies on the mechanism of action of clozapine: The dopamine-serotonin hypothesis of schizophrenia. Psychopharmacology 99: S18-S27.

Meltzer, H.Y. and Nash, J.F. (1991) Effects of antipsychotic drugs on serotonin receptors. Pharmacol Rev. 43: 587-604.

Meltzer, H.Y. and Stahl, S.M. (1976) The dopamine hypothesis of schizophrenia: A review. Schiz Bull. 2: 19-76.

Millan, M.J., Brocco, M., Rivet, J.M., Audinot, V., Newman-Tancredi, A., Maiofiss, L., Queriaux, S., Despaux, N., Peglion, J.L., Dekeyne, A. (2000a) S18327 (1-[2-[4-(6-fluoro-1, 2-benzisoxazol-3-yl)piperid-1-yl]ethyl]3- phenyl imidazolin-2-one), a novel, potential antipsychotic displaying marked antagonist properties at alpha(1)- and alpha(2)-adrenergic receptors: II. Functional profile and a multiparametric comparison with haloperidol, clozapine, and 11 other antipsychotic agents. J Pharmacol Exp Ther. 292: 54-66.

Millan, M.J., Gobert, A., Newman-Tancredi, A., Lejeune, F., Cussac, D., Rivet, J.M., Audinot, V., Adhumeau, A., Brocco, M., Nicolas, J.P., Boutin, J.A., Despaux, N., Peglion, J.L. (2000b) S18327 (1-[2-[4-(6-fluoro-1, 2-benzisoxazol-3-yl)piperid-1-yl]ethyl]3- phenyl imidazolin-2-one), a novel, potential antipsychotic displaying marked antagonist properties at alpha(1)- and alpha(2)-adrenergic receptors: I. Receptorial, neurochemical, and electrophysiological profile. J Pharmacol Exp Ther. 292: 38-53.

Moore, H., West, A.R., Grace, A.A. (1999) The regulation of forebrain dopamine transmission: Relevance to the pathophysiology and psychopathology of schizophrenia. Biol Psychiatry 46: 40-55.

Moran, P.M., Fischer, T.R., Hitchcock, J.M., Moser, P.C. (1996) Effects of clozapine on latent inhibition in the rat. Behav Pharmacol. 7: 42-48.

Moser, P.C., Moran, P.M., Frank, R.A., Kehne, J.H. (1996) Reversal of amphetamine-induced behaviours by MDL 100,907, a selective 5-HT2A antagonist. Behav Brain Res. 73: 163-7.

Murray, R.M. and Lewis, S.W. (1987) Is schizophrenia a nerodevelopmental disorder? Br Med J. 295: 681-682.

Nordstrom, A.L., Farde, L., Halldin, C. (1993) High 5-HT(2) receptor occupancy in clozapine treated patients demonstrated by PET. Psychopharmacology 110: 365-367.

Nuechterlein, K.H. and Dawson, M.E. (1984) Information processing and attentional functioning in the developmental course of the schizophrenic disorder. Schiz Bull. 10: 160-203.

O'Callaghan, E., Larkin, C., Kinsella, A., Waddington, J.L. (1991) Familial, obstetric, and other clinical correlates of minor physical anomalies in schizophrenia. Am J Psychiatry 148: 479-83.

O'Donnell, P. and Grace, A.A. (1998) Dysfunctions in multiple interrelated systems as the neurobiological bases of schizophrenic symptom clusters. Schiz Bull. 24: 267-83.

Oades, R.D. (1982) Attention and schizophrenia: Neurobiological bases. London: Pitman.

Oades, R.D. (1985) The role of noradrenaline in tuning and dopamine in switching between signals in the CNS. Neurosci Biobehav Rev. 9: 261-282.

Payne, R.W. (1966) The measurement and significance of overinclusive thinking and retardation in schizophrenic patients. In P. Hoch and J. Zubin, ed. Psychopathology of schizophrenia, New York: Grune and Stratton.

Pearce, J.M. and Hall, G. (1980) A model for Pavlovian learning: Variations in the effectiveness of conditioned but not of unconditioned stimuli. Psychol Rev. 87: 532-552.

Pennartz, C.M., Groenewegen, H.J., Lopes da Silva, F.H. (1994) The nucleus accumbens as a complex of functionally distinct neuronal ensembles: an integration of behavioural, electrophysiological and anatomical data. Prog Neurobiol. 42: 719-61.

Peters, S.L. and Joseph, M.H. (1993) Haloperidol potentiation of latent inhibition in rats: evidence for a critical role at conditioning rather than pre-exposure. Behav Pharmacol. 4: 183-186.

Phillips, R.G. and LeDoux, J.E. (1995) Lesions of the fornix but not the entorhinal or perirhinal cortex interfere with contextual fear conditioning. J Neurosci. 15: 5308-5315.

Pouzet, B., Veenman, C.L., Yee, B.K., Feldon, J., Weiner, I. (1999) The effects of radiofrequency lesion or transection of the fimbria- fornix on latent inhibition in the rat. Neuroscience 91: 1355-68.

Rao, M.L. and Moller, H.J. (1994) Biochemical findings of negative symptoms in schizophrenia and their putative relevance to pharmacologic treatment - a review. Neuropsychobiology 30: 160-172.

Rappaport, M., Silverman, J., Hopkins, H.K., Hall, K. (1971) Phenotiazine effects on auditory signal detection in paranoids and paranoid schizophrenics. Science 174: 723-725.

Redgrave, P., Prescott, T.J., Gurney, K. (1999) The basal ganglia: a vertebrate solution to the selection problem? Neuroscience 89: 1009-23.

Reilly, S., Harley, C., Revusky, S. (1993) Ibotanate lesions of the hippocampus enhance latent inhibition in conditioned taste aversion and increase resistance to extinction in conditioned taste preference. Behav Neurosci. 107: 996-1004.

Robbins, T.W. (1991) Cognitive deficits in schizophrenia and Parkinson's disease - neural basis and the role of dopamine. In P. Willner and J. Scheel-Kruger, ed. The mesolimbic dopamine system - from motivation to action, Chichester: John Wiley and Sons Ltd.

Robbins, T.W. and Everitt, B.J. (1982) Functional studies of the central catecholamines. Int Rev Neurobiol. 23: 303-365.

Robbins, T.W. and Koob, G.F. (1980) Selective disruption of displacement behaviour by lesions of the mesolimbic dopamine system. Nature 285: 409-12.

Robbins, T.W., Sahakian, B.J. (1983) Behavioural effects of psychomotor stimulant drugs: clinical and neuropsychological implications. In I. Creese, ed. Stimulants: neurochemical, behavioral and clinical perspectives, New York: Raven Press.

Robinson, G.B., Port, R.L., Stillwell, E.G. (1993) Latent inhibition of the classically conditioned rabbit nictitating membrane response is unaffected by the NMDA antagonist MK-801. Psychobiology 21: 120-124.

Rochford, J., Sen, A.P., Quirion, R. (1996b) Effect of nicotine and nicotinic receptor agonists on latent inhibition in the rat. J Pharmacol Exp Ther. 277: 1267-1275.

Rochford, J., Sen, A.P., Rousse, I., Welner, S.A. (1996a) The effect of quisqualic acid-induced lesions of the nucleus basalis magnocellularis on latent inhibition. Brain Res Bull. 41: 313-7.

Ruob, C., Elsner, J., Weiner, I., Feldon, J. (1997) Amphetamine-induced disruption and haloperidol-induced potentiation of latent inhibition depend on the nature of the stimulus. Behav Brain Res. 88: 35-41.

Ruob, C., Weiner, I., Feldon, J. (1998) Haloperidol-induced potentiation of latent inhibition: Interaction with parameters of conditioning. Behav Pharmacol. 9: 245-253.

Schmajuk, N., Lam, Y.W., Christiansen, B.A. (1994) Latent inhibition of the rat eyeblink response: effect of hippocampal aspiration lesions. Physiol Behav. 55: 597-601.

Schmajuk, N.A. and Moore, J.W. (1985) Real-time attentional models for classical conditioning and the hippocampus. Physiol Psychol. 13: 278-290.

Schmajuk, N.A., Moore, J.W. (1988) The hippocampus and the classically conditioned nictitating membrane response: A real-time attentional-associative model. Psychobiology 16: 20-35.

Schotte, A., Janssen, P.F.M., Gommeren, W., Luyten, W.H.M.L., Van Gompel, P., Lesage, A.S., De Loore, K., Leysen, J.E. (1996) Risperidone compared with new and reference antipsychotic drugs: In vitro and in vivo receptor binding. Psychopharmacology 124: 57-73.

Schroeder, U., Schroeder, H., Darius, J., Grecksch, G., Sabel, B.A. (1998) Simulation of psychosis by continuous delivery of PCP from controlled-release polymer implants. Behav Br Res. 97: 59-68.

Schultz, W. (1998) Predictive reward signal of dopamine neurons. J Neurophysiol. 80: 1-27.

Serban, G., Siegel, S., Gaffney, M. (1992) Response of negative symptoms of schizophrenia to neuroleptic treatment. J Clin Psychiatry 53: 229-234.

Shadach, E., Feldon, J., Weiner, I. (1999) Clozapine-induced potentiation of latent inhibition is due to its action in the conditioning stage: implications for the mechanism of action of antipsychotic drugs. Int J Neuropsychopharmacology 283-291.

Shadach, E., Gaisler, I., Schiller, D., Weiner, I. (in press) The latent inhibition model dissociates between clozapine, haloperidol and ritanserin. Neuropsychopharmacology.

Shakow, D. (1962) Segmental set: a theory of the formal psychological deficit in schizophrenia. Arch Gen Psychiatry 6: 17-33.

Shalev, U. (1998) A neurodevelopmental model of an attentional deficit: the effects of perinatal treatments and stress on latent inhibition. Dept Psychol, Tel-Aviv University.

Shalev, U., Feldon, J., Weiner, I. (1998) Gender- and age-dependent differences in latent inhibition following pre-weaning non-handling: implications for a neurodevelopmental animal model of schizophrenia. Int J Dev Neurosci. 16: 279-88.

Shervan-Schreiber, D., Cohen, J.D., Steingard, S. (1996) Schizophrenic deficits in the processing of context: A test of a theoretical model. Arch Gen Psychiatry 53: 1105-1113.

Snyder, S.H. (1976) The dopamine hypothesis of schizophrenia: focus on the dopamine receptor. Am J Psychiatry 133: 197-202.

Solomon, P., Kiney, C.A., Scott, D.R. (1978) Disruption of latent inhibition following systemic administration of parachlorophenylalanine (PCPA). Physiol Behav. 20: 265-271.

Solomon, P. and Moore, J.W. (1975) Latent inhibition and stimulus generalization of the classically conditioned nictitating membrane response in rabbits (Oryctolagus cuniculus) following dorsal hippocampal ablation. J Comp Physiol Psychol. 89: 1192-1203.

Solomon, P., Nichols, G.L., Kiernan, J.M.I., Kamer, R.S., Kaplan, L.J. (1980) Differential effects of lesions in medial and dorsal raphe of the rat: latent inhibition and septo-hippocampal serotonin levels. J Comp Physiol Psychol. 94: 145-154.

Solomon, P.R., Crider, A., Winkelman, J.W., Turi, A., Kamer, R.M., Kaplan, L.J. (1981) Disrupted latent inhibition in the rat with chronic amphetamine or haloperidol-induced supersensitivity: Relationship to schizophrenic attention disorder. Biol Psychiatry 16: 519-537.

Solomon, P.R. and Staton, D.M. (1982) Differential effects of microinjections of d-amphetamine into the nucleus accumbens or the caudate putamen on the rat's ability to ignore an irrelevant stimulus. Biol Psychiatry 17: 743-756.

Sotty, F., Sandner, G., Gosselin, O. (1996) Latent inhibition in conditioned emotional response: c-fos immunolabelling evidence for brain areas involved in the rat. Brain Res. 737: 243-54.

Spitzer, M., Braun, U., Hermle, L., Maier, S. (1993) Associative semantic network dysfunction in thought-disorded schizophrenic patients - direct evidence from indirect semantic priming. Biol Psychiatry 34: 864-877.

Surwit, R.S. and Poser, E.G. (1974) Latent inhibition in the conditioned elctrodermal response. J Comp Physiol Psychol. 86: 534-548.

Swerdlow, N.R., Braff, D.L., Hartston, H., Perry, W., Geyer, M.A. (1996) Latent inhibition in schizophrenia. Schiz Res. 20: 91-103.

Swerdlow, N.R. and Koob, G.F. (1987) Dopamine, schizophrenia, mania and depression: Toward a unified hypothesis of cortico-striato-pallido-thalamic function. Behav Brain Sci. 10: 215-217.

Taghzouti, K., Louilot, A., Herman, J., Le Moal, M., Simon, H. (1985a) Alternation behavior, spatial discrimination, and reversal disturbances following 6-hydroxydopamine lesions in the nucleus accumbens of the rat. Behav Neural Biol. 44: 354-63.

Taghzouti, K., Simon, H., Louilot, A., Herman, J.P., Le Moal, M. (1985b) Behavioral study after local injection of 6-hydroxydopamine into the nucleus accumbens in the rat. Brain Res. 344: 9-20.

Tai, C.T., Cassaday, H.J., Feldon, J., Rawlins, J.N.P. (1995) Both electrolytic and excitotoxic lesions of nucleus accumbens disrupt latent inhibition of learning in rats. Neurobiol Learn Memory 64: 36-48.

Tamminga, C. (1999) Glutamatergic aspects of schizophrenia. Br J Psychiatry 174 (Suppl. 37): 12-15.

Tandon, R. (1995) Expert commentary: Neurobiological substrate of dimensions of schizophrenic illness. J Psychiatr Res. 29: 255-260.

Tandon, R., Arbor, A., Kane, M.J., Oaks, G. (1993) Neuropharmacologic basis for clozapine's unique profile. Arch Gen Psychiatry 50: 158-159.

Tandon, R., Goldman, R.S., Goodson, J., Greden, J.F. (1990) Mutability and relationship between positive and negative symptoms during neuroleptic treatment in schizophrenia. Biol Psychiatry 27: 1323-1326.

Thornton, J.C., Dawe, S., Lee, C., Capstick, C., Corr, P.J., Cotter, P., Frangou, S., Gray, N.S., Russell, M.A., Gray, J.A. (1996) Effects of nicotine and amphetamine on latent inhibition in human subjects. Psychopharmacology 127: 164-73.

Torrey, E.F. (1991) A viral-anatomical explanation of schizophrenia. Schiz Bull. 17: 15-8.

Totterdell, S. and Meredith, G.E. (1997) Topographical organization of projections from the entorhinal cortex to the striatum of the rat. Neuroscience 78: 715-29.

Trimble, K.M., Bell, R., King, D.J. (1997) Enhancement of latent inhibition in the rat by the atypical antipsychotic agent remoxipride. Pharmacol Biochem Behav. 56: 809-816.

Trimble, K.M., Bell, R., King, D.J. (1998) Enhancement of latent inhibition in the rat at a high dose of clozapine. J Psychopharmacol. 12: 215-219.

Vaid, R.R., Yee, B.K., Shalev, U., Rawlins, J.N., Weiner, I., Feldon, J., Totterdell, S. (1997) Neonatal nonhandling and in utero prenatal stress reduce the density of NADPH-diaphorase-reactive neurons in the fascia dentata and Ammon's horn of rats. J Neurosci. 17: 5599-609.

Vaitl, D. and Lipp, V. (1997) Latent inhibition and autonomic responses: A psycholophysiological approach. Behav Brain Res. 88: 85-94.

Van den Bos, R. and Cools, A.R. (1989) The involvement of the nucleus accumbens in the ability of rats to switch to cue-directed behaviors. Life Sci. 44: 1697-1704.

Venables, P.H. (1984) Cerebral mechanisms, autonomic responsiveness and attention in schizophrenia. In W.D. Spaulding and J.K. Cole, ed. Theories of schizophrenia and psychosis, Lincoln: University of Nebraska Press.

Wagner, A.R. and Rescorla, R.A. (1972) Inhibition in Pavlovian conditioning: Application of a theory. In R.A. Boakes and M.A. Halliday, ed. Inhibition and Learning, New York: Academic Press.

Warburton, E.C., Joseph, M.H., Feldon, J., Weiner, I., Gray, J.A. (1994) Antagonism of amphetamine-induced disruption of latent inhibition in rats by haloperidol and ondansetron: implications for a possible antipsychotic action of ondansetron. Psychopharmacology 114: 657-64.

Weinberger, D.R. and Lipska, B.K. (1995) Cortical maldevelopment, anti-psychotic drugs, and schizophrenia: a search for common ground. Schiz Res. 16: 87-110.

Weiner, I. (1990) Neural substrates of latent inhibition: The switching model. Psychol Bull. 108: 442-461.

Weiner, I., Bernasconi, E., Broersen, L.M., Feldon, J. (1997a) Amphetamine-induced disruption of latent inhibition depends on the nature of the stimulus. Behav Pharmacol. 8: 442-57.

Weiner, I. and Feldon, J. (1987) Facilitation of latent inhibition by haloperidol in rats. Psychopharmacology 91: 248-53.

Weiner, I. and Feldon, J. (1992) Phencyclidine does not disrupt latent inhibition in rats: implications for animal models of schizophrenia. Pharmacol Biochem Behav. 42: 625-31.

Weiner, I. and Feldon, J. (1997) The switching model of latent inhibition: An update of neural substrates. Behav Brain Res. 88: 11-25.

Weiner, I., Feldon, J., Katz, Y. (1987a) Facilitation of the expression but not the acquisition of latent inhibition by haloperidol in rats. Pharmacol Biochem Behav. 26: 241-6.

Weiner, I., Feldon, J., Tarrasch, R., Hairston, I., Joel, D. (1998a) Fimbria-fornix cut affects spontaneous activity, two-way avoidance and delayed non matching to sample, but not latent inhibition. Behav Brain Res. 96: 59-70.

Weiner, I., Feldon, J., Ziv-Harris, D. (1987b) Early handling and latent inhibition in the conditioned suppression paradigm. Dev Psychobiol. 20: 233-40.

Weiner, I., Gal, G., Feldon, J. (1999) Disrupted and undisruptable latent inhibition following shell and core lesions. Ann N Y Acad Sci. 877: 723-7.

Weiner, I., Gal, G., Rawlins, J.N., Feldon, J. (1996a) Differential involvement of the shell and core subterritories of the nucleus accumbens in latent inhibition and amphetamine-induced activity. Behav Brain Res. 81: 123-33.

Weiner, I., Hairston, I., Shayit, M., Feldman, G., Joel, D. (1998b) Strain differences in latent inhibition. Psychobiology 26: 57-64.

Weiner, I., Izraeli-Telerant, A., Feldon, J. (1987c) Latent inhibition is not affected by acute or chronic administration of 6 mg/kg dl-amphetamine. Psychopharmacology. 91: 345-351.

Weiner, I., Kidron, R., Tarrasch, R., Arnt, J., Feldon, J. (1994) The effects of the new antipsychotic, sertindole, on latent inhibition in rats. Behav Pharm. 5: 119-124.

Weiner, I., Lubow, R.E., Feldon, J. (1981) Chronic amphetamine and latent inhibition. Behav Brain Res. 2: 285-286.

Weiner, I., Lubow, R.E., Feldon, J. (1984) Abolition of the expression but not the acquisition of latent inhibition by chronic amphetamine in rats. Psychopharmacology 83: 194-199.

Weiner, I., Lubow, R.E., Feldon, J. (1988) Disruption of latent inhibition by acute administration of low doses of amphetamine. Pharmacol Biochem Behav. 30: 871-878.

Weiner, I., Schnabel, I., Lubow, R.E., Feldon, J. (1985) The effects of early handling on latent inhibition in male and female rats. Dev Psychobiol. 18: 291-7.

Weiner, I., Shadach, E., Barkai, R., Feldon, J. (1997b) Haloperidol- and clozapine-induced enhancement of latent inhibition with extended conditioning: Implications for the mechanism of action of neuroleptic drugs. Neuropsychopharmacology 16: 42-50.

Weiner, I., Shadach, E., Tarrasch, R., Kidron, R., Feldon, J. (1996b) The latent inhibition model of schizophrenia: further validation using the atypical neuroleptic, clozapine. Biol Psychiatry 40: 834-43.

Weiner, I., Smith, A.D., Rawlins, J.N., Feldon, J. (1992) A neuroleptic-like effect of ceronapril on latent inhibition. Neuroscience 49: 307-15.

Weiner, I., Tarrasch, R., Bernasconi, E., Broersen, L.M., Ruttimann, T.C., Feldon, J. (1997c) Amphetamine-induced disruption of latent inhibition is not reinforcer- mediated. Pharmacol Biochem Behav. 56: 817-26.

Weiner, I., Tarrasch, R., Feldon, J. (1996c) Basolateral amygdala lesions do not disrupt latent inhibition. Behav Brain Res. 72: 73-81.

Williams, J.H., Wellman, N.A., Geaney, D.P., Cowen, P.J., Feldon, J., Rawlins, J.N. (1998) Reduced latent inhibition in people with schizophrenia: an effect of psychosis or of its treatment. Br J Psychiatry 172: 243-9.

Williams, J.H., Wellman, N.A., Geaney, D.P., Feldon, J., Cowen, P.J., Rawlins, J.N.P. (1997) Haloperidol enhances latent inhibition in visual tasks in healthy people. Psychopharmacology 133: 262-268.

Williams, J.H., Wellman, N.A., Geaney, D.P., Feldon, J., Rawlins, J.N., Cowen, P.J. (1996) Antipsychotic drug effects in a model of schizophrenic attentional disorder: A randomised trial of the effects of haloperidol on latent inhibition in healthy people. Biol Psychiatry 40: 1135-1143.

Willner, P. (1991) Behavioural models in psychopharmacology. In P. Willner, ed. Behavioural models in psychopharmacology: Theoretical, industrial and clinical perspectives, Cambridge: Cambridge University Press.

Wolkin, A., Sanfilipo, M., Wolf, A.P., Angrist, B., Brodie, J.D., Rotrosen, J. (1992) Negative symptoms and hypofrontality in chronic schizophrenia. Arch Gen Psychiatry 49: 959-965.

Yee, B.K., Feldon, J., Rawlins, J.N.P. (1995) Latent inhibition in rats is abolished by NMDA-induced neuronal loss in the retrohippocampal region but this lesion effect can be prevented by systemic haloperidol treatment. Behav Neurosci. 109: 227-240.

Young, A.M.J., Joseph, M.H., Gray, J.A. (1993) Latent inhibition of conditioned dopamine release in rat nucleus accumbens. Neuroscience 54: 5-9.

Zahm, D.S. (1999) Functional-anatomical implications of the nucleus accumbens core and shell subterritories. Ann N. Y. Acad Sci. 877: 113-28.

Zahm, D.S. and Brog, J.S. (1992) On the significance of subterritories in the "accumbens" part of the rat ventral striatum. Neuroscience 50: 751-767.

Zalstein-Orda, N. and Lubow, R.E. (1995) Context control of negative transfer induced by preexposure to irrelevant stimuli:latent inhibition in humans. Learn Motiv. 26: 11-28.

13 RAT LATENT INHIBITION AND PREPULSE INHIBITION ARE SENSITIVE TO DIFFERENT MANIPULATIONS OF THE SOCIAL ENVIRONMENT: A COMPREHENSIVE STUDY OF THE ENVIRONMENTAL APPROACH TO NEURODEVELOPMENTAL MODELS OF SCHIZOPHRENIA

Joram Feldon, Julia Lehmann, Christopher Pryce and Isabelle Weiss

INTRODUCTION

In the present chapter we review a series of rat studies conducted in our laboratory during the last five years, investigating the long-term consequences of manipulations of the social environment for behavioural processes which are widely recognised as being of direct relevance to psychosis, and in particular to schizophrenia. The ultimate aim of these studies is to ascertain the relevance and robustness of effects induced by manipulations of the rat's social environment as animal models of important symptoms and features of human psychosis. There are a number of potential advantages to the modelling approach we are taking. Firstly, our research work has been influenced by the evidence that many psychiatric disorders, and notably schizophrenia, emerge out of early developmental aberrations, and the theory that epigenetic changes induced by these early events express themselves later in the life span as clinical disorder (Weinberger, 1987). One approach to the animal modelling of this neurodevelopmental hypothesis of schizophrenia is to perform surgical lesions of specific brain structures in the early postnatal period and to monitor the behavioural consequences of these lesions long-term (Lipska, this volume). Our neurodevelopmental approach and that of some other laboratories is non-surgical, and involves specific manipulation of the social environment which, it is hypothesised, will expose the developing brain to events it is not expecting and/or deprive it of events that it is expecting, leading to long-term change in structure-function of specific brain areas. A neurodevelopmental animal model based exclusively on environmental manipulation, if demonstrated to possess robust face and predictive validity will, relative to lesion models, also possess a unique level of construct validity (Ellenbroek and Cools, 1998; Feldon and Weiner, 1992). Second, in contrast to the neurodevelopmental (lesion or environment) approach, the majority of the existing animal models of psychopathology rely heavily on drug-induced states; for example, the amphetamine- or phencyclidine-induced rat models of schizophrenia, or the reserpine-induced rat model of depression. The major disadvantage of such drug-induced models is that the examination of putative therapeutic agents *vis-a-vis* predictive validity is restricted to those that are antagonistic to the drug used to induce the behavioural change: For example, whilst the psychomotor effects (hyperlocomotion or stereotypy) induced by amphetamine or apomorphine can be antagonised by antipsychotic (neuroleptic) drugs with their universal characteristic of dopaminergic receptor blockade, this evidence does not necessarily advance our understanding of the aetiology or treatment of disorders characterised by psychomotor disturbance. A third advantage of a robust neurodevelopmental model based purely on the effects of environmental manipulation is that it allows for quantitative neurochemical and neurophysiological examination of the central nervous system in the absence of confounding surgical or pharmacological effects.

Fourth, with respect to the advantages of the environmental approach to neurodevelopmental animal models, the research in this area which preceded that conducted in this laboratory has provided some very interesting evidence in terms of environmental manipulations leading to behavioural changes reminiscent of the symptoms of schizophrenia. This is particularly true of the attentional processes of latent inhibition (LI) (Feldon et al., 1990; Feldon and Weiner, 1988; Weiner et al., 1985, 1987) and prepulse inhibition (PPI) (Geyer et al., 1993; Robbins et al., 1996). disturbance of which has been a central focus of theories of schizophrenia aetiology. As described below, both LI and PPI can be studied using very similar methodology in humans and their animal models; one interesting point which we would like to bring to the reader's attention here though, is that whereas LI was first studied in animals and then applied to humans, the opposite is true for PPI.

In LI, according to its simplest, two-stage working definition, repeated exposure to a stimulus (e.g., visual, auditory) not followed by meaningful consequences (Pre-exposure stage) renders this stimulus of reduced efficacy in terms of subsequent learning (Conditioning stage). LI is then defined as the stimulus-preexposed group learning the conditioned stimulus (CS)-unconditioned stimulus (US) association less or at least more slowly than the non-preexposed group. As such, LI is amenable to testing in a range of rodent classical and instrumental conditioning paradigms (Lubow, 1989), and can also be tested in human subjects using very similar parameters (Lubow and Gewirtz, 1995). Furthermore, LI, i.e., the ability to ignore irrelevant stimuli, is altered in schizophrenic patients, as well as in people scoring high on a schizotpy scale and volunteers exposed to low doses of amphetamine (for review see Weiner and Feldon, 1997). In the rat, LI is reduced following repeated low doses of amphetamine, but is unaffected by any dose of apomorphine or any selective dopamine agonist, or any NMDA antagonist. LI is potentiated by high doses of amphetamine (Feldon et al., 1995; Weiner and Feldon, 1997).

In their Tel Aviv Laboratory in the 1980's, Feldon and Weiner provided the first evidence that manipulation of the social environment in the rat can yield a robust neurodevelopmental animal model of impaired LI. Using Wistar rats, across postnatal days (PND) 1-21 male and female pups were either exposed to daily early handling (EH), constituting either 5 or 15 minutes of daily separation from the home cage, mother and litter mates, or to early non-handling (NH), constituting complete non-disturbance except for occasional supplementation of water and food. Following weaning at PND 21 and subsequent rearing in social groups, adult male NH rats demonstrated reduced or non-existent levels of LI relative to male EH, female EH and female NH rats, as a consequence of CS pre-exposure of NH male subjects failing to impair their subsequent conditioning relative to their non-preexposed counterparts (Weiner et al., 1985, 1987). It was then further demonstrated that LI in NH male adults is restored by the antipsychotic drug haloperidol (Feldon and Weiner, 1988). Based on these observations, Feldon and Weiner (1992) proposed that early non-handling in male rats constitutes an animal model of certain of the attentional dysfunctions presented in schizophrenia. That is, in the context of LI, NH actually represents the manipulation relative to EH. The same conclusion was drawn by Seymour Levine in the context of NH versus EH effects on development of fearfulness and stressor reactivity, with deprivation of sensory stimulation in NH pups being proposed as the mediating mechanism (Levine, 1960). Other research groups, most notably that of Meaney and colleagues, do not hold with this interpretation, and emphasise the effects of EH on maternal care as the mediator of NH-EH differences (e.g., Liu et al., 1997; Meaney et al., 1996). Recently, interest in pre-weaning environmental manipulations and LI has been renewed following the report that a manipulation of 24-hour maternal separation conducted at PND 10 – specifically comprising removal of the mother and maintenance of the pups as a litter at nest temperature – leads to an impairment of LI in the conditioned taste aversion paradigm (Ellenbroek and Cools, 1995). However, as reviewed in the current chapter, in addition to the original evidence for an LI deficit in NH males, we now have extensive evidence that, in general, manipulations of the pre-weaning social environment comprising various durations of maternal separation and performed across a range of PNDs, actually lead to *enhanced* LI in adulthood relative to normal-husbandry controls (Lehmann et al., 1998, in press-a; Weiss et al., submitted manuscript). Furthermore, we (Feldon et al., 1990; Weiss et al., submitted manuscript) and then Wilkinson et al., (1994) have both demonstrated that social isolation performed post-weaning does not affect LI in terms of either enhancement or impairment.

In PPI, the attenuation of the reflexive acoustic startle response (ASR) to a loud acoustic pulse stimulus occurs as a consequence of this stimulus being immediately preceded by an auditory or tactile stimulus, or prepulse, that is itself too weak to elicit the ASR. Whilst PPI itself comprises modulation of a reflex response, sensorimotor gating is the mechanism which is proposed to underlie this phenomenon, and it is possible that gating efficacy at this reflex level reflects gating efficacy of the same individual at higher levels of processing, including selective attention. Importantly, as with LI, PPI is deficient in schizophrenic patients; in human volunteers PPI is reduced following treatment with NMDA antagonists (Vollenweider et al., 2000). In rats, essentially in direct contrast to LI, PPI is disrupted severely by a variety of systemically-delivered direct (e.g., apomorphine, D_2-specific agonists) and indirect (e.g., amphetamine) DA agonists, as well as NMDA antagonists (e.g., PCP, MK-801, ketamine) (for review see Swerdlow and Geyer, 1998). With regard to the long-term response of rat PPI to environmental manipulations, it has been demonstrated that postnatal social isolation, versus normal-husbandry group rearing, leads to substantial attenuation of PPI, and that this attenuation can be reversed with typical or atypical antipsychotic drugs (Geyer et al., 1993). As stated above, the general evidence is that post-weaning isolation does not affect LI. The same research group which reported that 24-hour maternal separation reduces LI in adulthood has also reported that it reduces PPI in adulthood (Ellenbroek et al., 1998). However, as reviewed below, our comprehensive data set demonstrates categorically that pre-weaning environmental manipulations do not affect PPI (Lehmann et al., in press-b).

Therefore, the present chapter reviews our comprehensive studies of pre-weaning environmental manipulations of infants and post-weaning social isolation of pre-adults, in terms of their effects on LI and PPI in adulthood. In addition, given that spontaneous activity and amphetamine-induced activity are also considered to be indicative of the functional state of brain structures and neurotransmitter systems of relevance to animal models of psychosis, effects of these manipulations on activity measures are also presented. The relationships between the different behavioural effects of each manipulation are described with a view to elucidating their relative merits and limitations. To the extent that our findings are not in line with those reported by others, in the methods section we have highlighted important details of experimental design which are sometimes overlooked. Finally, here, in this chapter we concentrate on our studies conducted with males. Whilst many of these studies were conducted in females also, we and others have reported consistently that males are generally more responsive to environmental manipulations than are females (e.g., Feldon and Weiner, 1992; Lehmann et al., 1998, 1999; Weiss et al., 2000).

METHODOLOGY

The experiments reviewed in this chapter were conducted either on our own Wistar rat line or on the Sprague Dawley strain, with all subjects bred in-house. We have demonstrated that post-weaning social isolation has a less-robust effect on PPI in Wistar than in Sprague-Dawley rats (Domeney and Feldon, 1998; Weiss et al., 1999, in press); therefore, studies of isolation have been performed either with both Wistar and Sprague-Dawley or with the latter only. In our facility rats are maintained on a reversed 12 hr dark-light cycle with lights off between 07:00-19:00. For the provision of subjects, adult males and females were paired together for five days and males then removed; pregnant females were then allocated randomly to treatment groups. In the case of pre-weaning manipulations the procedures deployed were as follows with more detailed descriptions available in the publications cited:
1) Normal-husbandry controls (CON): on PND 1-21 subjects were handled briefly once per week for cage cleaning; they were kept in a room to which personnel were allowed unrestricted access (e.g., Lehmann et al., 1998).
2) Early handling (EH): on PND 1-21 subjects were isolated alone on sawdust in a small plastic container for 15 min, with handling pre- and post-isolation (Weiner et al., 1985).
3) Early non-handling (NH): on PND 1-21 subjects remained completely undisturbed with the litter mates and mother in the home cage, in a room entered only sporadically for food and water supplementation (Weiner et al., 1985).
4) Early isolation (EI): on PND 1-21 subjects were isolated alone on sawdust in a small plastic container for 4 hr at 28-30°C, with handling pre- and post-isolation.
5) Repeated maternal separation for 4x 6 hr (RMS 12-18): on PND 12, 14, 16 and 18, subjects were isolated from the mother but remained with the litter in an incubator at 25°C for 6 hr (Lehmann et al., 1998).

6) Single maternal separation for 1x 24 hr (MS): on PND 9, the mother was removed for 24 hr and subjects remained with the litter in the home cage which was placed on a heating pad at 36°C (Lehmann et al., in press-b).

At PND 21, all subjects were weaned and caged in groups of four subjects of the same sex and from different litters. EH and NH subjects were always bred simultaneously and tested against each other; EI subjects were bred simultaneously with and tested against CON, as were RMS 12-18 and MS subjects. The post-weaning environmental manipulation was:

7) Social isolation (ISO): on PND 1-21 subjects were treated as per CON (above) and on PND 21 subjects were weaned and subsequently reared alone until testing. The comparison group was CON subjects which post-weaning were reared in groups of four subjects of the same sex and from different litters (Domeney and Feldon, 1998; Weiss et al., 1999, in press). In addition, in one study pre-weaning EI versus no-EI and post-weaning ISO versus group-rearing (GRP) were combined according to a 2 (EI, no-EI) x 2 (ISO, GRP) design (Weiss et al., submitted manuscript).

In terms of behavioural paradigms, as stated above LI can be tested in the rat in a variety of classical and operant conditioning paradigms. We have studied the effects of environmental manipulations on LI in the paradigms of conditioned emotional response, conditioned taste aversion, and two-way active avoidance (e.g., Lehmann et al., 1998, in press-a). Here we focus on LI as interfaced with two-way active avoidance, which we have used with each of the manipulations given above. Briefly, rats are conditioned in 100 trials/day to avoid an electric foot shock (US) by jumping from one compartment of an avoidance chamber to the other during a 10s tone or flashing light (CS). In cases where an avoidance response is not performed within the 10s CS presentation, a 2s 0.5mA foot shock is delivered which in the majority of cases leads to an escape response. For the purposes of LI measurement, each treatment group is divided into two groups: on one or two days prior to conditioning, subjects in one group are placed in the avoidance chamber and preexposed to 50 presentations/day of the to-be-CS (preexposed, or PE group), and subjects in the other group are placed in the avoidance chamber for the same duration without CS preexposure (nonpreexposed, or NPE group). The results are presented below in terms of latency after CS onset to avoid/escape in 10 blocks of 10 consecutive trials. For each environmental manipulation separately, the performance of the NPE versus PE groups is presented alongside its respective control condition, thus providing a clear presentation of two-way avoidance acquisition and LI.

PPI of the ASR is measured according to the standard procedure established for the rat (Domeney and Feldon, 1998; Geyer et al., 1993). Startle pulses of 120 dB[A] white noise of 30ms duration are presented to determine basal ASR. The four different prepulses take the form of 20ms of white noise at the following intensities: 72, 76, 80, or 84 dB[A]; the time interval between the prepulse offset and the pulse onset is 80ms. Startle amplitude is measured in arbitrary units by an accelerometer during 100ms after startle pulse onset and percentage PPI induced by each prepulse intensity is calculated as: [100-(100 x startle amplitude at prepulse trial)/(startle amplitude at startle pulse alone trial)].

Locomotor activity is determined in the open field (Lehmann et al., 1999; Weiss et al., 1999). Spontaneous activity refers to the locomotor activity of subjects in the absence of any pharmacological manipulation and following a period of habituation to the test room *per se*. *d*-Amphetamine-induced activity refers to the locomotor activity of subjects following acute treatment with a low-moderate dose of this psychostimulant (1.0-1.5mg/kg). Typically, subjects are first tested for spontaneous activity in the novel open field and then, after a 1-2 week interval, for baseline activity in the now familiar open field followed by a test of activity in response to saline injection, and then activity in response to intra-peritoneal *d*-amphetamine.

Very importantly, our standard research design is based on unrelated subjects (for a detailed review see Lehmann and Feldon, in press). That is, when we perform environmental manipulation, littermates come through the manipulation together but when we perform tests in adulthood no two littermates are included on the same paradigm. For example, litters A-G are exposed to EH; only one subject from each of these litters will be tested for LI in active avoidance, and the same applies to PPI of the ASR, and spontaneous and *d*-amphetamine-induced activity in the open field. This methodology is the only one that yields independent subjects on each paradigm in which we are interested. Of course because we want to be able to analyse our data using parametric tests based on the general linear model then it is essential that we satisfy the major assumption of these tests, namely independence of subjects. If the "litter effect" is not controlled for then in the typical situation there will be reduction in within-treatment between-subject variance, which will increase the likelihood of obtaining statistically significant treatment effects. For example, a research design based on inclusion of two littermates as opposed to one already results in a 2-3-fold increase in the likelihood of a treatment effect yielding a statistically significant effect (Denenberg, 1977). Several laboratories that have reported studies on environmental manipulations have not controlled for "litter effect" (e.g., Ellenbroek et al., 1998; Liu et al., 1997).

RESULTS

Below we provide a summary of our results for the effects of environmental manipulations on LI, PPI and locomotor activity, as obtained with male Wistar and male Sprague-Dawley rats. Within each paradigm, our findings are presented in the order: EH versus NH, EI versus CON, RMS versus CON, MS versus CON, ISO versus CON, and EI/no-EI x ISO/GRP. Table 1 provides an overview of all of our findings.

In the case of LI in the active avoidance paradigm, all pre-weaning manipulations led to an effect on LI whereas post-weaning ISO did not affect LI. Beginning with EH versus NH, NH leads to a significant increase in avoidance latency in the NPE subjects ($p<0.05$), which might well reflect the increased fearfulness associated generally with this pre-weaning manipulation. As given in Figure 1, relative to NH subjects, in which LI is absent ($p>0.59$), EH results in increased LI ($p<0.002$), with an increase in avoidance latency in PE EH subjects as well as the decrease in NPE EH subjects contributing to this EH-NH difference. Relative to CON, EI does not alter avoidance latency in NPE subjects ($p>0.87$); EI does increase LI, with LI being non-significant in CON subjects ($p>0.30$) and significant in EI subjects as a result of retarded avoidance learning in PE EI subjects ($p<0.02$) (Figure 2). RMS 12-18 also does not affect avoidance latency relative to CON as measured in the NPE groups ($p>0.21$), but does increase LI, with once again an absence of LI in CON ($p>0.78$ in this study) and retarded avoidance learning in PE RMS subjects leading to clear LI ($p<0.05$) (Figure 3). MS on PND9 does not influence avoidance learning relative to CON according to response latency in the NPE subjects ($p>0.18$); again, LI is not statistically significant in the CON subjects ($p>0.11$ in this case), whereas there is a trend to significant LI in MS subjects ($p<0.07$) (Figure 4). Therefore, pre-weaning manipulations of the infant-mother environment lead in adulthood to increased LI in the active avoidance paradigm, regardless of whether the manipulation is EH versus NH, or EI, RMS or MS versus CON (Table 1). Furthermore, we have also demonstrated that RMS 12-18 increases LI in the paradigms of conditioned emotional response and conditioned taste aversion (Lehmann et al., 1998). Ellenbroek and Cools (1995), however, report that MS at PND 10 reduces LI in the latter paradigm.

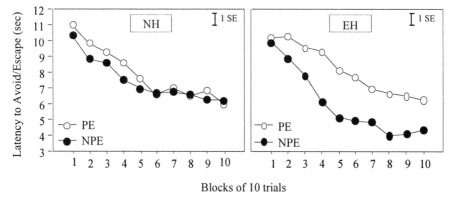

Figure 1. Effect of tone CS pre-exposure on avoidance latency in early handled ($p<0.002$) versus early nonhandled ($p>0.59$) male Wistar rats (N = 10 PE vs 10 NPE in both treatments). Values in Figures 1-6 represent mean latencies of 10 trials each. The 1 SE bar in each figure represents 1 standard error derived from the appropriate analysis of variance (ANOVA).

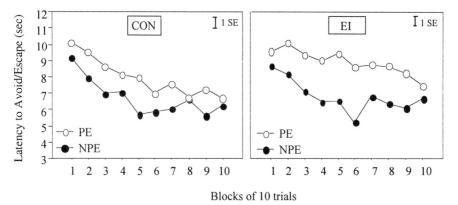

Figure 2. Effect of flashing light CS pre-exposure on avoidance latency in early isolated ($p<0.02$) versus normal-husbandry control ($p>0.30$) male Wistar rats (N = 6 vs 6).

238

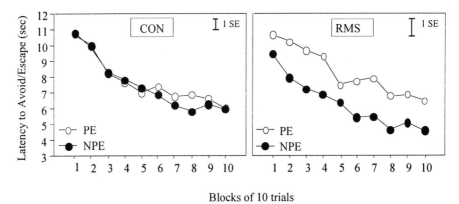

Blocks of 10 trials

Figure 3. Effect of tone CS pre-exposure on avoidance latency in repeated 6-hr maternal separation at PND 12, 14, 16, 18 ($p<0.05$) versus normal-husbandry control ($p>0.78$) male Wistar rats (N = 10 vs 10)

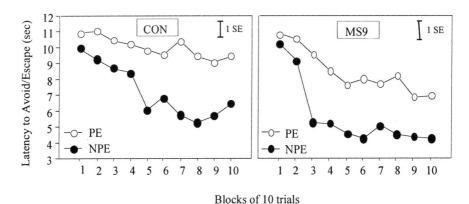

Blocks of 10 trials

Figure 4. Effect of tone CS pre-exposure on avoidance latency in 24-hr PND 9 maternally separated ($p<0.07$) versus normal-husbandry control ($p>0.11$) male Wistar rats (N = 4 vs 4).

Turning to the post-weaning manipulation of ISO, our studies demonstrate that this is without effect on LI (Weiss et al., submitted manuscript). Firstly, comparing ISO with GRP (identical in this case to CON in the above studies) in terms of NPE subjects, there is a significant difference in terms of avoidance latency, with ISO demonstrating impaired avoidance ($p<0.01$). LI, however, is not significant in either GRP ($p>0.19$) or ISO subjects ($p>0.13$) (Figure 5). When post-weaning ISO is studied using a 2 x 2 design with EI, there is no interaction effect of ISO and EI ($p>0.98$); EI+ISO subjects ($p<0.04$) and EI+GRP subjects ($p<0.05$) demonstrate significant and equivalent levels of LI (Figure 6). Importantly, therefore, there is no negating effect of ISO (Weiss et al., submitted manuscript) on the effect of EI, so that EI+ISO subjects demonstrate significant LI (Figure 6) whereas no-EI+ISO subjects do not (Figure 5). Note that the significant LI seen in EI+GRP (Figure 6 left panel) as compared with the lack of LI in the no-EI+GRP (Figure 5, left panel) constitutes a replication in Sprague-Dawley rats of the EI effect described above for Wistar rats (Figure 2).

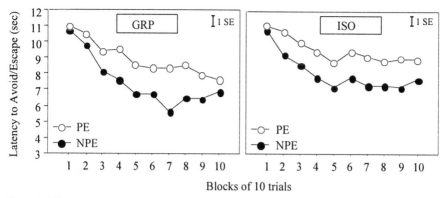

Figure 5. Effect of tone CS pre-exposure on avoidance latency in post-weaning socially isolated ($p>0.13$) versus group-reared control ($p>0.19$) male Sprague-Dawley rats (N = 8 vs 7).

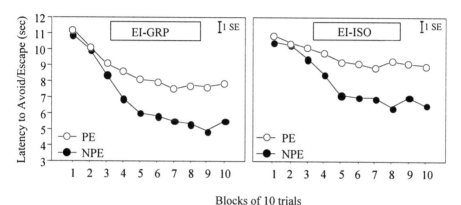

Blocks of 10 trials

Figure 6. Effect of tone CS pre-exposure on avoidance latency in early isolated and post-weaning socially isolated ($p<0.04$) versus early isolated and post-weaning group-reared ($p<0.05$) male Sprague-Dawley rats (N = 8 vs 7).

In the case of PPI, pre-weaning environmental manipulations are universally without effect, whereas ISO leads to reduced PPI. Beginning with EH versus NH rats, there is no significant difference in PPI ($p>0.62$; Figure 7A). This is also the case for EI versus CON ($p>0.44$; Figure 7B), RMS 12-18 versus CON ($p>0.92$; Figure 7C) (Lehmann et al., 2000), and MS at PND 9 versus CON ($p>0.92$; Figure 7D) (Lehmann et al., in press-b). As can be seen in Figures 7A-D inclusive, subjects exposed to each of these manipulations demonstrate the typical pattern in terms of PPI increasing as a function of prepulse intensity ($p<0.001$ in all cases). The absence of an effect of MS is in contrast to the report of Ellenbroek et al. (1998); it is certainly possible that "litter effect" could contribute to this contrasting finding. Rats exposed to ISO demonstrate a significant impairment in PPI of the ASR relative to rats maintained in groups as adults ($p<0.003$; Figure 8). In this 2 x 2 study, there is no significant effect of EI on PPI ($p>0.15$), replicating the finding in Wistar rats (Figure 7B). Furthermore, there is no interaction effect of EI and ISO ($p>0.81$): both no-EI+ISO and EI+ISO demonstrate reduced PPI relative to GRP subjects. Importantly, therefore, there is no negating effect of EI on the effect of ISO.

240

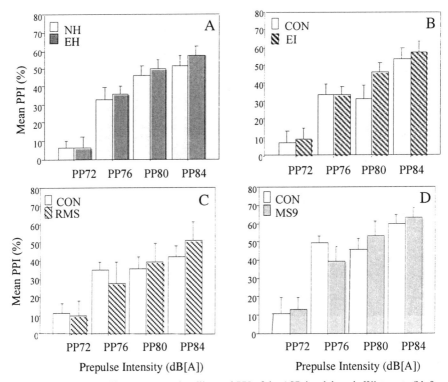

Figure 7. (A) Early handling versus non-handling and PPI of the ASR in adult male Wistar rats (N=8 vs 8) (F(1,14)=0.25, p>0.62). (B) Early isolation versus normal-husbandry controls and PPI of the ASR in adult male Wistar rats (N=8 vs 8) (F(1,14)=0.52, p>0.51). (C) Repeated 6-hr maternal separation versus normal-husbandry controls and PPI of the ASR in adult male Wistar rats (N=16 vs 16) (F(1,28)=0.01, p>0.92). (D) PND 9 maternally separation versus normal-husbandry controls and PPI of the ASR in adult male Wistar rats (N=8 vs 8) (F(1,14)=0.01, p>0.92). All values are means±SEMs.

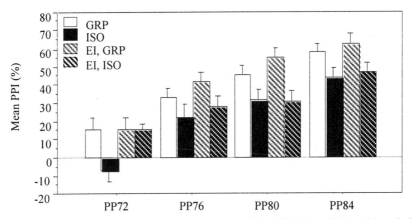

Figure 8. Effects of post-weaning ISO and pre-weaning EI on PPI of the ASR in adult male Sprague-Dawley rats. ISO leads to a PPI deficit versus subjects maintained in groups as adults (F(1,56)=9.89, p<0.03); this effect is not in interaction with EI (N=15/treatment) (F(1,56)=0.05, p>0.81).

As stated in the Introduction, there is a general expectation that treatments yielding an effect on LI and/or PPI will also yield effects in terms of psychomotor activity, either spontaneous or following dopaminergic challenge. In addition to our conclusive demonstration that pre-weaning environmental manipulations affect LI and not PPI and that post-weaning isolation affects PPI and not LI, we have found that an effect of an environmental manipulation on spontaneous activity does not necessarily translate into an additional effect on psychomotor response to d-amphetamine. Our findings on the effects of environmental manipulations on psychomotor activity are as follows (see also Table 1): Beginning again with EH versus NH, EH tends to increase spontaneous locomotor activity ($p \leq 0.08$) and increases the locomotor response to acute d-amphetamine ($p < 0.05$). In Wistar rats, EI leads to no effect on spontaneous locomotion versus CON and to increased locomotion following d-amphetamine ($p < 0.04$); in Sprague-Dawley rats relative to GRP subjects, EI does not affect either spontaneous ($p > 0.29$) or amphetamine-induced ($p > 0.13$) locomotion. In RMS 12-18 rats relative to CON, there is an absence of effect on either spontaneous or amphetamine-induced locomotion (Lehmann et al., 1998), and the same is true of subjects experiencing 24-h MS at PND 9 (Lehmann et al., 1999). ISO increases spontaneous activity in the open field whilst leaving the amphetamine response unaffected in Wistar rats (Domeney and Feldon, 1998; Weiss et al., 1999), and is without effect on spontaneous activity and actually reduces the amphetamine response in Sprague-Dawley rats. Referring to Table I, the final major finding of our studies as reviewed here is that there is no consistent, predictive relationship between the effect of an environmental manipulation on LI or PPI and its effects on psychomotor behaviour in the open field, neither spontaneous nor following d-amphetamine challenge.

Table 1. Summary of effects of environmental manipulations on LI, PPI, activitty

Manipulation	Strain	LI	PPI	Locomotor Activity Spontaneous	Amphetamine
Pre-weaning					
EH vs NH	Wistar	↑	0	↑	↑
EI vs CON	Wistar	↑	0	0	↑
	Spr-Daw	↑	0	0	0
RMS12-18 vs CON	Wistar	↑	0	0	0
MS PND9 vs CON	Wistar	↑	0	0	0
Post-weaning					
ISO vs GRP (CON)	Wistar	0	↓	↑	0
	Spr-Daw	0	↓	0	↓
Pre-weaning + Post-weaning					
EI+ISO vs No-EI+ISO	Spr-Daw	↑	0	0	0
EI+ISO vs EI+GRP	Spr-Daw	0	↓	0	0
EI+ISO vs No-EI+GRP	Spr-Daw	↑	↓	0	0

↑ = increase, ↓ = decrease, 0 = no effect, versus respective control group.

DISCUSSION

Clearly, therefore, manipulations of the social environment of the rat at distinct stages early on in its life span exert a marked impact on behavioural processes which are altered in schizophrenia, and as such can make an important contribution to our understanding of the neurobiology of this mental disorder. Schizophrenic patients demonstrate atypical LI in that it is either reduced or persistent (Weiner and Feldon, 1997; Williams et al., 1998), and atypical PPI in that it is reduced (Swerdlow and Geyer, 1998). An animal model which, via a single manipulation, induces effects in terms of both LI and PPI would represent the "ideal situation" in terms of face validity. We have demonstrated in this extensive series of studies that neither a pre-weaning nor a post-weaning environmental manipulation leads to effects on both LI and PPI. Rather, pre-weaning manipulations as varied as 15-min daily isolation to a single 24-h maternal separation all result in persistent LI without affecting PPI, whilst post-weaning social isolation leaves LI unaffected and reduces PPI. However, in our most recent study, as described above, where we have combined pre-weaning 4-h early isolation at PND 1-21 with post-weaning social isolation beginning at PND 21 in Sprague-Dawley rats, we have demonstrated that the respective effects of EI and ISO on LI and PPI are maintained in the presence of each other (Weiss et al., submitted manuscript). This combined pre-weaning/post-weaning environmental manipulation represents an animal model of combined altered LI and PPI. Given that these effects are achieved entirely via environmental manipulations in the absence of surgical or pharmacological manipulation, then the model is characterised by all the advantages of this approach as presented in the Introduction. These include potential construct validity in terms of underlying pathophysiology and neurobiology, and maintenance of a nervous system which can be studied meaningfully at the neurochemical, neuroanatomical and electrophysiological levels.

The universal ability of pre-weaning environmental manipulations to potentiate LI, most notably due to persistence of the CS-no contingency relationship, is striking. This apparent perseveration of attentional processes is consistent with cognitive inflexibility, an important negative symptom of schizophrenia (Murphy et al., 2000), and may also have important parallels with the re-emergence of LI in schizophrenics as a function of the chronicity of their illness (Weiner and Feldon, 1997). A discussion of the putative cortico-limbic-striatal changes underlying such potentiated LI is provided in the switching model of Weiner and Feldon (1997). What is clear is that some aspect(s) of the LI neural circuitry that matures during pre-weaning development is altered and that it is already immune from environmental modification early post-weaning. It is noteworthy that both pre-weaning early isolation (Hall et al., 1999) and post-weaning social isolation (Jones et al., 1992) lead to increased dopaminergic activity in the nucleus accumbens in adulthood. This would suggest that there are processes additional to dopaminergic ones that are also involved in LI mediation and are differentially sensitive to the pre- and post-weaning environment. Robbins and co-workers have proposed that effects on serotonin pathways, for example, should certainly be taken into account in the study of the inter-relationships between environmental manipulations, neurobiological effects, and behavioural, including attentional, processes (Robbins et al., 1996).

Inhibition of sensorimotor gating, like LI and the inhibition/potentiation thereof, is underlain by a complex cortico-limbic-striatal circuitry (Swedlow and Geyer, 1998). Our finding that this circuitry is not susceptible to long-term change as a consequence of disruption of pre-weaning homeostasis is very important, particularly in combination with the evidence from this and other laboratories that rats maintained in post-weaning social isolation do demonstrate reduced PPI. Neuroleptics act to increase PPI in socially-isolated subjects, indicating that social isolation may induce changes in central dopaminergic mechanisms, but certainly not excluding the involvement of other neurotransmitter systems; serotonergic, glutamatergic and cholinergic systems all influence sensorimotor gating (Swerdlow and Geyer, 1998). Furthermore, the evidence that early isolation increases amphetamine-induced dopamine release in the nucleus accumbens (Hall et al., 1999) but does not impair PPI, also argues for the involvement of either altered dopaminergic activity in other brain regions or additional neurotransmitters, in the regulation of sensorimotor gating.

Our evidence for a dissociation between the effects of environmental manipulations on LI or PPI and their effects on spontaneous and amphetamine-induced locomotion, also points strongly to the involvement of changes beyond increased dopaminergic activity in the nucleus accumbens in the neurodevelopment of atypical latent inhibition and sensorimotor gating. As stated above, one of the major advantages of environmental manipulations is that this approach to animal modelling results in a brain that is free of surgical and pharmacological intervention, and that can be investigated systematically in order to identify the neurotransmitters and neural substrates involved in neurodevelopment of the marked and specific behavioural effects which we have demonstrated.

ACKNOWLEDGEMENTS

We sincerely thank the Swiss Federal Institute of Technology, Zurich, Switzerland, and F. Hoffmann La Roche AG, Basel, Switzerland, for the funding and support which made this research possible. Daniela Bettschen provided excellent assistance with the running of some of the studies described, and Annette Domeney and Thomas Stöhr contributed significantly to this research program.

REFERENCES

Denenberg, V.H. (1977) Assessing the effects of early experience. In R.D. Myers, ed. Methods in Psychobiology, Vol III (pp. 127-147). New York: Academic Press.

Domeney, A.M. and Feldon, J. (1998) The disruption of prepulse inhibition by social isolation in the Wistar rat: How robust is the effect? Pharmacol Biochem Behav 59: 883-890.

Ellenbroek, B.A. and Cools, A.R. (1995) Maternal separation reduces latent inhibition in the conditioned taste aversion paradigm. Neurosci Res Comm, 17: 27-33.

Ellenbroek, B.A. and Cools, A.R. (1998) The neurodevelopment hypothesis of schizophrenia: clinical evidence and animal models. Neurosci Res Comm 22: 127-136.

Ellenbroek, B.A., van den Kroonenberg, P.T.J.M., Cools, A.R. (1998) The effects of an early stressful life event on sensorimotor gating in adult rats. Schizophrenia Res 30: 251-260.

Feldon, J., Avnimelech-Gigus, N., Weiner, I. (1990) The effects of pre- and postweaning rearing conditions on latent inhibition and partial reinforcement extinction effect in male rats. Behav Neural Biol 53: 189-204.

Feldon, J., Shalev, U., Weiner, I. (1995) "Super" latent inhibition (LI) with high dose of amphetamine. Soc Neurosci Abstracts 21: 1230.

244

Feldon, J. and Weiner, I. (1988) Long-term attentional deficit in nonhandled males: possible involvement of the dopaminergic system. Psychopharmacol 95: 231-236.

Feldon, J. and Weiner, I. (1992) From an animal model of an attentional deficit towards new insights into the pathophysiology of schizophrenia. J Psychiatry Res 26: 345-366.

Geyer, M.A., Wilkinson, L.S., Humby, T., Robbins, T.W. (1993) Isolation rearing of rats produces a deficit in prepulse inhibition of acoustic startle similar to that in schizophrenia. Biol Psychiat 34: 361-372.

Hall, F.S., Wilkinson, L.S., Humby, T., Robbins, T.W. (1999) Maternal deprivation of neonatal rats produces enduring changes in dopamine function. Synapse 32: 37-43.

Jones, G.H., Hernandez, T.D., Kendall, D.A., Marsden, C.A., Robbins, T. W. (1992) Dopaminergic and serotonergic function following isolation rearing in rats: study of behavioural responses and post-mortem and in-vivo neurochemistry. Pharmacol Biochem Behav 43: 17-35.

Lehmann, J. and Feldon, J. (in press) Long-term bio-behavioural effects of maternal separation in the rat: consistent or confusing? Rev Neurosci.

Lehmann, J., Stöhr, T., Schuller, J., Domeney, A., Heidbreder, C., Feldon, J. (1998) Long-term effects of repeated maternal separation on three different latent inhibition paradigms. Pharmacol Biochem Behav 59: 873-882.

Lehmann, L., Pryce, C.R., Bettschen, D., Feldon, J. (1999) The maternal separation paradigm and adult emotionality and cognition in male and female Wistar rats. Pharmacol Biochem Behav 64: 705-715.

Lehmann, J., Stöhr, T., Feldon, J. (2000) Long-term effects of prenatal stress experience and postnatal maternal separation on emotionality and attentional processes. Behav Brain Res 107: 133-144.

Lehmann, J., Logeay, C., Feldon, J. (in press-a) Long-term effects of a single 24 hour maternal separation on three different latent inhibition paradigms. Psychobiol.

Lehmann, J., Pryce, C.R., Feldon, J. (2000) Lack of effect of an early stressful life event on sensorimotor gating in adult rats. Schizophr Res 41: 365-371.

Levine, S. (1960). Stimulation in infancy. Sci Amer 202: 81-86.

Liu, D., Diorio, J., Tannenbaum, B., Caldji, C., Francis, D., Freedman, A., Sharma, S., Pearson, D., Plotsky, P. M., and Meaney, M.J. (1997) Maternal care, hippocampal glucocorticoid receptors, and hypothalamic-pituitary-adrenal responses to stress. Science 277: 1659-1662.

Lubow, R.E. (1989) Latent Inhibition and Conditioned Attention Theory. Cambridge, U.K.: CUP.

Lubow, R.E. and Gewirtz, J.C. (1995) Latent inhibition in humans: data, theory, and implications for schizophrenia. Psychol Bull 117: 87-103.

Meaney, M.J., Diorio, J., Francis, D., Widdowson, J., LaPlante, P., Caldji, C., Sharma, S., Seckl, J.R., Plotsky, P.M. (1996) Early environmental regulation of forebrain glucocorticoid receptor gene expression: Implications for adrenocortical responses to stress. Dev Neurosci 18: 49-72.

Murphy, C.A., Heidbreder, C., Feldon, J. (2000) Cocaine sensitization enhances latent inhibition of a conditioned fear response. Schizophr Res 41: 247 (abstract).

Robbins, T.W., Jones, G.H., Wilkinson, L.S. (1996) Behavioural and neurochemical effects of early social deprivation in the rat. J Psychopharmacol 10: 39-47.

Swerdlow, N.R., Braff, D.L., Taaid, N., Geyer, M.A. (1994) Assessing the validity of an animal model of deficient sensorimotor gating in schizophrenic patients. Arch Gen Psychiatry 51: 139-154.

Swerdlow, N.R. and Geyer, M.A. (1998) Using an animal model of deficient sensorimotor gating to study the pathophysiology and new treatments of schizophrenia. Schizophr Bull 24: 285-301.

Vollenweider, F.X., Umbricht, D., Geyer, M., Hell, D. (2000) Effects of NMDA-antagonists and 5-HT2A-agonists on prepulse inhibition in human volunteers. Schizophr Res 41: 147 (abstract).

Weinberger, D.R. (1987) Implications of normal brain development for the pathogenesis of schizophrenia. Arch Gen Psychiatry 44: 660-669.

Weiner, I. and Feldon, J. (1997) The switching model of latent inhibition: an update of neural substrates. Behav Brain Res 88: 11-25.

Weiner, I., Feldon, J., Ziv-Harris, D. (1987) Early handling and latent inhibition in the conditioned suppression paradigm. Develop Psychobiol 20: 233-240.

Weiner, I., Schnabel, I., Lubow, R.E., Feldon, J. (1985) The effects of early handling on latent inhibition in male and female rats. Devel Psychobiol 18: 291-297.

Weiss, I.C., Feldon, J., Domeney, A. M. (1999). Isolation rearing-induced disruption of prepulse inhibition: further evidence for fragility of the response. Behav Pharmacol 10: 139-149.

Weiss, I.C., Domeney, A.M., Feldon, J. (2000) Sex differences in the effects of maternal separation and/or social isolation on sensorimotor gating in adult rats. Schizophr Res 41: 59 (abstract).

Weiss, I.C., Di Iorio, L., Feldon, J., Domeney, A. (2000) Strain differences in the isolation-induced effects on prepulse inhibition of the acoustic startle response and on locomotor activity. Behav Neurosci 114:364-373.

Weiss, I.C., Domeney, A.M., Moreau, J-L., Russig, H., Feldon, J. Dissociation between the effects of pre-weaning and/or post-weaning social isolation on prepulse inhibition and latent inhibition in adult Sprague-Dawley rats. Submitted to Behav Neurosci.

Wilkinson, L.S., Killcross, S.S., Humby, T., Hall, F.S., Geyer, M.A., Robbins, T.W. (1994). Social isolation in the rat produces developmentally specific deficits in prepulse inhibition of the acoustic startle response without disrupting latent inhibition. Neuropsychopharmacol 10: 61-72.

Williams, J.H., Wellman, N.A., Geaney, D.P., Cowen, P.J., Feldon, J., Rawlins, J.N.P. (1998) Reduced latent inhibition in people with schizophrenia: an effect of psychosis or of its treatment. Br J Psychiatry 172: 243-249.

14 ANIMAL MODELS OF SET-FORMATION AND SET-SHIFTING DEFICITS IN SCHIZOPHRENIA

Trevor W. Robbins

ABSTRACT

Schizophrenia is associated with a specific profile of cognitive impairments that is related to psychotic symptoms and stress-related deficits in a complex manner. Many of these cognitive deficits resemble those observed following frontal or temporal lobe dysfunction. We have developed several computerized tests that can be used in both experimental animals and humans, in the so-called CANTAB battery. Thus we have devised a computerized analogue of the Wisconsin Card Sorting Test (WCST) for testing non-human primates that is sensitive to impairment in neurosurgical patients with frontal lobe excisions and schizophrenia. This analogue breaks the WCST down into simpler components, including intra-dimensional and extra-dimensional shifts, and reversal learning, which have been found to be differentially sensitive to lesions to different parts of the prefrontal cortex in monkeys, and also to differential neurochemical lesions of these regions. The extra-dimensional shift discrimination is among the most sensitive tests we have used for revealing deficits in high-functioning schizophrenics, but chronic patients also exhibit significant difficulties with the intra-dimensional shift, possibly indicative of impairments in abstraction. In first episode patients diagnosed with schizophrenia by contrast, the deficit on the WCST analogue, while qualitatively similar to that of chronic hospitalized patients with schizophrenia, is relatively mild in comparison with performance on other tests such as spatial working memory. On retest a year later however, performance on the WCST analogue appears to deteriorate further, whereas performance on other tests often improves. The deterioration in performance on the WCST analogue seems unlikely to represent effects of medication, as it is more prevalent in patients with greater durations of untreated psychosis. The utility of the WCST analogue as a method for establishing close relationships between specific cognitive deficits in schizophrenia and certain cortical regions is noted. Its capacity for modification for use in rodents as experimental subjects, allowing a much more powerful means of manipulating certain key factors implicated in the aetiology of schizophrenia, is also explored. Both primate and rodent models are concluded to be necessary for modelling different facets of the cognitive dysfunction syndrome in schizophrenia.

INTRODUCTION

Cognitive deficits in schizophrenia are typically heterogeneous and wide-ranging, depending on factors whose precise importance is still unresolved, such as age and severity of illness, the chronicity of symptoms, the duration of untreated psychosis, the occurrence of stress and the precise medication regimen. The relationship of cognitive deficits to psychotic symptoms is still unclear (Figure 1), virtually all causal relationships plausibly operating. For example, core cognitive problems, such as the failure to monitor willed intentions, could conceivably cause delusions; alternatively, the psychotic symptoms may arise by analogy with epileptic phenomena to distort normal cognitive functions. These interactions in turn may be affected by such fluctuating influences as stress, triggered for example by life events or dysfunctional social relationships. The neuropsychological nature of the cognitive deficits in schizophrenia suggests several foci, including both frontal and temporal lobe impairments, which may be magnified by neuromodulatory influences (e.g., via dopaminergic activity) operating either at a cortical level, or within the striatum, where somewhat independent streams of information processing emanating from distinct cortical regions are relayed. The importance of understanding the cognitive deficit in schizophrenia is the increasing realization that its effective treatment is crucial for the social rehabilitation of schizophrenic individuals.

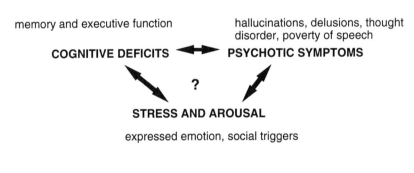

Figure 1. Putative causal relationships between the main contributory components of the cognitive syndrome in schizophrenia, including psychotic symptoms. The reciprocating arrows indicate that we cannot be sure of the direction of causal influences between these three constructs. Putative neural bases of the constructs are also shown.

Prominent among the cognitive impairments in schizophrenia are deficits in tests of executive function, commonly associated with frontal lobe damage. Such deficits are characterized by impairments in planning, maintenance of goal-directed behavior and cognitive flexibility. The latter is often assessed using the WCST, in which subjects initially have to deduce a rule for sorting compound stimuli according to a particular perceptual dimension (such as shape or color), and then to shift to alternative rule on the basis of changing feedback. It is this shift which is so problematic for patients with frontal lobe damage (Milner, 1963). In general, the results indicate that patients with schizophrenia achieve fewer sorting categories than controls and display significantly more perseverative errors, a failing itself suggestive of frontal lobe dysfunction. Indeed, Weinberger and colleagues (Weinberger and Berman, 1996) have used this test most effectively as a challenge for frontal lobe function in schizophrenic individuals in a functional imaging context. Such a challenge initially could be employed to probe for 'hypofrontality' in subjects diagnosed with schizophrenia, although this hypothesis entails certain problems of interpretation, including the possibility that the hypofrontality is an effect rather than a cause of impaired performance on the WCST (Frith, 1996). Resolution of the critical debate, however, seems to indicate that the WCST may well produce aberrant frontal activation in schizophrenic subjects that is distinct from that produced by other forms of psychopathology (Weinberger and Berman, 1996). An important residual question, however, is whether the nature of the WCST deficit is really comparable to that seen following frontal lobe dysfunction.

AN ANALOGUE OF THE WCST FOR HUMANS AND EXPERIMENTAL ANIMALS

In our own work, we have striven to attempt a functional decomposition of the WCST, which in reality is a complex sequence of discrimination learning tasks that can be understood within the framework of animal and human learning theory. This functional decomposition, therefore, comprises a suite of visual discrimination learning tasks that can be solved on the basis of trail and error feedback (Figure 2). The decomposition of the WCST into simpler components has the further attraction of reducing what is in reality a very complex task to more basic and readily analysed task contingencies. In fact, an analysis based on animal and human learning theory reduces the core component of the WCST to an extra-dimensional shift (eds, i.e. the shifting of behavioral control from one perceptual dimension of a stimulus compounded of multiple elements to another dimension, Roberts et al., 1988). One problem in the analysis of shifting from one stimulus to another is the associative interference that builds up if the same exemplar stimuli are used. Therefore, to avoid the intrusion of this lower-order process, novel exemplars of the compound stimuli are employed that utilise the same stimulus dimensions. Thus, in our procedure (Figure 2), subjects (both monkeys and humans) are invited to discriminate first say, between different *shapes*, one of which is consistently associated with reinforcement, and the other of which is consistently not related to reinforcement. Exactly similar stimuli are used for the human, as well as non-human, primates. Following simple discrimination, further control by the shape dimension, as distinct from a particular exemplar, is achieved by having the subject perform in a reversal learning procedure, in which the previously reinforced exemplar becomes non-reinforced, and *vice versa* (Figure 2). Subsequently, an alternative perceptual dimension is introduced. Two examples of superimposed *lines* may occur with either shape, but are only randomly associated with positive feedback. At a critical stage, one of the lines becomes reinforced, whereas the shapes are now only randomly associated with reinforcement. This is an example of an extra-dimensional shift. An important control is necessary to ensure that the animal or human is in fact exhibiting selective control by one stimulus dimension and not merely learning by rote which stimuli are rewarded on a configural basis (i.e., learning that each of two compound stimuli is correct). This control is provided by an intra-dimensional (ids) shift, in which new exemplars of the shape and line dimensions are again introduced, but the previously reinforced dimension (say shape) remains correct. This is called the 'total change' design (see Roberts et al., 1988 for discussion). If the subjects were attending to the stimuli on a configural basis, this would predict that performance should be equivalent for intra- and extra-dimensional shifting. If they were attending selectively to one of the dimensions only, then an intra-dimensional shift should be easier than an extra-dimensional shift, as measured by the number of errors or trials it takes to reach criterion. In fact, both for human and non-human primates (marmosets and rhesus monkeys), extra-dimensional shifting is always more difficult than intra-dimensional shifting (Roberts et al., 1988; Weed et al., 1999), even though the species, perhaps unsurprisingly, take progressively longer to learn either type of shift in relation to their phylogenetic status.

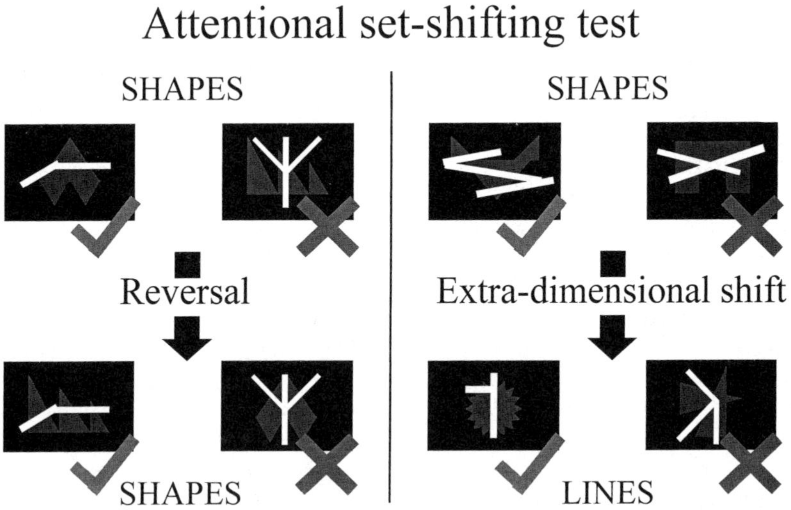

Attentional set-shifting test

Figure 2. Shows 2 different stages in the intra-dimensional/extra-dimensional visual discrimination paradigm. On the left hand side, reinforcement is switched between two compound stimuli comprising shapes and lines (which can occur in any combination across trials). The shape is reinforced, regardless of which line it occurs with. On reversal, it is the alternate shape that is now reinforced, again irrespective of its pairing with line. On the right hand side, shape is initially again the reinforced dimension. On the shift, novel exemplars are provided, but now one of the lines is consistently reinforced and the shape dimension is now irrelevant. This is an extra-dimensional shift. An intra-dimensional shift (not shown) also requires novel exemplars but the shape dimension continues to be the reinforced one. Reproduced with permission from Robbins (1998).

Somewhat remarkably, rats also tested on a touch sensitive screen were able eventually to learn the intra-dimensional shift task, although no rat has ever attained criterion on the extra-dimensional stages of the visual discrimination task (Bussey et al., 1994; Robbins, 1998), possibly because it is beyond the cognitive capacity of this species. It is an important point to consider whether rats would fail *all* forms of extra-dimensional shifts, as there is evidence that they can achieve extra-dimensional shifts under certain circumstances (Shepp and Eimas, 1964; Rowe et al., 1996). For example, given their basic sensory capacities, it would be plausible that they could effect extra-dimensional shifts with olfactory stimuli. Such evidence has recently become available from Birrell and Brown (2000) who have used an olfactory ids/eds discrimination learning paradigm to demonstrate a role for the medial prefrontal cortex in extradimensional shifting in the rat. The argument that rats cannot perform this shift because of limitations of cognitive capacity imposed by a relatively poorly developed prefrontal cortex thus appears dubious. What is remarkable, however, is the clear convergence of evidence, cross-species that implicates the prefrontal cortex in extra-dimensional shifting in rats, marmosets and humans (see below).

Further construct validation at the behavioral level may be achieved by studying other task manipulations. For example, there is some evidence that marmosets may find learning more difficult when discriminating or shifting to the line dimension. Native villagers in Venezuela apparently also have such difficulties which are overcome in part by prior training on the line dimension (J. Iddon, personal communication). An additional theoretical issue of interest concerns the possible use of language in human subjects to mediate performance of this task. Recently, it has been suggested that the WCST contains an important working memory component based on the phonological slave system (Dunbar and Sussman, 1995). This was demonstrated by the disruptive effects in normal subjects of blockade of this phonological 'loop' by articulatory suppression (repeated utterance of words such as 'the' or 'see-saw'). The experiment emphasises a potentially important constraint on animal models of cognitive functions because of the confounding effects of linguistic strategies. We have, however, used this same manipulation of articulatory suppression on subjects performing our intra-dimensional/extra-dimensional set-shifting task and found no deficits to date, perhaps because our stimuli are less readily or usefully verbally labelled.

The other criterion we have applied in testing for functional homology is to show that the various components of the attentional set-shifting paradigm are mediated by similar neural systems across human and non-human primates. Thus, studies in humans (Owen et al., 1991) and marmosets (Dias et al., 1996,1997) have established that damage to the prefrontal cortex can produce selective deficits at the extra-dimensional shifting stage. In the study by Dias et al. (1996), excitotoxic lesions of the lateral prefrontal cortex were effective in this regard (see Figure 3). By contrast, similar excitotoxic lesions of the orbitofrontal cortex impaired reversal learning (Dias et al., 1996), a result also found in humans with orbitofrontal damage caused by closed head injury (Rolls et al., 1994) or by dementia of the frontal type (or 'lobar atrophy') (Rahman et al., 1998a,b). Recent evidence obtained using functional neuroimaging with PET (Rogers et al., 2000) has also confirmed that reversal learning and intra- and extra-dimensional shifting engages some overlapping, but also distinct circuitries. While there is further evidence that the extra-dimensional shift activates selective regions of the human prefrontal cortex, we have only found subcortical activation to date following reversal learning.

Reversal does, however, engage the ventral striatum, which forms part of the same cortico-striatal 'loop' as the orbitofrontal cortex. This evidence will therefore predict deficits in reversal learning of this type following lesions of the ventral striatum in monkeys.

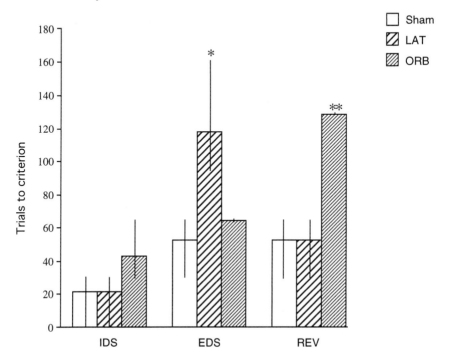

Figure 3. Double dissociation of the effects of orbital and lateral lesions of the marmoset prefrontal cortex on intra-dimensional set-shifting, extra-dimensional set-shifting and reversal learning (based on data reported in Dias et al., 1996).

As patients with basal ganglia disorders such as Parkinson's (PD) (Downes et al., 1989) and Huntington's diseases (Lawrence et al., 1998), as well as patients with schizophrenia, are all impaired on the extra-dimensional shift (as well as the WCST), this provides a possibly useful animal model of this type of cognitive deficit in these groups. We have capitalized on this by investigating the effects of relatively selective cholinergic or dopaminergic depletions from the prefrontal cortex in marmosets in order to determine if such depletion, which is known to form part of the neuropathological picture in PD patients, could be responsible for their impairments in 'cognitive flexibility.' In fact, the evidence collected thus far suggests that this is not the case (in fact, the prefrontal depleted monkeys are apparently better than normal at the extra-dimensional shift, though impaired on the delayed response task, Roberts et al., 1994). The finding is consistent with evidence of inverse correlations of WCST performance with fluorodopa binding in the cortex of PD patients (Leenders, 1993). However, dopamine depletion from the caudate nucleus in marmosets fails to produce simple deficits in extra-dimensional shifting, but rather produces impairment when the animals are required to shift back towards a previously learned attentional 'set' (Collins et al., 2000). Moreover, further analysis of the apparently facilitated performance in the prefrontally dopamine depleted marmosets has revealed a possible reason for their anomalous performance. It appears that the lesioned marmosets do not come under equivalent levels of stimulus control as the sham-operated animals. Specifically, they may fail at certain stages of the visual discrimination tasks if the prefrontal dopamine depletion is effected prior to extensive compound discrimination training. Thus marmosets with prefrontal dopamine loss are more severely disrupted by the introduction of an irrelevant novel dimension to replace a previously irrelevant one, suggesting that these animals were still inappropriately monitoring the alternative dimension, and had not established fully effective sets. This hypothesis was substantiated by further demonstrations of impaired intra-dimensional shift learning in prefrontal dopamine depleted monkeys under certain conditions.

Recent human psychopharmacological findings have shown that whereas the catecholamine indirect agonist methylphenidate enhances the propensity to exhibit extra-dimensional shifting, the dopamine D2 receptor antagonist sulpiride impairs extra-dimensional shifting on a more complex 3-dimensional variant of the task in normal volunteers (Mehta et al., 1999). This result is potentially significant in the interpretation of findings with medicated schizophrenic groups who are typically treated with neuroleptic drugs having D2 receptor antagonist properties. The findings with dopamine depleted marmosets are also relevant for the interpretation of WCST deficits in schizophrenia, which have been related by some workers to reduced prefrontal DA function.

PERFORMANCE OF PATIENTS WITH SCHIZOPHRENIA ON TESTS OF ATTENTIONAL SET FORMATION AND SHIFTING

The ids/eds attentional set-shifting paradigm and its variants have so far yielded striking but clear results when used to test groups of schizophrenic patients. In one recent study, Pantelis et al. (1999) utilized a group of 51 patients with chronic schizophrenia. Those with relatively high IQ (n=24) were compared with patients with lesions in the prefrontal cortex (n=22) and with normal control subjects (n=18), the groups being well-matched for age, sex and IQ, as indexed by the National Adult Reading Test. The schizophrenic group showed a significantly higher attrition at the intra-dimensional shift stage of learning compared with the other two groups. Even those schizophrenic subjects who were able to achieve criterion at this stage performed it significantly worse than the other groups in terms of errors committed. This relative selectivity of deficit at the ids stage is of considerable interest, as it has not been exhibited in such a consistent way by any of the several other forms of psychopathological groups that have been tested using this procedure, including Huntington's disease, Parkinson's disease, frontal lobe damage and dementia of the frontal type. The nature of the deficit suggests an impairment of abstracting ability, i.e., the ability to generalize a rule beyond the specific exemplars for which it had been acquired, which emancipates the normal volunteer from concrete forms of responding. Such a deficit is consistent with what is observed clinically in schizophrenia in terms of symptoms, and may be relevant to the classical thought disorder. In neural terms, these problems of intra-dimensional shifting and abstracting ability are generally not considered to be indicative of dysfunction limited to frontal regions. The PET functional imaging study of Rogers et al. (2000) reported that intra-dimensional shift learning was characterized by quite a wide range of neural activations, including the temporal, as well, as the frontal lobes. The deficit in intra-dimensional shift learning is consistent with data from a PET study of normal volunteers suggestive of a fronto-temporal framework for this form of learning. The patients doing particularly badly at the ids stage tended to respond too quickly, and also tended to score low on clinical scales of bradykinesia, and high on scales of behavioral disorganization.

At the eds stage, both the frontal group and the schizophrenic sub-group showed greater attrition than controls. The schizophrenic subjects failing the eds stage had higher levels of negative symptomatology such as flattened affect and poverty of speech. However, this impairment was overshadowed in this group by the profound impairments at the ids stage. An earlier study (Elliott et al., 1995, 1998) found evidence for a much more specific deficit at the eds stage. These studies employed a variant of the eds task in which it was possible to determine whether deficits reflected perseveration of responses to the previously reinforced dimension or a failure to engage attention to the previously irrelevant dimension (a form of learned irrelevance, related to latent inhibition, see Weiner, this volume). Elliott et al. (1998) found highly specific deficits in attrition at the eds stage for the perseveration condition that resembled, but far out-stripped in magnitude, what was found for patients with frontal lobe excisions. By comparison with the Pantelis et al. study patients were more mildly affected by the disease, typically being outpatients rather than chronically hospitalized individuals. Overall, both the Pantelis et al. and Elliott et al. studies showed that the level of impairment on the ids/eds paradigm could not be simply related to IQ. In the Pantelis et al. study, attrition was simply shifted to the left in the low IQ compared with high IQ sub-groups, but the two sub-groups exhibited qualitatively similar forms of deficit (see Figure 4). The overall conclusion from these studies is that schizophrenics are poor at intra-dimensional, as well as extra-dimensional shifts, a pattern consistent with a rather wider stage of deficits rather than simply frontal impairment. These impairments are specific however, in the sense that they are not simply related to IQ or to indices of dementia. Elliott et al. (1998) also showed specificity of cognitive deficits in terms of relative magnitude across a range of cogntive functions. The patients with schizophrenia were impaired in virtually every test, but the magnitude of the deficit in terms of standardized scores was by far the greatest for the test of extra-dimensional shifting. The patients with attentional set formation and shifting deficits in the study by Pantelis et al. (1999) also had a much broader range of cognitive impairments, including several aspects of visuospatial memory and planning function also shown to be sensitive to prefrontal cortical damage (see Pantelis et al., 1997).

DEFICITS IN INTRA-DIMENSIONAL AND EXTRA-DIMENSIONAL SHIFTING IN THE STAGING OF COGNITIVE DEFICITS IN SCHIZOPHRENIA

One way of discerning the importance of different aspects of the cognitive syndrome in schizophrenia is to study the cognitive profile in a longitudinal manner, from the first episodes of psychosis. This has been achieved in recent studies from Eileen Joyce's laboratory at Imperial College, which has characterized a large group of first episode schizophrenics and then followed them over many months (Hutton et al., 1998). These patients were administered a large battery of standard and more experimental tests, including the ids/eds visual discrimination paradigm. The important results on initial entry to the programme were that performance on the ids/eds test was actually superior to that attained in several other parts of the battery, particularly in tests of spatial working memory and various forms of paired associate learning and semantic memory, which are known to be severely deficient in chronic schizophrenia. Although the first episode patients were significantly impaired in relation to age and IQ matched controls, the nature of the impairment did not, again, indicate a specific impairment in extra-dimensional shifting, as errors were increased proportionately in both the ids and eds stages. Thus, the same tendency to be impaired at the ids stage in chronic schizophrenia is seen even in the earliest stages of presentation. However, the specific and profound impairment seen in the eds test (Elliott et al., 1998) was not at all present in this first episode group.

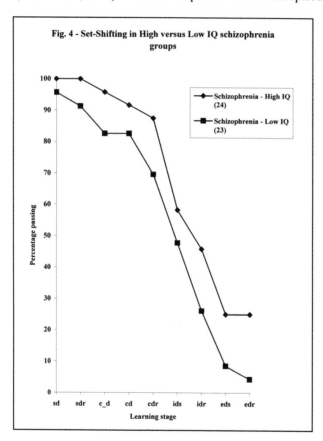

Figure 4. Relative performance of low and high IQ schizophrenic groups on the visual discrimination ids/eds paradigm. The attrition of both groups is shown in reaching the learning criterion at each stage. sd=simple discimination, c_d=compound discrimination (separate lines and shapes), cd=compound discrimination (superimposed lines and shapes), cdr=compound discrimination reversal (see also fig. 2, left hand side), ids=intradimensional shift, idr =intradimensional shift reversal, eds =extradimensional shift, edr=extradimensional shift reversal. Note the relatively steady attrition in both groups across the various stages, especially and unusually at the intra-dimensional stage. Typical performance of control subjects matched for age and IQ is not shown, but in this study over 90% successfully passed the entire sequence of learning stages. Reproduced from Pantelis et al., 1999, with permission.

Of even greater significance is that on retest 12 months later, the deficit on the ids/eds task became greater at a time when the patients had been stabilized on anti-psychotic medication (Joyce et al., 2000). It is of course plausible that this worsening of performance could be attributed to anti-psychotic medication, as the anti-psychotic drug sulpiride has been shown to impair extra-dimensional shifting (Mehta et al., 1999). However, while a possible effect of medication remains a distinct possibility, it is pertinent that performance on many of the other tests showed considerable improvement. These improvements are unlikely to be caused by practice effects a year later – in fact, if anything, practice might be expected most to benefit extra-dimensional shift performance. The possibility that the ids/eds test is somehow more susceptible to impairment by neuroleptic drugs is diminished by the observation that this deficit was found to be greatest in those patients who had the longest periods of untreated psychosis (Joyce et al., 2000). Thus, these data are consistent with the hypothesis of a progressively deteriorating cognitive state that is exacerbated by delay in treatment with anti-psychotic drugs. These observations suggest that performance on the ids/eds test might be useful for indicating prognosis with respect to possible rehabilitation strategies. Of course, much work remains to be done, for example, in understanding the neural correlates of evolving performance on the ids/eds procedure. Published observations have suggested that successful eds performance in normal subjects is related to an activation in the dorsolateral and rostrolateral prefrontal cortex (Brodmann area 10), in the ventral putamen, and deactivations in the temporal lobe (Rogers et al., 2000). Thus, in general terms, the impaired performance of the schizophrenic patients probably reflects changes in this circuitry.

IMPLICATIONS FOR MODELS OF SCHIZOPHRENIA

The term 'model' can be used in different ways, for example, as a way of exploring possible aetiological factors in a disorder, as well as simulating some of its key elements. In this brief chapter we have not tried to advance performance on the ids/eds task as a 'model' for schizophrenia. Instead we have tried to understand in greater detail the nature of the cognitive deficit in schizophrenia, by studying one aspect of its complex symptomatology. This process of modelling distinct symptoms is a useful one, given the complexity of such symptoms in schizophrenia. Given that schizophrenics are so unsuccessful in performing tasks such as these, it makes sense to use them to explore the neural as well as the cognitive underpinnings of schizophrenia. This can be achieved in part by suitable experiments with animals, as well as by adopting procedures for functional neuroimaging to define the necessary circuitry for this type of capacity. It is not yet clear which aetiological factors will turn out to be the most important in the expression of schizophrenia, but the validation of any model of this type, as well as effective and objective means for cognitive improvement, will require sophisticated tests such as these. A possible limitation derives from the fact that rats are not especially competent at the extradimensional shift task (although reasonably good ids performance is quite feasible). This would render the ids/eds task difficult to use for rats in assessing, for example, manipulations such as exposure to toxins during early development, or to deprivation of social contact, which may affect relevant cortical, as well as striatal regions. Such manipulations are of course much more difficult to implement in primates. However, the recent demonstration of an homologous form of extra-dimensional shifting in rats as in primates (Birrell and Brown, 2000) does suggest that the use of aetiological models might also be greatly enhanced by these improved methods. It may well be possible to simulate one small, but important part of the cognitive deficit syndrome in schizophrenia. This may be used either to gain further understanding of the neuropsychological picture in schizophrenia, or even as sophisticated and well-validated 'assay' to explore and assess effects of relevant genetic, social or developmental factors.

ACKNOWLEDGEMENTS

This work was supported by a Wellcome Trust Programme grant, awarded to TWR, BJ Everitt, BJ Sahakian and A. Roberts, and completed within the MRC Brain, Behavior and Neuropsychiatry Co-operative group.

REFERENCES

Birrell J. and Brown V.J. (2000) Medial frontal cortex mediates perceptual attentional set shifting in the rat. Submitted Ms.

Bussey, T.J., Muir, J.L., Robbins, T.W. (1994) A novel automated touchscreen procedure for assessing learning in the rat using computer graphic stimuli. Neuroscience Research Communications 15, 103-110.

Collins, P., Wilkinson, L.S., Everitt, B.J., Robbins, T.W., Roberts, A.C. (2000) The effect of dopamine depletion from the caudate nucleus of the common marmoset on tests of prefrontal cognitive function. Behavioral Neuroscience, in press.

Dias, R., Roberts, A., Robbins, T.W. (1996) Dissociation in prefrontal cortex of affective and attentional shifts. Nature, 380, 69-72.

Dias, R., Robbins, T.W., Roberts, A.C. (1997) Dissociable forms of inhibitory control within prefrontal cortex with an analogue of the Wisconsin card sort test: restriction to novel situations and independence from 'on-line' processing. Journal of Neuroscience. 17, 9285-9297.

Downes, J.J., Roberts, A.C., Sahakian, B.J., Evenden, J.L., Robbins, T.W. (1989) Impaired extra-dimensional shift performance in medicated and unmedicated Parkinson's disease: evidence for a specific attentional dysfunction. Neuropsychologia, 27, 1329-1344.

Dunbar K. and Sussman D. (1995) Toward a cognitive account of frontal-lobe deficits in normal subjects. Ann NY Acad Sci 769, 289-304

Elliott, R., McKenna, P.J., Robbins, T.W., Sahakian, B.J. (1995) Neuropsychological evidence for fronto-striatal dysfunction in schizophrenia. Psychological Medicine, 25, 619-630.

Elliott, R., McKenna, P.J., Robbins, T.W., Sahakian, B.J. (1998) Specfic neuropsychological deficits in schizophrenic patients with preserved intellectual function. Cognitive Neuropsychiatry 3, 45-70.

Frith C.D. (1996) The role of the prefrontal cortex in self-consciousness: the case of auditoryhallucinations. Philosophical Transactions of the Royal Society B 351 1505-1514.

Hutton, S.B., Puri, B.K., Duncan, L.J., Robbins, T.W., Barnes T.R.E., Joyce, E. M. (1998) Executive function in first-episode schizophrenia. Psychological Medicine. 28, 463-473.

Joyce, E.M., Hutton, S.B., Robbins, T.W., Barnes, T.R.E. (2000) Changes in executive function during the early stages of schizophrenia and the relationship to untreated psychosis. Submitted ms.

Lawrence, A.D., Hodges, J.R., Rosser, A.E., Kershaw, A., ffrench-Constant, C., Rubinsztein, D.C., Robbins, T.W., Sahakian, B.J. (1998) Evidence for specific cognitive deficits in preclinical Huntington's disease. Brain. 121, 1329-1341

Leenders KL (1993) Mental dysfunction in patients with Parkinson's disease. In Mental Dysfunction in Parkinson's Disease, (ed EC Wolters and P. Scheltens) pp133-139 Amsterdam, Vrije Univesity Press.

Mehta, M.A., Sahakian, B.J., McKenna, P.J., Robbins, T.W. (1999) Systemic sulpiride in young adult volunteers simulates the profile of cognitive deficits in Parkinson's disease. Psychopharmacology. 146, 162-174.

Milner B (1963) Effects of different brain lesions on card-sorting: the role of the frontal lobes. Archives of Neurology 9, 100-110.

Owen, A.M., Roberts, A.C., Polkey, C.E., Sahakian, B.J., Robbins, T.W. (1991) Extra-dimensional versus intradimensional set shifting performance following frontal lobe excision, temporal lobe excision or amygdalo-hippocampectomy in man. Neuropsychologia, 29, 993-1006.

258

Pantelis, C., Barnes, T.R.E., Nelson, H.E., Tanner, S., Weatherley, L., Owen, A.M., Robbins, T.W. (1997) Frontal-striatal cognitive deficits in patients with chronic schizophrenia. Brain, 120, 1823-1843.

Pantelis, C., Barber, E.Z., Barnes, T.R.E., Nelson, H.E., Owen, A.M., Robbins, T.W. (1999) A comparison of set-shifting ability in patients with schizophrenia and frontal lobe damage. Schizophrenia Research. 37, 251-270.

Rahman, S., Sahakian, B.J., Robbins, T.W. (1998a) Comparative studies of frontal lobe function: what they may reveal about possible therapeutic strategies in frontotemporal dementia. Dementia and Geriatric Cognitive Disorders. 10 (suppl) 15-28.

Rahman, S., Sahakian, B.J., Hodges, J.R., Rogers, R.D., Robbins, T.W. (1998b) Specific cognitive deficits in mild frontal variant frontotemporal dementia. Brain. 122, 1469-1493

Robbins, T.W. (1998) Homology in behavioral pharmacology: an approach to animal models of human cognition. Behavioral Pharmacology, 9, 509-520.

Roberts, A., Robbins, T.W., Everitt, B.J. (1988) Extra- and Intra-dimensional shifts in man and marmoset. Q.J. exp. Psychol. 40B, 321-342.

Roberts, A.C., De Salvia, M.A., Wilkinson, L.S., Collins, P., Muir, J.L., Everitt, B.J., Robbins, T.W. (1994) 6-hydroxydopamine lesions of the prefrontal cortex in monkeys enhance performance on an analogue of the Wisconsin Card Sorting test: Possible interactions with subcortical dopamine. J. Neuroscience 14, 2531-2544.

Rogers, R.D., Andrews, T.C., Grasby, P.M., Brooks, D., Robbins, T.W. (2000) Contrasting cortical and sub-cortical PET activations produced by reversal learning and attentional-set shifting in humans. Journal of Cognitive Neuroscience. In Press.

Rowe, J., Saunders, J.R. , Durantou, F., Robbins, T.W. (1996) Systemic idazoxan impairs performance in a non-reversal shift test: implications for the role of the central noradrenergic systems in selective attention. Journal of Psychopharmacology, 10, 188-194.

Rolls E.T., Hornak J., Wade, D., McGrath, J. (1994) Emotion-related learning in patients with social and emotional changes associated with frontal lobe damage. Journal of Neurology, Neurosurgery and Psychiatry. 57, 1518-1524.

Shepp B.E. and Eimas, P.D. (1964) Intradimensional and extradimensional shifts in the rat. Journal of Comparative and Physiological Psychology 57, 357-361.

Weed M.R., Taffe, M.A., Polis, I., Roberts, A.C., Robbins, T.W., Koob, G.F., Bloom, F.E., Gold, L.H. (1999) Performance norms for a rhesus monkey neuropsychological testing battery; acquisition and long-term performance.Cognitive Brain Research 8, 185-201.

Weinberger D.R. and Berman K. F. (1996) Prefrontal function in schizophrenia:confounds and controversies. Philosophical Transactions of the Royal Society B351, 1495-1503.

15 EARLY DISRUPTION OF CORTICOLIMBIC CIRCUITRY AS A MODEL OF SCHIZOPHRENIA

Barbara K. Lipska and Daniel R. Weinberger

INTRODUCTION

The main problem with modeling schizophrenia has been a lack of knowledge about its etiology and basic neurobiology. This problem has precluded modeling aspects other than a rather limited number of phenomena. Most traditional models of schizophrenia reproduce primarily phenomena linked to dopamine, because the dopaminergic system has been strongly, although indirectly, implicated in this disorder (all effective antipsychotic drugs are antagonists of dopamine receptors, and dopamine agonists induce symptoms that resemble psychosis) (Kornetsky and Markowitz, 1978; McKinney and Moran, 1981; Ellenbroek and Cools, 1990; Costall and Naylor, 1995). Some dopamine-based models involve behavioral paradigms that were inspired by antipsychotic (i.e., antidopaminergic) pharmacology but bear no resemblance to schizophrenia (e.g., antagonism of apomorphine-induced emesis). Others reproduce phenomena analogous to selected features of schizophrenia such as motor behaviors (e.g., dopamimetic-induced stereotypies) and information processing deficits (e.g. apomorphine-induced prepulse inhibition of startle (PPI) abnormalities) (for review see, Costall and Naylor, 1995). These dopamine-linked behaviors, although not specific or unique for schizophrenia, can be at least detected and precisely evaluated in non-human species and were useful in screening drugs with a predicted mechanism of action (e.g., dopamine blockade). Their predictive validity might be expected given that the models were based on changing dopamine function. However, as "dopamine-in, dopamine-out" models (i.e., models based on direct pharmacological manipulation of the dopaminergic system and testing behavioral outcome related to this disruption), they precluded exploring other than dopamine-based mechanisms of the disease and discovering novel antipsychotic therapies. Consequently, drugs that emerged as a result of such models all exerted antidopaminergic efficacy. Antidopaminergic drugs, however, although ameliorative of some of the symptoms of schizophrenia, do not cure the disease. It has become increasingly clear that models based on manipulations of the dopamine system may have exhausted their heuristic potential and that new strategies need to be developed to provide novel targets for the development of more effective therapeutic agents.

NOVEL HEURISTIC MODELS OF SCHIZOPHRENIA

In the context of our current limited knowledge about schizophrenia, the principal goal of heuristic models is to test the plausibility of theories derived from the emerging research data about the disorder, to uncover novel mechanisms of schizophrenia-like phenomena and suggest potential new treatments. Recently, interest in schizophrenia research has shifted from a principal focus on dopamine to other theories, the most prominent of which are theories of abnormal neurodevelopment, dysfunction of cortical glutamatergic neurons, and genetic susceptibility. Animal models have followed a similar trend. These novel models are either non-pharmacological or based on pharmacological manipulation of a neurotransmitter other than dopamine. Thus, they offer the potential of elucidating non-dopamine mechanisms of disease and treatment. However, despite their non-dopaminergic origin, the face and predictive validity of this new generation of models still strongly depends, at least in part, on how closely they reproduce certain dopamine-related phenomena (e.g., enhanced locomotion, stereotyped behaviors, deficits in sensorimotor gating and responsiveness to antidopaminergic drugs, see Table 1).

Table 1. Clinical Aspects of Schizophrenia and Relevant Behavioral Changes in Animals

Schizophrenia: Clinical Phenomena	Animal Models: Behavioral Changes
1. Psychotic symptoms	Behaviors related to increased dopaminergic transmission: i) Dopamimetic-induced hyperlocomotion ii) Reduced haloperidol-induced catalepsy
2. Stereotypic behaviors	Dopamimetic-induced stereotypies
3. Worsening of psychotic symptoms by NMDA-antagonists	NMDA antagonists-induced locomotion
4. Vulnerability to stress	Stress-induced hyperlocomotion
5. Information processing deficits	Sensorimotor gating (PPI, P50)
6. Attentional deficits	Deficits in latent inhibition
7. Cognitive deficits	Impaired performance in delayed alternation and spatial memory tests
8. Social withdrawal	Reduced contacts with unfamiliar partners

A major problem in evaluating any model of schizophrenia is a lack of a straightforward "litmus test" of fidelity. This is because there is no valid genotype, cellular phenotype or other biological marker that is characteristic of and unique for the disorder. The choice of validation criteria is often subjective, reflecting a researcher's preference about what is important and what can be modeled in an animal. However, as new findings about the pathophysiology of schizophrenia emerge, new models may be expected to focus on certain cell or tissue phenotypes selected behavioral characteristics, as well as time-honored effects on dopamine related function (Table 1).

Many of the proposed new models test specific hypotheses that schizophrenia is caused by a subtle defect in cerebral development (Lillrank et al., 1995). They are based on experimentally induced disruption of brain development that becomes evident in an adult animal in the form of altered brain neurochemistry and aberrant behavior (neurodevelopmental models) and test whether the effects of early brain damage could remain inconspicuous until after a considerable delay, as appears to be the case in the human condition (Weinberger, 1986, 1987; Murray and Lewis, 1987; Bloom, 1993). Some of these neurodevelopmental models test the plausibility of various etiological hypotheses of schizophrenia, including malnutrition (Susser and Lin, 1992), obstetric complications (Woerner et al., 1973; DeLisi, 1988; Hultman et al., 1997; Dalman et al., 1999; Brake et al., 1997b,c; El-Khodor and Boksa, 1997, 1998), viral infections (Mednick et al., 1988; Kendell and Kemp, 1989; O'Callaghan et al., 1991; Adams et al., 1993; Rott et al., 1985; Waltrip et al., 1995; Solbrig et al., 1994, 1996a,b; Fatemi et al., 1999), and early postnatal stress implicated in the onset of the disorder (Liu et al., 1997, Jones et al., 1992; Geyer et al., 1993; Wilkinson et al., 1994). Other models do not attempt to reproduce specific putative causative factors implicated in schizophrenia, but mimic cellular aberrations that presumably follow a disruption of early cortical development analogous to what has been described in the human postmortem studies (Akbarian et al., 1993). These conditions are modeled by gestational irradiation or in-utero exposure to a mitotic toxin, methylazoxymethanol acetate (MAM) (Rakic, 1996; Mintz et al., 1997; Johnston et al., 1988; Talamini et al., 1998). Still another approach is represented by lesion models that reproduce a putative defect in schizophrenia by chemical or surgical destruction of brain regions or neurotransmitter systems implicated in the disorder (Lipska et al., 1993; Brake et al., 1997; Chambers et al., 1996; Wan et al., 1996; Grecksch et. al. 1999; Saunders et al., 1998; Rajakumar et al., 1996; Bardgett et al., 1996; Flores et al., 1996a,b; Lipska et al, 1998a). As models of developmental pathology, they represent a rather crude technique, but provide important information about the function of restricted brain areas and neural connections between them. Characteristically, a majority of these new models, despite a diversity of inducing factors, target in various ways components of a common neural circuitry frequently implicated in schizophrenia, i.e., the temporolimbic cortices – nucleus accumbens/striatal complex – thalamus – prefrontal cortex.

In the following sections, we will focus on the model involving developmental disruption of the temporolimbic cortex, and show that this early insult results in the dysfunction of a wide circuitry implicated in schizophrenia, including the dopamine system and brain regions engaged in cognitive functions.

NEONATAL HIPPOCAMPAL LESION MODEL

A number of studies have focused on neonatal damage of restricted brain regions in rats (Lipska et al., 1993; Brake et al., 1997; Flores et al., 1996a; Chambers et al., 1996; Wan et al., 1996; Grecksch et al., 1999) and in monkeys (Saunders et al., 1998) as potential novel neurodevelopmental models of schizophrenia. The main objective of these studies is to damage the hippocampus, a brain area consistently implicated in human schizophrenia (Falkai and Bogerts,

1986; Jeste and Lohr, 1989; Bogerts, 1990; Harrison and Eastwood, 1998; Suddath et al., 1990; Eastwood and Harrison, 1995; Weinberger, 1999), and thus disrupt development of the widespread cortical and subcortical circuitry in which the hippocampus participates. The timing of damage was chosen to roughly correspond to the second/third trimester of gestation in humans, a developmental period implicated in schizophrenia. As the rat brain at birth is at a less mature developmental stage than the brain of the human neonate (approximately the 12-13-day-old rat pup's brain corresponds in terms of the degree of maturation to the full-term newborn human infant (Romijn et al., 1991), rats were lesioned in the hippocampus at very early postnatal ages (days 3-7).

The results of our studies demonstrated that neonatal (postnatal days 3-7) excitotoxic lesions of the ventral portion of the rat hippocampus (VH) produce a temporally specific pattern of abnormalities (emergence in adolescence) in a number of dopamine related behavioral paradigms. The neonatal VH lesions result in postpubertal onset of abnormal behaviors, such as hyperlocomotion in a novel environment and after d-amphetamine, enhanced stereotypy after apomorphine, diminished catalepsy after haloperidol, and deficits in prepulse inhibition of startle (PPI) (Lipska et al., 1993; Lipska and Weinberger, 1993, 1994a, 1995; Lipska et al., 1995a; Flores et al., 1996a; Wan et al., 1996; Brake et al., 1999; Black et al., 1998; Le Pen et al., 1999), phenomena reminiscent of schizophrenia in terms of a temporal profile of changes (emergence in early adulthood) and neurotransmitter systems engaged (dopamine hyperactivity). Consistent with observations in schizophrenia, abnormal behaviors can be reversed by neuroleptics (Lipska and Weinberger, 1994a). Moreover, this developmental lesion interacts with genetic and environmental factors (Lipska and Weinberger, 1995) that can alter a profile of emergent behaviors. For instance, Fisher344 rats, a highly stress-responsive strain, show particularly high susceptibility to the behavioral effects of neonatal hippocampal damage. Lewis rats, on the other hand, bred for low stress responsiveness, appear to be resistant to the behavioral consequences of identical lesions (Lipska and Weinberger, 1995). Involvement of a genetic component in this model is particularly important because it addresses another aspect of the disease, i.e., that schizophrenia is a highly heritable disorder that probably involves multiple genes with small effects across large populations (Kendler et al., 1996).

VH Lesion Disrupts PFC Function

In a large series of studies we and other investigators have shown that the neonatal ventral hippocampal lesion results in a constellation of behavioral changes that emerge in adolescence, a time coincident with sexual maturation. It raised the possibility that hormonal changes during puberty might be responsible for the emergent abnormalities. However, emergence in adolescence of behavioral disruptions does not seem to be dependent on the surge of gonadal hormones as evidenced by the results of the study in which we tested lesioned rats that had been castrated prior to puberty (Lipska and Weinberger, 1994b). These rats showed a similar pattern of abnormal behaviors as their non-castrated lesioned counterparts. Thus, we have posited that changes in behavior appear in these rats in adolescence because neonatal insult altered development and function of the component(s) of neural circuitry in which the VH participates and that are critical for these behaviors at maturity. The prefrontal cortex (PFC) is a strong candidate as an anatomical substrate for such changes because it receives VH projections, matures late, participates in complex behaviors, and has been implicated as a prominent site of pathology in schizophrenia (Weinberger, 1999). We have then set out to determine if indeed function of PFC is compromised in the neonatally hippocampally lesioned animals, and if the type of abnormalities is reminiscent of changes observed in the human disorder.

Changes in complex behaviors

In a series of experiments we have demonstrated that the neonatal VH lesion disrupts complex behaviors (cognitive behaviors and social interactions) that engage PFC, a brain region interconnected with VH and posited to develop abnormally in the context of missing hippocampal afferents. Changes in these behaviors are considered key negative symptoms of schizophrenia.

Cognitive changes were evaluated in a T-maze forced-trial delayed alternation test (Moghaddam et al., 1999). This test is used to assess working memory in rodents and is sensitive to the integrity of the PFC (Freeman and Stanton, 1992). Rats were presented with a randomly chosen forced run that was rewarded, followed by choice runs (delay 1, 10 or 40 sec between the runs) rewarded if alternation occurred. At all delays, the neonatally lesioned rats performed significantly worse than controls. However, rats lesioned in adulthood were not impaired in this task. This suggests that neonatal but not adult damage of the VH impairs working memory, and that this abnormality may be reflective of impaired function of the PFC (Fuster, 1995; Yang et al., 1999). This finding supported our hypothesis that PFC develops aberrantly if devoid of normal hippocampal input from early in life.

Social behaviors were assessed at two ages: pre- and postpuberty. Two unfamiliar rats of the same lesion status (sham or lesion) were placed in a large open field and videotaped (Sams-Dodd et al., 1997). Frequency and types of contacts between rats were then evaluated. Neonatally lesioned rats made less social contacts than controls. In contrast to dopamine related behaviors that emerged late in development, this impairment was present prepuberty and lasted into adulthood. Moreover, it has subsequently been shown that social behaviors are not disrupted by the adult VH lesion (Becker et al., 1999), the finding that again supported the notion of unique alterations in the development of brain regions critical for these behaviors after neonatal VH damage.

Another behavior disrupted by the neonatal VH lesion is hypersensitivity to N-methyl-D-aspartate (NMDA) antagonists, observed in schizophrenic patients and consistent with the hypothesis of compromised cortical glutamatergic function in schizophrenia (Krystal et al., 1994; Jentsch and Roth, 1999; Moghaddam et al., 1997). In another cohort of rats, we tested the motor response to MK-801, a non-competitive NMDA antagonist. As hypothesized, the neonatally lesioned rats showed exaggerated hyperlocomotion and enhanced stereotypic behaviors in response to various doses of MK-801 (0.05-0.2 mg/kg); these abnormal behaviors emerged only in adolescence (day 56), lasted into adulthood (day 105), and were reversed by neuroleptics (haloperidol and clozapine) (Al-Amin et al., submitted). As shown before for other types of behaviors, adult VH lesioned animals did not exhibit these abnormalities. The fact that the analogous lesion in adult rats did not impair cognitive function, social behaviors or responsiveness to MK-801 suggested that loss of VH projections per se is not sufficient to disrupt these behaviors.

We hypothesized that if indeed aberrant function of PFC is responsible for abnormal behaviors, then removal of presumably dysfunctional PFC in adult rats with neonatal VH lesions will normalize some of the behavioral abnormalities (Lipska et al., 1998a). Obviously, we would not expect that behaviors critically dependent on the PFC (such as cognition) would be normalized by its removal but rather those that are abnormally modulated by aberrantly developed PFC, such as locomotor behaviors in response to stress or stimulants. Consistent with our prediction, rats with double excitotoxic lesions (neonatal VH and adult PFC) did not show exaggerated hyperlocomotion in response to d-amphetamine as compared to controls.

To address the specificity of the effects, we tested whether direct damage to the PFC in neonates produces similar changes as the VH lesion, and whether there is a critical temporal window for the VH lesion to occur in order to exert delayed hyperactivity syndrome. The PFC lesion was produced on postnatal day 7 and involved the area that receives direct projections from the VH, i.e., the prelimbic/infralimbic subregion. We showed that direct neonatal damage of the PFC did not result in hyperlocomotor activity in response to amphetamine, stress of novelty or MK-801, as did neonatal damage of the VH (Lipska et al., 1998a). These data suggest that at least some of the abnormal phenomena observed in the animals with the neonatal VH damage depend on the presence of intrinsic PFC neurons that developed in the context of abnormal temporal-limbic connections, and cannot be induced by complete loss of the PFC neurons. We then asked whether there is a critical time window for the VH lesion to exert presumed changes in the PFC connectivity that would result in this unique profile of responses, i.e., initial sparing followed by behavioral hyperactivity. Rats received identical excitotoxic VH lesions at 3, 7 and 14 days of age. Motor responses to novelty, d-amphetamine and apomorphine were tested in juveniles (day 35), adolescent (day 56) and adult rats (day 86). Rats lesioned at day 3 resembled animals with lesions at day 7, i.e. displayed motor hyperactivity after a period of relative normalcy, around the time of puberty. In contrast, rats lesioned at day 14, showed a profile of changes reminiscent of adult lesioned rats (Lipska et al., 1992). Thus, excitotoxic damage of the VH in infant rats results in a different profile of behavioral changes depending upon the age at which it occurred; at day 14 the rat brain has already developed in such a way that it precludes transient sparing. Our findings from the behavioral studies demonstrate that excitotoxic damage of the VH, but not of the PFC, restricted to early postnatal period (before 14 days of age), provides a heuristic model of many aspects of schizophrenia, including PFC malfunction.

Molecular changes in the cortex

The results of behavioral studies strongly suggested that PFC function is compromised as a result of early VH lesion. We have then explored potential molecular substrates of this dysfunction.

Somewhat surprisingly, tissue levels of dopamine, serotonin and their metabolites in the PFC of the lesioned rats pre- and post-puberty were not changed. However, measurements of 3-methoxytyramine (3-MT), a marker of extracellular dopamine, revealed that PFC of the VH lesioned rats responded to stress with significantly attenuated dopamine release (Lipska et al., 1995b). Subsequently, we have obtained similar results with microdialysis; neonatally VH lesioned rats showed as adults attenuated release of dopamine during restraint stress and after amphetamine as compared with controls (Lillrank et al., 1996a). Basal levels of dopamine were not altered in these experiments. Thus, dopamine input to PFC seems to be altered under stressful conditions, although the direction of changes (attenuation) was unexpected in light of enhanced behavioral responsiveness. On the other hand, these changes are similar to those observed in animals chronically stressed or chronically exposed to psychostimulants (Vanderschuren et al., 1999; Gambarana et al., 1999).

Other components of the dopamine system, e.g., dopamine receptors, were not altered as shown in binding (using ^{3}H-raclopride and ^{3}H-YM-09151-2) and in situ hybridization studies (Knable et al., 1994; Lipska et al., 1997). There were no changes in cortical 5-HT2A (using ^{3}H-ketanserin) (Black et al., 1998), a subtype of a serotonin receptor implicated in the action of antipsychotic drugs

We evaluated also glutamatergic and γ-aminobutyric acid (GABA)-ergic systems, as they play a crucial role in regulating cortical function and cortical regulation of dopamine release (Mathe et al., 1999; Yang et al., 1999), and found that the expression of an essential subtype of the NMDA receptor NR1 was not changed (Shannon Weickert et al., 1999)), but cortical expression of the neuronal glutamate transporter EAAC1 mRNA (localized postsynaptically primarily on glutamatergic neurons, but also found in GABAergic cells and glia (Conti et al., 1998; Kugler and Schmitt 1999) was significantly reduced (Bertolino et al., 1999), suggesting subtle changes in cortical neurons. Others have shown that extracellular glutamate/aspartate levels in the cortex of the VH lesioned rats are not altered in vivo in response to high K+ stimulation (but are reduced in a slice preparation (Schroeder et al., 1999)), nor is the expression of GluR1 or GluR2 mRNA, subunits of AMPA (α-amino-3-hydroxy-5-methyl-4-isoxazolepropionic acid) receptor (Stine et al., 1997). We then found that glutamate decarboxylase-67 (GAD67) mRNA, a synthetic enzyme for GABA, was reduced, suggesting attenuated GABAergic inhibition (Mathe et al., 1998), a possibility that is currently being investigated in our laboratory. The reduction in GAD67 mRNA may be consistent with reduced dopamine in PFC, as cortical GABAergic interneurons are under tonic stimulatory control by ventral tegmental area (VTA) dopamine neurons (Retaux et al., 1994), and mimics a recent finding in schizophrenia (Akbarian et al., 1995). Alternatively, reduced GAD67 mRNA may also suggest reduced glutamatergic tone as glutamate, through its interaction with NMDA receptors, exerts a stimulatory effect on GAD67 mRNA expression (Qin et al., 1994). Thus, although the exact mechanisms underlying these changes need to be elucidated, findings from the animal model suggest that aberrant cortical dopamine/glutamate/GABA interactions may (at least in part) underlie cortical dysfunction, and that EAAC1 and GAD67 may represent potential markers for testing in human genetic and postmortem studies.

Because of signs of behavioral disinhibition and possible attenuated inhibition of cortical neurons, we hypothesized that the signal transduction mechanisms sensitive to stimulation may be altered. We focused on two transcription factors, c-fos, an immediate early gene, that is expressed acutely after stimulation but the response is lost upon repeated stimulation, and ΔFosB, a chronic Fos-related antigen (FRA), that accumulates in the brain (including PFC) after chronic perturbations (e.g., stress, repeated drug exposure, seizures) (Nestler et al.,

1999). Expression of c-fos mRNA was significantly reduced in the cortex of the VH lesioned rats in response to a high dose of amphetamine suggesting development of tolerance to stimulation (Lillrank et al., 1996b), a phenomenon observed also in rats showing behavioral sensitization to amphetamine (Feldpausch et al., 1998). ΔFosB levels were measured by evaluating immunoreactivity of N-terminus directed antibody (FosB(N) recognizing FosB and ΔFosB) over a C-terminus directed antibody (FosB(C) recognizing only FosB). As there was only a minimal FosB(C) signal, FosB(N) immunoreactivity likely reflected ΔFosB levels that were markedly elevated in cortical regions of the neonatally lesioned rats; this increase was unique to the neonatal VH lesion as adult lesioned animals did not differ from controls (Lee et al., 1998). As the VH lesioned animals do not display seizures, these changes support the notion of other ongoing processes in the cortex of neonatally VH lesioned rats such as stress-induced changes (increased corticotropin releasing factor (CRF) also leads to widespread c-fos induction) and functional adaptations to the lesion. The enhanced ΔFosB expression likely has implications for cortical regulation of second order target genes, some of which are now being identified (Nestler et al., 1999). ΔFosB provides another candidate gene to be tested in the human postmortem tissue, although long-term medication may confound the results in human studies (as prolonged drug treatment might be expected to increase ΔFosB expression).

As a number of data gathered so far suggested that the neonatally VH lesioned rats show many characteristics of "overstimulation" similar to those described in chronic stress and in models of chronic exposure to stimulants (i.e., behavioral hyperresponsiveness, prolonged hypothalamo-pituitary-adrenocortical (HPA) axis response, reduced c-fos, enhanced ΔFosB, attenuated dopamine release (Imperato et al., 1996)), we measured cortical expression of trophic factors, brain derived neurotrophic factor (BDNF) and fibroblast growth factor (FGF), as these molecules also are affected by chronic stress (Nibuya et al., 1999) and play a role in maturational (regulation of synaptic sprouting particularly of pyramidal cortical neurons (McAllister et al., 1997)), and recovery from injury processes, as well as other molecules involved in plasticity (neuronal growth-associated protein-43 (GAP-43), limbic system-associated membrane protein (LAMP), synaptophysin). No changes were found in adult rats with neonatal VH lesions, except for BDNF mRNA whose expression tended to be lower in PFC of the lesioned rats at baseline and after restraint stress (Khaing et al., 1999; Molteni et al., 1999). Subsequently, others showed that BDNF mRNA was significantly reduced in PFC of the lesioned rats after exposure to swim stress as compared to stressed control rats (Ashe et al., 1999). These data support the notion that the neonatally VH lesioned rats might experience chronic stress that may account for reduced BDNF (Smith et al., 1995; Nibuya et al., 1999), and suggest abnormal modulation of cortical glutamatergic neurons (McAllister et al., 1997). They also support a recent observation of a small reduction of BDNF mRNA expression in the PFC of patients with schizophrenia (Brouha et al., 1996).

To test the hypothesis emerging from the clinical studies that N-acetylaspartate (NAA) signal reflecting regional neuronal activity (Moffett et al., 1991; Simmons et al., 1991) is reduced in regionally defined neuronal populations, we have evaluated NAA in PFC of the living animal with proton magnetic resonance spectroscopy (^{1}H-MRS) (4.7 Varian NMR scanner using a STEAM pulse sequence). Spectra were acquired in the PFC and striatum at 35 and 57 days of age in rats with the neonatal (day 7) VH lesions. Reduced levels of NAA were seen in PFC (but not in striatum) at 57 (but not 36 days) of age (Bertolino et al., 1999). The results of this study provide evidence of adolescent emergence of neuronal deficits in response to the neonatal VH lesion that are unique for the PFC. These findings are consistent with the ^{1}H-MRS studies of adult monkeys following neonatal temporo-limbic removals (Bertolino et al., 1997) and recent studies in untreated and medicated patients with schizophrenia (Bertolino et al., 1998).

VH Lesion Disrupts Subcortical Dopamine System

We hypothesized that abnormal cortical function would result in aberrant regulation of subcortical dopamine neurotransmission and tested this by assessing various indices of the dopamine system (release, receptors, transporter). Mechanisms through which PFC and VH interact with subcortical dopamine release are complex and largely unclear (Shim et al., 1996). They may involve direct action of glutamate released from cortical (PFC and VH) terminals on dopamine terminals in dopamine target areas (n. accumbens, striatum) as well as regulation of midbrain neurons through cortical synaptic contacts directly onto the midbrain cells (Murase et al., 1993; Taber et al., 1995). Both increased and reduced activity of midbrain dopamine neurons was reported in response to PFC damage depending on specific circumstances (type of damage, stress, anesthesia, etc.).

In our studies, the behavioral changes and their reversal by neuroleptics strongly suggest that the subcortical dopamine system is overactive in adult rats with neonatal VH lesions. Dopamine release, however, is not increased in these animals but reduced in response to stress and amphetamine in the n. accumbens and striatum as shown in our 3-MT (Lipska et al., 1995) and microdialysis studies (Lillrank et al., 1999a). Although counterintuitive, these data are remarkably similar to those obtained in animals repeatedly treated with amphetamine (Imperato et al., 1996; Castner et al., 2000), again suggesting that the neonatally VH lesioned rats share many characteristics with the amphetamine sensitization model in which behavioral responses are dissociated from dopamine release (Kuczenski et al., 1991). Serotonin release shows a similar albeit less pronounced reduction in our rats (Lillrank et al., 1999a). Some investigators confirmed our findings using voltammetry in the stressed VH lesioned animals (Brake et al., 1999), but others found no change after amphetamine by microdialysis (Wan et al., 1996) or an increase in dopamine metabolites when cerebrospinal fluid (CSF) was sampled during stress (Wan et al., 1998).

We asked whether behavioral changes suggestive of dopamine hyperactivity may be caused by supersensitivity of striatal dopamine receptors but found that the densities of postsynaptic dopamine receptors D1, D2 or D3 are not increased either in binding studies (Lillrank et al., 1999b) or by in situ mRNA hybridization (Lipska et al., 1997). Instead, a slight but significant reduction in striatal expression of D2 mRNA was detected. These findings were confirmed by Black et al., 1998 and partially supported by Flores et al., 1996a, who found, however, a decrease in D3 binding in the limbic striatum. We found no changes in the levels of expression of neuropeptides, enkephalin or neurotensin, and an increase in dynorphin mRNA expression, an opioid peptide co-localized with D1 receptor and shown to be elevated in response to behavioral sensitization (Steiner and Gerfen, 1998).

We demonstrated in several independent experiments that expression of the dopamine transporter (DAT) mRNA, a critical component in the regulation of dopaminergic transmission involved in the clearance of synaptic dopamine (Jones et al., 1998), was reduced in the midbrain neurons of the neonatally lesioned rats but not in rats with identical adult lesions (Lipska et al., 1998b, 1999). Although reduced expression of DAT would lead to longer lasting action of the neurotransmitter, and possibly behavioral consequences reminiscent of a hyperdopaminergic state, it remains yet to be clarified if DAT is indeed responsible for the apparent behavioral hyperresponsiveness in the neonatally lesioned rats, reflects a compensatory mechanism for attenuated dopamine release, or otherwise compromised function of midbrain dopamine neurons. The fact, however, that dopamine release is attenuated suggests rather the latter possibility of overall reduced activity of dopaminergic neurons (interestingly, however, tyrosine hydroxylase (TH) mRNA or protein is not altered in VTA or SN of the lesioned rats). The finding of reduced DAT mRNA is again similar to the sensitization paradigm (Burchett and Bannon, 1997), although in some studies on chronic exposure to stimulants increased DAT mRNA (Shilling et al., 1997) or no change (Frey et al., 1997) has also been reported.

Finally, as sensitization involves changes in the second messenger systems and signal transduction mechanisms rather than changes at the presynaptic or postsynaptic receptor level (Duman et al., 1988; Nestler, 1993; Nestler and Aghajanian, 1997), we have measured ΔFosB in the n. accumbens (as described above in the cortex), and found a significant increase in the VH lesioned rats, indicating again a similarity between mechanisms underlying these two paradigms. However, ΔFosB expression in the n. accumbens (unlike in PFC) did not differ between the neonatally and adult lesioned animals.

CONCLUSION

In recent years, we have witnessed remarkable changes in the approach to studying the etiology and pathophysiology of schizophrenia at the level of animal neurobiology. Schizophrenia had long been regarded as a social or psychological illness, not a brain disorder with a particular neurobiological cause. This situation has changed rapidly in light of mounting evidence linking schizophrenia to certain neuropathological processes in the brain, although their origin is still unclear. Heuristic animal models may prove to be important tools in testing new theories about the origin and mechanisms of this disorder. In particular, some of the recent models have confirmed the plausibility of neurodevelopmental insults having long lasting effects on the dopamine system and behaviors relevant to schizophrenia, and supported the notion that targeting other than dopaminergic neurotransmitter systems (e.g., glutamatergic) may lead to new approaches to treatment.

REFERENCES

Adams, W., Kendell., R.E., Hare, E.H., Munk-Jorgensen, P. (1993) Epidemiological evidence that maternal influenza contributes to the aetiology of schizophrenia: an analysis of Scottish, English and Danish data. Br. J. Psychiat. 163 : 169-177.

Akbarian, S., Bunney, W.E., Jr., Potkin, S.G., Wigal, S.B., Hagman, J.O., Sandman, C.A., Jones, E.G. (1993) Altered distribution of nicotinamide-adenine dinucleotide phosphate-diaphorase cells in frontal lobe of schizophrenics implies disturbances of cortical development. Arch. Gen. Psychiat. 50:169-177.

Akbarian, S., Kim, J.J., Potkin, S.G., Hagman, J.O., Tafazzoli, A., Bunney, W.E. Jr., Jones, E.G. (1995) Gene expression for glutamic acid decarboxylase is reduced without loss of neurons in prefrontal cortex of schizophrenics. Arch Gen Psychiatry 52: 258-66.

Al-Amin, H.A., Weinberger, D.R., Lipska, B.K. Exaggerated MK-801-induced motor hyperactivity in rats with the neonatal lesion of the ventral hippocampus. Submitted. Behav Pharm

Ashe, P., Chlan-Fourney, J., Juorio, A.V., Li, X.-M., Boulton, A.A. (1999) Brain-derived neurotrophic factor mRNA in rats with neonatal ibotenic acid lesions of the ventral hippocampus. Soc Neurosci Abstract 635.11.

Bardgett, M.A. and Csernansky, J.G. (1996) Schizophrenia-like limbic-cortical neuropathology in rats: delayed effect of a developmental lesion. Soc Neurosci Abstract 22: 1189.

Becker, A., Grecksch, G., Bernstein, H.-G., Hollt, V., Bogerts, B. (1999) Social behavior in rats lesioned with ibotenic acid in the hippocampus: quantitative and qualitative analysis. Psychopharmacology 144: 333-338.

Bertolino, A., Saunders, R.C., Mattay, V.S., Bachevalier, J., Frank, J.A., Weinberger, D.R. (1997) Altered development of prefrontal neurons in rhesus monkeys with neonatal mesial temporo-limbic lesions: A proton magnetic resonance spectroscopic imaging study. Cereb Cortex 7: 740-748.

Bertolino, A. Callicott, J.H., Elman, I., Mattay, V.S., Tedeschi, G., Frank, J.A., Breier, A., Weinberger, D.R. (1998) Regionally specific neuronal pathology in untreated patients with schizophrenia: a proton magnetic resonance spectroscopic imaging study. Biol Psychiatry 43: 641-648.

Bertolino, A., Roffman, J.L., Lipska, B.K., Van Gelderen, P., Olso,n A., Weinberger, D.R. (1999) Postpubertal emergence of prefrontal neuronal deficits and altered dopaminergic behaviors in rats with neonatal hippocampal lesions. Soc Neurosci Abstract 520.8.

Black, M.D., Lister, S., Hitchcock, J.M., Giersbergen, P., Sorensen, S.M. (1998) Neonatal hippocampal lesion model of schizophrenia in rats: sex differences and persistence of effects into maturity. Drug Dev Res 43: 206-213.

Bloom, F.E. (1993) Advancing a neurodevelopmental origin of schizophrenia. Arch. Gen. Psychiat. 50: 224-227.

Bogerts, B., Ashtar, M., Degreef, G., Alvir, J.M.J., Bilder, R.M., Lieberman, J.A. (1990) Reduced temporal limbic structure volumes on magnetic resonance images in first-episode schizophernia. Psychiatr. Res.: Neuroimaging 35 : 1-13.

Brake, W.G., Sullivan, R.M., Flores, G., Srivastava L., Gratton, A. (1997a) Effects of neonatal ventral hippocampal lesions on the nucleus accumbens dopamine response to stress in adult rats. Soc Neurosci Abstract 23 : 1928.

Brake, W., Noel, M.B., Boksa, P., Gratton, A. (1997b) Infuence of perinatal factors on the nucleus accumbens dopamine response to repeated stress during adulthood: An electrochemical study in rat. Neuroscience 77: 1067-76.

Brake, W.G., Boksa, P., Gratton, A. (1997c) Effects of perinatal anoxia on the locomotor response to repeated amphetamine administration in adult rats. Psychopharmacology 133: 389-395.

Brake, W.G., Sullivan, R.M., Flores, G., Srivastava, L., Gratton, A. (1999) Neonatal ventral hippocampal lesions attenuate the nucleus accumbens dopamine response to stress: an electrochemical study in the rat. Brain Res 831: 25-32.

Brouha, A.K., Weickert, C.S., Hyde, T.M., Herman, M.M., Murray, A.M., Bigelow, L.B., Weinberger, D.R., Kleinman, J.E. (1996) Reductions in brain derived neurotrophic factor mRNA in the hippocampus of patients with schizophrenia. Soc Neurosci Abstract 22: 1680.

Burchett, S.A. and Bannon, M. (1997) Serotonin, dopamine and norepinephrine transporter mRNAs: heterogeneity of distribution and response to 'binge' cocaine administration. Brain Res Mol Brain Res 49: 95-102.

Castner, S.A., Al-Tikriti, M.S., Baldwin, R.M., Seibyl, J.P., Innis, R.B., Goldman-Rakic, P.S. (2000) Behavioral changes and [123I]IBZM equilibrium SPECT measurement of amphetamine-induced dopamine release in rhesus monkeys exposed to subchronic amphetamine. Neuropsychopharmacology 22: 4-13

Chambers, R.A., Moore, J., McEvoy, J.P., Levin, E.D. (1996) Cognitive effects of neonatal hippocampal lesions in a rat model of schizophrenia. Neuropsychopharmacology 15: 587-594

Conti, F., DeBiasi, S., Minelli, A., Rothstein, J.D., Melone, M. (1998) EAAC1, a high-affinity glutamate transporter, is localized to astrocytes and gabaergic neurons besides pyramidal cells in the rat cerebral cortex. Cereb Cortex 8: 08-16.

Costall, B. and Naylor, R.J. (1995) Animal neuropharmacology and its prediction of clinical response. In: S.R. Hirsch and D.R. Weinberger, eds. pp. 401-424. Blackwell Science Ltd, Oxford.

Dalman, C., Allebeck, P., Cullberg, J., Grunewald, C., Koster, M. (1999) Obstetric complications and the risk of schizophrenia: a longitudinal study of a national birth cohort. Arch. Gen. Psychiatry 56:234-40.

DeLisi, L.E., Dauphinais, I.D., Gershon, E.S. (1988) Perinatal complications and reduced size of brain limbic structures in afmilial schizophrenia. Schizophr. Bull. 14:185-191.

Duman, R.S., Tallman, J.F., Nestler, E.J. (1998) Acute and chronic opiate-regulation of adenylate cyclase in brain: specific effects in locus coeruleus. J Pharmacol Exp Ther 246:1033-9

Eastwood, S.L. and Harrison, P.J. (1995) Decreased synaptophysin in the medial temporal lobe in schizophrenia demonstrated using immuno-utoradiography. Neuroscience 69:339-43.

El-Khodor, B.F. and Boksa, P. (1997) Long-term reciprocal changes in dopamine levels in prefrontal cortex versus nucleus accumbens in rats born by Cesarean section compared to vaginal birth. Exp. Neurol. 145: 118-129.

El-Khodor, B.F., and Boksa, P. (1998) Birth insult increases amphetamine induced responses in the adult rat. Neuroscience 87: 893-904.

Ellenbroek, B.A., and Cools, A.R. (1990) Animal models with construct validity for schizophrenia. Behav. Pharm. 1: 469-490.

Falkai, P., and Bogerts, B. (1986) Cell loss in the hippocampus of schizophrenics. Eur. Arch. Psychiatry Neurol. Sci. 236: 154-61.

Fatemi, S.H., Emamian, E.S., Kist, D., Sidwell, R.W., Nakajima, K., Akhter, P., Shier, A., Sheikh, S., Bailey, K. (1999) Defective corticogenesis and reduction in Reelin immunoreactivity in cortex and hippocampus of prenatally infected neonatal mice. Mol. Psychiatry 4:145-54.

Feldpausch, D.L., Needham, L.M., Stone, M.P, Althaus, J.S., Yamamoto, B.K., Svensson, K.A., Merchant, K.M (1998) The role of dopamine D4 receptor in the induction of behavioral sensitization to amphetamine and accompanying biochemical and molecular adaptations. J Pharmacol Exp Ther 286: 497-508.

Flores, G., Barbeau, D., Quirion, R., Srivastava, L.K. (1996a) Decreased binding of dopamine D3 receptors in limbic subregions after neonatal bilateral lesion of rat hippocampus. J. Neurosci. 16: 020-2026.

Flores, G., Wood, G.K., Liang, J.-J., Quirion, R., Srivastava, L.K. (1996b) Enhanced amphetamine sensitivity and increased expression of dopamine D2 receptors in postpubertal rats after neonatal excitotoxic lesions of the medial prefrontal cortex. J. Neurosci. 16:7366-7375.

Freeman, J.H., Jr. and Stanton, M.E. (1992) Medial prefrontal cortex lesions and spatial delayed alternation in the developing rat: recovery or sparing? Behav Neurosci 106: 924-932.

Frey, K., Kilbourn, M., Robinson, T. (1997) Reduced striatal vesicular monoamine transporters after neurotoxic but not after behaviorally-sensitizing doses of methamphetamine. Eur J Pharmacol 334: 273-279.

Fuster, J.M. (1995) Memory in the Cerebral Cortex : An Empirical Approach to Neural networks in the Human and Nonhuman Primate. Cambridge, MA, The MIT Press.

Geyer, M.A., Wilkinson, L.S., Humby, T., Robbins, T.W. (1993) Isolation rearing of rats produces a deficit in prepulse inhibition of acoustic startle similar to that in schizophrenia. Biol. Psychiatry 34: 361-372.

Gambarana, C., Masi, F., Tagliamonte, A., Scheggi, S., Ghiglieri, O., De Montis, M.G. (1999) A chronic stress that impairs reactivity in rats also decreases dopaminergic transmission in the nucleus accumbens: a microdialysis study. J Neurochem 72: 2039-46.

Greck sch, G., Bernstein, H.G., Becker, A., Hollt, V., Bogerts, B. (1999) Disruption of latent inhibition in rats with postnatal hippocampal lesions. Neuropsychopharmacology 20: 525-32.

Hultman, C.M., Ohman, A., Cnattingius, S., Wieselgren, I.M., Lindstrom, L.H. (1997) Prenatal and neonatal risk factors for schizophrenia. Br. J. Psychiatry 170 : 128-133.

Imperato, A., Obinu, M.C., Carta, G., Mascia, M.S., Casu, M.A., Gessa, G.L. (1996) Reduction of dopamine release and synthesis by repeated amphetamine treatment: role in behavioral sensitization. Eur J Pharmacol 317: 231-237.

Jentsch, J.D. and Roth, R.H. (1999) The neuropsychopharmacology of phencyclidine: from NMDA receptor hypofunction to the dopamine hypothesis of schizophrenia. Neuropsychopharmacology 20: 201-25.

Jeste, D.V. and Lohr, J.B. (1989) Hippocampal pathologic findings in schizophrenia: a morphometric study. Arch. Gen. Psychiat. 46, 1019-1024.

Johnston, M.V., Barks, J., Greenmyre, T., Silverstein, F. (1988). Use of toxins to disrupt neurotransmitter circuitry in the developing brain. Prog. Brain Res. 73: 425-446.

Jones, G.H., Hernandez, T.D., Kendall, D.A., Marsden, C.A., Robbins, T.W. (1992) Dopaminergic and serotonergic function following isolation rearing in rats: Study of behavioral responses and postmortem and in vivo neurochemistry. Pharm. Biochem. Behav. 43: 17-35.

Jones, S.R., Gainetdinov, R.R., Jaber, M., Giros, B., Wightman, R.M., Caron, M.G. (1998) Profound neuronal plasticity in response to inactivation of the dopamine transporter. Proc Natl Acad Sci U S A 95: 4029-4034.

Harrison, P.J., and Eastwood, S.L. (1998) Preferential involvement of excitatory neurons in medial temporal lobe in schizophrenia. Lancet 352: 1669-1673.

Kendell, R.E. and Kemp, I.W. (1989) Maternal influenza in the etiology of schizophrenia. Archiv. Gen. Psychiat. 46 : 878-882.

Kendler, K.S., MacLean, C.J., O'Neill, F.A., Burke, J., Murphy, B., Duke, F., Shinkwin, R., Easter, S.M., Webb, B.T., Zhang, J., Walsh, D., Straub, R.E. (1996) Evidence for a schizophrenia vulnerability locus on chromosome 8p in the Irish study of high-density schizophrenia families. Am. J. Psychiatry 153: 1534-1540.

Khaing, Z.Z., Molteni, R., Valentine, M.G., Shannon Weickert, C., Weinberger, D.R., Lipska, B.K. (1999) Antipsychotics downregulate BDNF mRNA expression in the rat hippocampus. Soc Neurosci Abstract 200.5

Knable, M.B., Murray, A.M., Lipska, B.K., Karoum, F., Weinberger, D.R. (1994) D2/D3 and D4 receptor densities are not altered in rats with neonatal hippocampal damage. Soc Neurosci Abstr 20:1260.

Kornetsky, C. and Markowitz, R. (1978) Animal models of schizophrenia. In: M.A. Lipton, A. DiMascio, K.F. Killam, eds. Psychopharmacology: A Generation of Progress, pp. 583-593. Raven Press, New York.

Krystal, J.H., Karper, L.P., Seibyl, J.P., Freeman, G.K., Delaney, R., Bremmer, J.D., Heninger, G.R., Bowers, M.B. Jr, Charney, D.S. (1994). Subanesthetic effects of noncompetitive NMDA receptor antagonist, ketamine, in humans: Psychotomimetic, perceptual, cognitive, and neuroendocrine responses. Arch Gen Psychiat 51:199-214.

Kuczenski, R., Segal, D.S., Aizenstein, M.L. (1991) Amphetamine, cocaine, and fencamfamine: relationship between locomotor and stereotypy response profiles and caudate and accumbens dopamine dynamics. J Neurosci 11: 2703-2712.

Kugler, P., Schmitt, A. (1999) Glutamate transporter EAAC1 is expressed in neurons and glial cells in the rat nervous system. Glia 27: 129-142.

Lee, C.J., Binder, T., Lipska, B.K., Zhu, Y., Weinberger, D.R., Nakabeppu, Y., Robertson, G.S. (1998) Neonatal ventral hippocampal lesions produce an elevation of delta-FosB-like protein(s) in the rodent neocortex. Soc Neurosci Abstract 24: 489.

Le Pen, G., Grottick, A., Higgins, G., Ballard, T., Martin, J., Jenck, F., Moreau, J.-L. (1999) Cognitive impairment induced by neonatal excitotoxic hippocampal damage in rats : further evaluation of an animal model of schizophrenia. Soc Neurosci Abstract 635.16.

Lillrank, S.M., Lipska, B.K., Weinberger, D.R. (1995) Neurodevelopmental animal models of schizophrenia. Clin. Neurosci. 3: 98-104.

Lillrank, S.M., Lipska, B.K., Kolachana, B.S., Weinberger, D.R. (1996a) Extracellular levels of dopamine and 5-HIAA are decreased in rats with a neonatal ventral hippocampal lesion. Soc Neurosci 22:1675.

Lillrank, S.M., Lipska, B.K., Bachus, S., Wood, G.K., Weinberger, D.R. (1996b) Amphetamine-induced c-fos mRNA expression is reduced in rats with neonatal ventral hippocampal lesions. Synapse 23: 182-191.

Lillrank, S.M., Lipska, B.K., Weinberger, D.R., Fredholm, B.B., Fuxe, K., Ferre, S. (1999a) Adenosine and dopamine receptor antagonist binding in the rat ventral and dorsal striatum: lack of changes after neonatal bilateral lesion of the ventral hippocampus. Neurochem Int 34: 235-244.

Lillrank, S.M., Lipska, B.K., Kolachana, B., Weinberger, D.R. (1999b) Altered levels of extracellular dopamine and 5-HIAA after restraint stress and amphetamine in rats with neonatal ventral hippocampal damage. An in vivo microdialysis study in awake rats. J Neur Transm, 106:183-196.

Lipska, B.K. and Weinberger, D.R. (1993) Delayed effects of neonatal hippocampal damage on haloperidol-induced catalepsy and apomorphine-induced stereotypic behaviors in the rat. Dev. Brain Res. 75: 13-222.

Lipska, B.K. and Weinberger, DR. (1994a) Subchronic treatment with haloperidol or clozapine in rats with neonatal excitotoxic hippocampal damage. Neuropsychopharmacology 10: 199-205.

Lipska, B.K. and Weinberger, D.R. (1994b) Gonadectomy does not prevent novelty- or drug-induced hyperresponsiveness in rats with neonatal excitototxic hippocampal damage. Dev. Brain Res. 78: 253-258.

Lipska, B.K. and Weinberger, D.R. (1995) Genetic variation in vulnerability to the behavioral effects of neonatal hippocampal damage in rats. Proc. Natl. Acad. Sci. USA 92: 8906-8910.

Lipska, B.K., Jaskiw, G.E., Chrapusta, S.J., Karoum, F., Weinberger, D.R. (1992) Ibotenic acid lesion of the ventral hippocampus differentially affects dopamine and its metabolites in the nucleus accumbens and prefrontal cortex in the rat. Brain Res 585: 1-6.

Lipska, B.K., Jaskiw, G.E., Weinberger, D.R. (1993) Postpubertal emergence of hyperresponsiveness to stress and to amphetamine after neonatal hippocampal damage: A potential animal model of schizophrenia. Neuropsychopharmacology 9: 67-75.

Lipska, B.K., Swerdlow, N.R., Geyer, M.A., Jaskiw, G.E., Braff, D.L., Weinberger, D.R. (1995a) Neonatal excitotoxic hippocampal damage in rats causes postpubertal changes in prepulse inhibition of startle and its disruption by apomorphine. Psychopharmacology 122: 35-43.

Lipska, B.K. Chrapusta, S.J., Egan, M.F., Weinberger, D.R. (1995b) Neonatal excitotoxic ventral hippocampal damage alters dopamine response to mild chronic stress and haloperidol treatment. Synapse 20: 125-130.

Lipska, B.K., Al-Amin, H.A., Khaing, Z.Z., Lerman, D.N., Lillrank, S.M., Weinberger DR (1997) Effects of acute and chronic neuroleptic treatment on expression of D2 and D3 receptors, neurotensin and enkephalin mRNA in rats with neonatal lesions of the ventral hippocampus. Soc Neuroci Abstract 23:1361.

Lipska, B.K., Al-Amin, H.A., Weinberger, D.R. (1998a) Excitotoxic lesions of the rat medial prefrontal cortex: effects on abnormal behaviors associated with neonatal hippocampal damage. Neuropsychopharmacology 19: 451-464.

Lipska, B.K., Khaing, Z.Z., Lerman, D.N., Weinberger, D.R. (1998b) Neonatal damage of the rat ventral hippocampus reduces expression of a dopamine transporter. Soc Neurosci Abstract 24, 365.

Lipska, B.K., Khaing, Z.Z., Lerman, D.N., Akil, M., Weinberger, D.R. (1999) Regulation of tyrosine hydroxylase and dopamine transporter mRNA by antipsychotic drugs in a rat model of schizophrenia. Soc Neurosci Abstract 29:67.5.

Liu, D., Diorio, J., Tannenbaum, B., Caldji, C., Francis, D., Freedman, A., Sharma, S., Pearson, D., Plotsky, P.M., Meaney, M.J. (1997) Maternal care, hippocampal glucocorticoid receptors, and hypothalamic- pituitary-adrenal responses to stress. Science 277: 1659-1662.

Mathe, J.M., Nomikos, G.G., Schilstrom, B., Svensson, T.H. (1998) Non-NMDA excitatory amino acid receptors in the ventral tegmental area mediate systemic dizocilpine (MK-801) induced hyperlocomotion and dopamine release in the nucleus accumbens. J. Neurosci. Res. 51 : 583-592.

Mathe, J.M., Nomikos, G.G., Blakeman, K.H., Svensson, T.H. (1999) Differential actions of dizocilpine (MK-801) on the mesolimbic and mesocortical dopamine systems: role of neuronal activity. Neuropharmacology 38: 121-128.

McAllister, A.K., Katz, L.C., Lo, D.C. (1997) Opposing roles for endogenous BDNF and NT-3 in regulating cortical dendritic growth. Neuron 18: 767-778.

McKinney, W.T. and Moran, E.C. (1981) Animal models of schizophrenia. Am. J. Psychiatry 138: 478-483.

Moffett, J.R., Namboodiri, M.A., Cangro, C.B., Neale, J.H. (1991) Immunohistochemical localization of N-acetylaspartate in rat brain. Neuroreport 2:131-134.

Mednick, S.A., Machon, R.A., Huttunen, M.O., Bonett, D. (1988) Adult schizophrenia following prenatal exposure to influenza epidemic. Arch. Gen. Psychiat. 45: 189-192.

Mintz, M., Youval, G., Gigi, A., Myslobodsky, M.S. (1997) Rats exposed to prenatal gamma-radiation at day 15 of gestation exhibit enhanced perseveration in T-maze. Soc Neurosci Abstract, 23: 1365.

Moghaddam, B., Adams, B., Verma, A., Daly, D. (1997) Activation of glutamatergic neurotransmission by ketamine: a novel step in pathway from NMDA receptor lockade to dopaminergic and cognitive disruptions associated with the prefrontal cortex. J. Neurosci. 17: 2921-2927.

Moghaddam, B., Aultman, J., Weinberger, D.R., Lipska, B.K. (1999) neonatal damage of the rat ventral hippocampus impairs acquisition of a working memory task. Soc Neurosci Abstract 25: 1891.

Molteni, R., Lipska, B.K., Figini, A., Khaing, Z.Z., Weinberger, D.R., Racagni, G., Riva, M.A. (1999) Developmental and stress-induced changes of neurotrophic factor expression in an animal model of schizophrenia. Soc Neurosci Abstract 200.4.

Murase, S., Mathe, J.M., Grenhoff, J., Svensson, T.H. (1993) Effects of dizocilpine (MK-801) on rat midrain dopamine cell activity: differential actions on firing pattern related to anatomical localization. J. Neur. Transm. [Gen.Sect.] 91: 13-25.

Murray, R.M. and Lewis, S.W. (1987) Is schizophrenia a neurodevelopmental disorder? Br. Med. J. 295: 681-682.

Nestler, E.J. and Aghajanian, G.K. (1997) Molecular and cellular basis of addiction. Science 278: 58-63.

Nestler, E.J. (1993) Cellular responses to chronic treatment with drugs of abuse. Crit Rev Neurobiol 7: 23-39.

Nestler, E.J., Kelz, M.B., Chen, J. (1999) DeltaFosB: a molecular mediator of long-term neural and behavioral plasticity. Brain Res 835: 10-17.

Nibuya, M., Morinobu, S., Duman, R.S. (1995) Regulation of BDNF and trkB mRNA in rat brain by chronic electroconvulsive seizure and antidepressant drug treatments. J Neurosci 15: 7539-7547.

Nibuya, M., Takahashi, M., Russell, D.S., Duman, R.S. (1999) Repeated stress increases catalytic TrkB mRNA in rat hippocampus. Neurosci Lett 267: 81-84.

O'Callaghan, E., Sham, P., Takei, N., Glover, G., Murray, R.M. (1991) Schizophrenia after prenatal exposure to 1957 A2 influenza epidemic. Lancet 337: 1248-1250.

Qin, Z.H., Zhang, S.P., Weiss, B. (1994) Dopaminergic and glutamatergic blocking drugs differentially regulate glutamic acid decarboxylase mRNA in mouse brain. Brain Res Mol Brain Res 21: 293-302.

Rajakumar, N., Williamson, P.C., Stoessl, J.A., Flumerfelt, B.A. (1996) Neurodevelopmental pathogenesis of schizophrenia. Soc Neurosci Abstract 22: 1187.

Rakic, P. (1996) Experimental deletion of specific cortical neurons: relevance to schizophrenia. 35th ACNP Annual Meeting, Abstract, 35: 91.

Retaux, S., Trovero, F., Besson, M.J. (1994) Role of dopamine in the plasticity of glutamic acid decarboxylase messenger RNA in the rat frontal cortex and the nucleus accumbens. Eur J Neurosci 6:1782-1791.

Romjin, H.J., Hofman, M.A., Gramsbergen, A. (1991) At what age is the developing cerebral cortex of the rat comparable to that of the full-term newborn human baby? Early Hum Dev 26: 61-67.

Rott, R., Herzog, S., Fleischer, B., Winokur, A., Amsterdam, J., Dyson, W., Koprowski, H. (1985) Detection of serum antibodies to Borna disease virus in patients with psychiatric disorders. Science 228: 755-756.

Sams-Dodd, F., Lipska, B.K., Weinberger, D.R. (1997) Neonatal lesions of the rat ventral hippocampus result in hyperlocomotion and deficits in social behaviour in adulthood. Psychopharmacology 132: 303-310.

Saunders, R.C., Kolachana, B.S., Bachevalier, J., Weinberger, D.R. (1998) Neonatal lesions of the temporal lobe disrupt prefrontal cortical regulation of striatal dopamine. Nature 393: 169-171.

Schroeder, H., Grecksch, G., Becker, A., Bogerts, B., Höllt, V. (1999) Alterations of the dopaminergic and glutamatergic neurotransmission in adult rats with postnatal ibotenic acid hippocampal lesion. Psychopharmacology 145: 61-66.

Shannon Weickert, C., Khaing, Z.Z., Weinberger, D.R., Lipska, B.K. (1999) Regulation of NMDAR1 mRNA by antipsychotic drugs in a rat model of schizophrenia. Soc Neurosci Abstract 683.10.

Shilling, P.D., Kelsoe, J.R., Segal, D.S. (1997) Dopamine transporter mRNA is up-regulated in the substantia nigra and the ventral tegmental area of amphetamine-sensitized rats. Neurosci Lett 236:131-134.

Shim, S.S., Bunney, B.S., Shi, W.X. (1996) Effects of lesions in the medial prefrontal cortex on the activity of midbrain dopamine neurons. Neuropsychopharmacology 15: 437-41.

Simmons, M.L., Frondoza, C.G., Coyle, J.T. (1991) Immunocytochemical localization of N-acetyl-aspartate with monoclonal antibodies. Neuroscience 45: 37-45.

Smith, M.A., Makino, S., Kvetnansky, R., Post, R.M. (1995) Stress and glucocorticoids affect the expression of brain-derived neurotrophic factor and neurotrophin-3 mRNAs in the hippocampus. J Neurosci 151: 1768-1777.

Solbrig, M.V., Koob, G.F., Fallon, J.H., Lipkin, W.I. (1994) Tardive dyskinetic syndrome in rats infected with Borna disease virus. Neurobiol. Dis 1: 111-119.

Solbrig, M.V., Koob, G.F., Joyce, J.N., Lipkin, W.I. (1996a) A neural substrate of hyperactivity in Borna disease: changes in brain dopamine receptors. Virology 222: 332-338.

Solbrig, M.V., Koob, G.F., Fallon, J.H., Reid, S., Lipkin, W.I. (1996b) Prefrontal cortex dysfunction in Borna disease virus (BDV)-infected rats. Biol. Psychiatry 40: 629-636.

Suddath, R.L., Christisin, G.W., Torrey, E.F., Casanova, M., Weinberger, D.R. (1990) Anatomical abnormalities in the brains of monozygotic twins discordant for schizophrenia. N. Eng. J. Med. 322: 789-794.

Susser, E.S., and Lin, S.P. (1992) Schizophrenia after prenatal exposure to the Dutch Hunger Winter of 1944-1945. Arch. Gen. Psychiat. 49: 983-988.

Steiner, H. and Gerfen, C.R. (1998) Role of dynorphin and enkephalin in the regulation of striatal output pathways and behavior. Exp Brain Res 123: 60-76.

Stine, C.D., Xue, C. J., Wolf, M.E. (1997) Microdialysis studies of excitatory amino acid transmitters in a rat model of schizophrenia. Soc Neurosci Abstract 22: 1675.

Taber, M.T., Das, S., Fibiger, H.C. (1995) Cortical regulation of subcortical dopamine release: mediation via the ventral tegmental area. J Neurochem 65: 1407-1410.

Talamini, L.M., Koch, T., Ter Horst, G.J., Korf, J. (1998) Methylazoxymethanol acetate-induced abnormalities in the entorhinal cortex of the rat; parallels with morphological findings in schizophrenia. Brain Res. 789,:293-306.

Vanderschuren, L.J., Schmidt, E.D., De Vries, T.J., Van Moorsel, C.A., Tilders, F,J., Schoffelmeer, A.N. (1999) A single exposure to amphetamine is sufficient to induce long-term behavioral, neuroendocrine, and neurochemical sensitization in rats. J Neurosci 19: 9579-9586.

Waltrip, R.W. 2nd, Buchanan, R.W., Summerfeld, A., Breier, A., Carpenter, W.T., Jr., Bryant, N.L., Rubin, S.A., Carbone, K.M. (1995) Borna disease virus and schizophrenia. Psychiatr. Res. 56: 33-44.

Wan, R.Q., Giovanni, A., Kafka, S.H., Corbett, R. (1996) Neonatal hippocampal lesions induced hyperresponsiveness to amphetamine: behavioral and in vivo microdialysis studies. Behav Brain Res 78: 211-223.

Wan, R.Q., Hartman, H., Corbett, R. (1998) Alteration of dopamine metabolites in CSF and behavioral impairments induced by neonatal hippocampal lesions. Physiol Behav 65: 429-436.

Weinberger, D.R. (1986) The pathogenesis of schizophrenia: a neurodevelopmental theory. In: H.A. Nasrallah and D.R. Weinberger, eds. The Neurology of Schizophrenia, pp. 397-406. Elsevier, Amsterdam.

Weinberger, D.R. (1987) Implications of normal brain development for the pathogenesis of schizophrenia. Archiv. Gen. Psychiatr. 44, 660-669.

Weinberger, D.R. (1999) Cell biology of the hippocampal formation in schizophrenia. Biol. Psychiat. 45 (in press).

Wilkinson, L.S., Killcross, S.S., Humby, T., Hall, F.S., Geyer, M.A., Robbins, T.W. (1994) Social isolation in the rat produces developmentally specific deficits in prepulse inhibition of the acoustic startle response without disrupting latent inhibition. Neuropsychopharmacology 10: 61-72.

Woerner, M.G., Pollack, M., Klein, D.F. (1973) Pregnancy and birth complications in psychiatric patients: a comparison of schizophrenic and personality disorder patients with their siblings. Acta Psychiat. Scand. 49: 712-721.

Yang, C.R., Seamans, J.K., Gorelova, N. (1999) Developing a neuronal model for the pathophysiology of schizophrenia based on the nature of electrophysiological actions of dopamine in the prefrontal cortex. Neuropsychopharmacology 21:161-194.

16 COPING WITH UNCERTAINTY: WHAT WOULD AN ANIMAL MODEL OF SCHIZOPHRENIA LOOK LIKE?

Loring J. Ingraham and Michael Myslobodsky

INTRODUCTION

In our field, where the clinical, genetic, psychophysiological, biochemical and psychopharmacological characterization of "schizophrenia" is incomplete, there has been limited success in investigating schizophrenia with the help of animal models. Nevertheless, there have been a number of putative models proposed to address individual features of the disorder. Below we review some of the models that have been suggested as being applicable to schizophrenia, outline some of the critical features required for successfully modeling schizophrenia-like behavioral features, and propose an empirically useful model of neurodevelopment and behavioral teratogenesis.

One popular approach to modeling schizophrenia has been to reproduce cognitive deficits associated with schizophrenic psychopathology. Disorders of attention have been a favorite candidate and have an extensive literature. It is clear, however, that disordered attention in any of its forms is not sufficient to define schizophrenia nor is it specific to that disorder. It is noteworthy that attention disorder syndromes have been presented either as models of schizophrenia (Mirsky, Ingraham and Kugelmass, 1995) or as models of petit mal epilepsy (Myslobodsky and Mirsky, 1988).

Similar limitations are true for models of memory. A decade of research has demonstrated that schizophrenia is frequently associated with memory deficits, particularly with deficient working memory (Fleming et al., 1997; Goldberg et al., 1998). Yet, notwithstanding an interest in creating a laboratory model of deficient working memory, such an effort would hardly create *ipso facto* a model of schizophrenia.

A convincing model of the syndrome of schizophrenia – rather than a model of part of a specific failing cognitive domain – might reasonably be expected to emulate much of what we know empirically about schizophrenia: a condition characterized by interpersonal incompetence, withdrawal and isolation, deficient drive and volition. Ideally, such a model should be consistent with empirical evidence of both genetic and environmental contributions to schizophrenia, and reflect as well growing evidence for the role of prenatal influences in the risk of adult pathology (De Bellis, Baum, et al. 1999; De Bellis, Keshavan, et al. 1999).

In many areas of medicine, animal model research has focused on a common laboratory animal – the rat. To many, a rodent model of schizophrenia judged against the human outcome of schizophrenic psychopathology may seem as irrelevant as a rodent model of dyslexia. After all, schizophrenia is Kraepelin's concept whose identification requires uniquely human characteristics. It does not have such indisputable behavioral identifiers as motor and/or electrographic seizures which can be so convincingly reproduced in experimental animals. While animals can certainly be made to appear 'psychotic' in that their behavior becomes punctuated by periods of excessive fear, reduced responsivity to environmental cues and extreme aggressiveness, these are distinct paroxysms typically produced by brain stimulation or neurotoxins, often as a sign of postictal or interictal states (Myslobodsky et al., 1981; Myslobodsky and Valenstein, 1980; Stevens, 1973). However interesting in their own right, they hardly emulate schizophrenia.

Perhaps a useful approach to modeling schizophrenia may be to start by reproducing the effect of putative causal factors, rather than by attempting to model some of the eventual sequelae of those causes, which may be non-specific and have multiple determinants. Given that there are likely to be multiple contributory factors to schizophrenia, a defendable alternative for model building is to begin by focusing on emulation of specific etiological factors.

Reports (Mednick et al., 1988, Hollister, Laing and Mednick, 1996; Susser and Lin, 1996) describing a variety of prenatal insults associated with schizophrenia in later life have made it clear that a proportion of schizophrenia may be associated with prenatal interference with normal neurodevelopmental processes. An animal model investigating environmental influences on prenatal development may accurately reflect the action of environmental factors in the pathogenesis of human disease. Alternatively, such a model may reproduce characteristic features of schizophrenia through an etiology different from that associated with human illness, a so called phenocopy (Goldschmidt, 1935). Rather than being a nuisance to the study of the genetics of schizophrenia, an experimentally induced phenocopy which mimicked the timing and effect of genetically determined prenatal insults and subsequent neuropathology and behavioral disturbances would be a considerable advance. Of course, the contributions of other empirically demonstrated influences on the development and course of schizophrenia, particularly the role of genes, must also be accounted for in a successful model.

WHAT IS AN ADEQUATE MODEL OF SCHIZOPHRENIA A MODEL OF?

Admittedly, no laboratory model of aberrant behavior survives when measured by the yardstick of schizophrenia. As an example, it is important to recall early attempts by McKinney and Bunney (1969) to recommend such yardsticks for a model of depression. The reasons why these otherwise sound requirements are so difficult to apply in the case of schizophrenia are revealing:

(1) Similarity of (Presumed) Inducing Conditions

This is a crucial requirement for it imposes a set of etiologic conditions, however hypothetical, prior to secondary cognitive deficits which are shared by other disorders. Regrettably, with regard to schizophrenia, this condition remains much too elusive to have been taken in the past as a mandatory pathfinder. Assuming that genetic factors affect an embryo, making it excessively sensitive to even minor environmental variations (Fraser, 1959) one can marginally comply with the requirement of the etiologic relevance of a variety of environmental factors. Yet, even if we suspected some factors as plausibly etiologic the strength of their association with the outcome has yet to be established with a required degree of accuracy. Also, any casual model imposes a number of questions of its own: How necessary and specific are these factors? At what strength are they relevant? When do they afflict the brain? How are they combined (e.g., Stein, Kline, and Kharrazi, 1984)?

(2) Resemblance of Behavioral States

Given that no behavioral state encountered in laboratory animals is recognizably 'schizophrenic,' rats' behavior is checked by a series of tests to confirm the presence of an anomaly. But one seldom decides *a priori* what are the components of such laboratory psychopathology syndromes and whether the outcomes are expected to be aggregated or singular. When injury inflicted to a brain structure is presumed to manifest aberrant behaviors the relevance of such deviance is not convincingly affirmed. Thus, rodents with hippocampal damage are generally noted for hyperactivity even though it is not clear what feature of psychopathology enhanced locomotion must emulate. As a result, in general, 'focal damage theories' have deservedly received rather poor welcome.

(3) Commonalty of Underlying Neurobiological Mechanisms

Despite the tremendous explosion of data on the nature of schizophrenia its pathophysiology remains elusive. The gist of what we learn of its neurobiological mechanisms is that they may not be what we though they were a few years ago.

(4) Alleviation by Clinically Useful Medication

This is the most ancient of all requirements, perhaps, deep-seated in the medieval 'diagnosis ex-juvantibus.' It is unfortunate, perhaps, that traditional neuroleptics bind so avidly to dopamine receptors. The elegant and oft reproduced curve of receptor binding and antipsychotic efficacy may have blinded us to the complexity of the neurochemistry of the disorder. Conversely, the tragedy of tardive dyskinesia may turn out to have been the necessary impetus for the discovery of novel classes of psychopharmacological agents, agents which have convincingly shattered the myth of a single neurotransmitter for each form of psychopathology. Thus, the third and fourth conditions are likewise problematic or rather circular, being determined by choices of isomorphic features of the disorder.

WHERE DO WE WISH TO GO?

Prospective Models

These models draw attention to studies indicating that prenatal insults including (a) Nutritional deficiency (Susser and Lin, 1996); (b) severe maternal stress during pregnancy (Huttunen and Niskanen, 1978); (c) exposure to influenza in the second trimester of fetal life (Mednick et al., 1988); (d) exposure to rubella (Lim et al. 1995); and Rh factor incompatibilities (Hollister, Laing and Mednick, 1996) all may be etiological factors for schizophrenia.

In the case of genetic factors in schizophrenia, a preliminary answer is known: Some heritable genetic factor is likely to be necessary for all but a fraction of schizophrenia. Despite the long history of analyses of family history positive and family history negative samples, there is limited evidence that such a distinction is useful (McGuffin et al, 1987; Farmer et al., 1990), especially given the confounds of the number of family members assessed for determining familiality and the reduced frequency of schizophrenia patients having children. In order to assert that small families with only one affected member represent a distinct non-familial subtype of schizophrenia, one must be prepared to at the same time argue that the distribution of such non-familial cases does not vary across populations: most studies of the familial distribution of schizophrenia find similar risks of illness among relatives of individuals with schizophrenia, which would be the case only if the relative proportion of familial and non-familial cases were stable across studies as well, implying that such non-familial factors do not vary in prevalence.

The recognition of the fact that a heritable factor is not sufficient has considerable implications in requiring other factors in models of schizophrenia. Simply stated, discordance for schizophrenia among identical twins, with identical risk to the offspring of affected and unaffected twins (Gottesman and Bertelsen, 1989) indicates that unexpressed genotypes exist, and may be relatively common. Further, the demonstration that the most common psychopathology among the relatives of individuals with schizophrenia is not schizophrenia, but rather a similar but less severe illness (Ingraham, 1995, 1999) suggests that genetic factors alone are not necessarily sufficient.

Are the genetic factors specific to schizophrenia? As indicated above, schizophrenia related diagnoses are more common than chronic schizophrenia among the relatives of individuals with schizophrenia. However, the genetic factor is not a general liability to all forms of psychopathology, as evidenced by the absence of an increased risk for anxiety or affective disorders among the relatives of schizophrenia patients (Kety et al., 1994).

The molecular expression of the genetic liability remains to be elucidated. Whether the relevant gene(s) affect the brain proximally in altered expression of receptor subtypes or more distally as alteration is immune response to viral challenge remains unknown. Further, the separation between genetic and environmental contributions can be problematic: genes influence environments and vice-versa.

A final note about genetic factors and their interaction with other factors in a model of a disorder is necessary. When environments are stable, with little variance, variability in outcome will be primarily genetically influenced. Where environments vary greatly, but genes little, environmental factors will be the major source of variability in outcome. Thus some understanding of the amount of variability present in both genes and environments is necessary to interpret the role each plays in a specific population.

Retrospective Models

By contrast, attempts at reconstructing the mechanism of the final pattern of the disorder are guided by the 'outcome,' or retrospective (pathophysiological) models. The strategy of reconstructive modeling is dominated by the exploration of complex behaviors that change in a specific direction following injury, or specific functions (e.g., ocular motility, attention, memory, skilled locomotion patterns, pleasure-seeking behaviors, etc.) which depend on complex interactions of numerous brain areas (Hirsch and Weinberger, 1995). A limitation of these models is a tendency towards nominating deficits that could conceivably be traced to their origin rather than focusing on those that are typical of schizophrenia. That does not mean that outcome models do not have predictive (etiological) value, whereas pathophysiological models are lacking in etiological insights. Mednick (1970) proposed combining a prospective model with retrospective features. His etio-pathophysiological scenario of schizophrenia included: (a) unspecified genetic components that predispose to at least some forms of schizophrenia; (b) pre- and/or perinatal injury with the hippocampus nominated as the most vulnerable brain target of such insult; (c) a consequent failure to inhibit ACTH secretion thereby leading to a state of permanent hyperexcitability, again attributed to the anoxic damage to the Sommer's Sector (CA1 field).

Ever since Mednick's initial paper, etiological models have made assumptions about pathophysiology whereas pathophysiological models speculate on the origin of imposed deficits (e.g., Schmajuk, 1987). The other reason why the division between etiologic and pathophysiological modeling is not orthogonal, as pointedly noted by Matthysse (1987), is that "all severe disorders, as they progress, gradually become etiologic factors in their own right."

SCHIZOPHRENIA AS A CASE OF BEHAVIORAL TERATOGENESIS

The scenario postulated by Mednick (1970) firmly placed schizophrenia, however implicitly, in the realm of mammalian teratogenesis. Regrettably, the research efforts in the field of experimental embryology were infrequently focused on psychopathology in general and schizophrenia, in particular (e.g., Rakic, 1988). Even such suggestive outcomes of prenatal irradiation as reduced head circumference was juxtaposed with reduced IQ and/or epilepsy (Otake and Schull, 1998), but not schizophrenia.

Teratogens are commonly viewed as factors or agents capable of causing gross anatomical damage via the disruption of the developmental processes between conception and birth of the progeny. Not all points on the journey from a conceptus to a newborn are equally relevant to specific outcomes. According to Wilson (1973), teratogenic manifestations appear in four categories: embryolethality, malformations, growth abnormalities, and functional deficit depending upon the time of prenatal injury. Behavioral (functional) teratogens have a narrow time window, limiting the period of vulnerability to organogenesis and the fetal time period.

The boundary between the functional as opposed to structural teratogenesis is fuzzy. There is no threshold effect for labeling one as opposed to the other. The rule of thumb for attributing a case to the functional teratogenesis is an absence of detectable pathology which could be easily violated with an increased resolution when behavioral aberrations could be associated with changes in the rate of apoptosis and some subtle anomalies in the connectivity of the neuronal network (Auroux, 1997; Kimler, 1998). Auroux (1997, p. 143) maintains that "teratogenic factors probably will be integrated into a continuum which will include macroscopic, microscopic, ultrastructural and finally molecular malformations."

However attractive the notion of schizophrenia as a case of behavioral teratogenesis may be, several objections are clear.

A teratogenic effect in schizophrenia is not definite in the sense that it does not produce an effect as reliable as cretinism with iodine deficiency or microcephaly with early prenatal ionizing radiation. When teratogens act at the early stage in development of the blastocyst they are likely to produce various neurological and/or somatic malformations or growth abnormalities (Wilson, 1973; Rugh, 1962; Auroux, 1997) and thus do not model a later onset disorder such as schizophrenia. When they act at the period of organogenesis or during the fetal period their association with the outcome may appear rather meager so as to convey a false impression of their low relevance. A current example of the latter is the demonstration of behavioral teratogenesis following modest levels of ethanol consumption by pregnant mothers (Streissguth et al., 1994) and the report of the association of maternal attitude towards pregnancy with development of schizophrenia in later life (Myhrman et al., 1996).

Most teratogenic factors are chronic in nature. That impeaches single-stage injury models targeting the structures with prolonged development (e.g., hippocampus, cerebellum). In view of the foregoing, the philosophy of a single brain area impairment (e.g., hippocampal damage) appears fallacious even when a definite teratogen is employed. The vulnerability of a system is related to the duration of the period of neurogenesis of its neurons. Assuming that the stressor is short lasting, such structures as the hippocampus or cerebellum have a better chance to resist damage due to their reserve of proliferative cells. The fact that they are implicated in schizophrenia suggests that one has to look for an agent that lasts long enough to drain the reserve of the proliferative pools.

Finally, some definitive human teratogens may be ineffective in laboratory animals; species vulnerable to some teratogens may be resistant to others. No explanation is available regarding within- and between-species variance in teratogenic sensitivity (Nishimura and Sirota, 1975).

While any single postulated prenatal environmental antecedent of schizophrenia may be found to be associated with only a fraction of adult cases of the disorder and may require large samples to demonstrate reliable effects, aggregating across similarly acting stressors may allow for reasonable power in more limited sample sizes. Additionally, models that accommodate the joint action of genetic, prenatal and postnatal effects, perhaps through multiple regression, increase the power of our studies. Multiple regression models allow for continuously distributed variables rather than the simple presence or absence of putative antecedents and provide estimates of the percentage of variance accounted for by each component such that relative importance can be compared. The neurobehavioral sequelae of various environmental toxins, such as lead and ethanol, have been elucidated with such models (Bellinger et al., 1992, Streissguth et al., 1994)

Prenatal Injury and 'Pandysmaturation'

Perhaps, neurologically oriented investigators might feel more comfortable with the modeling criteria which emphasize disordered pattern of acquisition of milestones ("pandysmaturation" of Fish, 1977; Fish et al., 1992); poor "cuddliness" in neonates (Benenson et al., 1999); inadequate motor coordination (Walker and Lewine, 1990; Cannon et al., 1999); and efficient information processing (attention deficit) (Mirsky et al., 1995).

The requirement of poor cuddliness is particularly relevant. The tendency to withdraw from reality and socially cohesive groups is an essential element for the clinical diagnosis of childhood schizophrenia. Among the "Sick Group" of patients described by Mednick (1970), 50% were passive, shy, guarded, lonely individuals, often with extreme signs of withdrawal. It is of interest that Mednick (1970) describes several "most important characteristics distinguishing the Sick Group," but withdrawal was not explicitly mentioned. Although the importance of testing social behavior and social isolation in psychiatry has been acknowledged it is surprising that this major trend of a patient to loneliness and extreme withdrawal has been absent from the scripts of experimental modeling of the disorder. Only more recently have Lipska and her colleagues (Lipska, Jaskiw and Weinberger, 1993; Lipska and Weinberger, 1993; this volume, for review) begun to test whether prenatal hippocampal lesions in neonatal rats have an effect on social behavior in adulthood. Another interesting example was given by Kim and Kirkpatrick (1996), who have investigated a highly social species (prairie voles) characterized by tight family bonds and a strong response to separation.

The disordered pattern of acquisition of milestones is typical of prenatal injury. In general, by throwing out of step some elements which otherwise would have developed in precisely coordinated harmony, this could conceivably either repress or exaggerate the pace of development of the whole constellation of behavior and cognition. Ever since Stockard (1921) it has been accepted that prenatal stressors act in the direction of the reducing of the developmental rate of animals: "For the past ten years I have claimed that all types of monsters not of hereditary origin are to be interpreted simply as *developmental arrests* (ital. added)" (Stockard, 1921, p. 117). Consequently, the resulting deformity was conceived of as secondary to their impeded rate of development. It remains uncertain how such processes would affect brain functions in adulthood and in what way they could predispose to psychopathology.

However, prenatal stressors are also capable of accelerating the pace of maturation and aging (Mintz and Myslobodsky, this volume). The acceleration of maturation may be deleterious for brain plasticity. The more mature the region the less likely it to benefit from repair by a reserve of immature cells available during gestation. An increased rate of maturation of the damaged tissue may also convey a false signal of the functional readiness and potentially encourage a more zealous apoptosis. The latter possibility is suggested by the dependence of survival of neurons upon their target organs (e.g., other cells, a muscle) which is a source of certain chemical signals promoting survival of connecting neurons (Oppenheim and Nunez, 1982). By preventing synaptic stimulation of the target (e.g., by neuromuscular blockade) it was possible to arrest motor neuron death (Pittman and Oppenheim, 1978). Assuming that central neurons, too, are deleted when connected with hyperactive elements one might suggest that an onset of neuronal activity in prematurely functioning neurons must trigger apoptosis thereby reducing the synaptic field.

THE "WHAT" AND "WHEN" OF STRESSORS

There is an extensive literature detailing the consequences of developmental stressors in laboratory animals. Given that neuronal cells are highly vulnerable at the period of their rapid multiplication and migration, virtually any stressor administered prenatally as well as prenatal infections or malnutrition could alter brain development and contribute to behavioral teratogenicity. The pattern of damage inflicted in embryogeny is thus to a considerable degree nonspecific in the sense that diverse maneuvers may lead to a similar range of deficient functions. The major factors in their action are the time of exposure and the strength (dose) of the damaging agent.

Time of Exposure

When neuroblasts of the germinal (ventricular) layer begin to migrate from the matrix to occupy their eventual destined locations in various brain regions they become highly vulnerable targets for a host of environmental stressors, compared to immature ependymal cells and mature neurons. The presence of the time-shift (developmental heterochronicity) for the departure of migrating cellular tides leaving the germinal matrix creates different, even if overlapping, time-windows of vulnerability for a variety of neuronal populations. Stockard (1921) was apparently the first to maintain that "when an important organ is entering its initial stage of rapid proliferation or budding, a serious interruption of the developmental process often causes decided injuries to this particular organ, while only slight or no ill effects may be suffered by the embryo in general" (p. 139). He has designated these sensitive periods as "critical moments." Thus, stressors, when relatively mild cannot cause a uniform damage to the whole embryo. Occasionally, such stressors are able to selectively damage cellular populations destined for certain locations, leaving relatively intact those of them that either already have occupied their place or have yet to initiate their migration. In this regard, critical periods permit a variety of inductors and stressors to override developmental events initiated by intrinsic (gene-controlled) programs.

Given that this programmed chronology of development is similar in all mammals it is possible to make a few relatively safe predictions as to whether an injury in humans has been inflicted at the period of intrauterine development and even guess when this might have happened, and when an analogous period of development in another animal would be. If epidemiological data indicate that individuals are at risk for schizophrenia when exposed to stressors during the second trimester, then an analogous stress should be delivered to a newborn rat which is believed to be developmentally equivalent to a 150-day old human embryo (second trimester) (Ojeda and Urnaski, 1994). Dobbing and Sands (1979) conclude that any species could potentially become an acceptable model of experimental embryology research if the equality of timing, severity and proportional duration of potential stressors are observed. Poorly defined timing is paramount to obtaining false negatives regarding the systems affected.

Which Animal to Choose

On the basis of the proportion of the brain development at a specific stage, Dobbing and Sands (1979) subdivided animals into "prenatal", "perinatal" and "postnatal" brain developers. If "postnatal brain developers" are defined as species who attain 30% or less of their brain maturity prenatally then humans will be found in a company of "postnatal" rodents, cats, and pigs. By contrast, rhesus monkeys will find themselves in a company of the sheep and Guinea pigs (Holt et al., 1981). Cats are comparable in the pace of growth to humans. However, they are polytoceous animals which makes them particularly sensitive to a different set of stressors. This leads to an important point: pups of the same litter may differ in size. A small size of the pup is not necessarily determined by a bad gene, but a bad place in utero. This misfortune may be further exaggerated by prenatal stressors and postnatal fights for survival. Birth into a sizable litter is a stressful event, particularly for a pup of a small size who needs to fight for its mothers warmth and milk.

PRENATAL EXPOSURE TO IONIZING RADIATION (A NEGLECTED MODEL)

It follows from the foregoing that any credible model of schizophrenia should fulfill several diverse requirements:
Allow that specific populations of cells are altered in schizophrenia and allow for neuronal damage in schizophrenia that is either ab initio or progressive;
  • Show that the timing and duration of prenatal insults is critical in determining their contribution to schizophrenia;
  • Provide evidence that pre- and perinatal insults to the CNS may be mildly expressed during development and more severely expressed as schizophrenia in adults;
  • Comply with findings that specific regions of the brain are anatomically altered and functionally compromised;
  • Permit an explanation of some paradoxical immunological concomitants of schizophrenia.
  • Demonstrate the relevance of a deficient dopaminergic system in the reproduced condition.

We have been impressed that progeny of animals exposed prenatally to ionizing irradiation answer a number of these requirements. The effects of ionizing radiation are merely summarized here; for detailed information, the reader is referred to the reviews and symposia on prenatal irradiation (Brent et al., 1987; Hicks, 1958; Hicks and D'Amato, 1978; Norton et al., 1991; Rugh, 1962; Schull et al., 1990; EULEP Symposium, 1984; GSF Symposium, 1986). An animal model using experimental exposure to ionizing radiation permits the avoidance of potential confounds, such as mother's age, obstetric complications, previous miscarriages, drug use and diseases, marital stressors, length of pregnancy, and others. Its major advantage is in easy dosing as well as the fact that beyond certain doses, central effects (structural, behavioral, and electrophysiological) are highly reproducible (Hicks, 1958; Hicks and D'Amato, 1978; Myslobodsky, 1976; Shofer et al., 1964). In this regard, ionizing irradiation seems an especially fitting alternative for producing a permanent insult during intrauterine development (Hicks and D'Amato, 1978; Rakic, 1988). It is a very useful, but little used, technique which answers the requirement of modeling environmental precipitants (Crow, 1987) and focuses on selecting the time and dose of exposure. This leads us to the next point.

Structural brain injury

The list of presumably developmental, cytoarchitectural findings in schizophrenia is impressive (Kovelman and Scheibel, 1984; Conrad et al., 1991; Jacob and Beckman, 1986; Benes et al., 1991; Benes and Bird, 1987; Akbarian, Bunney et al., 1993; Akbarian, Vinuela, et al., 1993). They are hardly pathognomic to schizophrenia and may be found in other disorders with inauspicious prenatal history. For example, a recent study by Belichenko et al. (1994) of biopsy material obtained from cortical epileptogenic zone in patients with temporal lobe epilepsy showed a high incidence of ectopic neurons in layer I, atypical apical and basilar dendrites in layers II-VI, and increased amount of neurons in the white matter. However, collectively these data have brought increasing structure to the field by suggesting that prenatal injury may be a sine qua non in experimental attempts at reproducing the pathophysiology of schizophrenia.

The strength of prenatal exposure to ionizing radiation as an experimental model is that it reproduces virtually all neuropathological findings reported in schizophrenia. These are reduced thickness of the cortex, ventriculomegaly, cortical atrophies, hypoplastic corpus callosum, hypoplastic vermis, ectopic islets of neurons, and abnormal cell orientation (Hicks, 1958; Hicks and D'Amato, 1978; Rakic, 1988). Typically, ectopic neurons are expected to be eliminated by cell death (Clarke and Cowan, 1975). Yet on a closer examination using the light and electron microscopy such islets of ectopic cortex seem to contain functional cells and viable synapses (Donoso and Norton, 1982).

Motivation deficit ('Anhedonia')

The study exploring hedonistic behavior in adult rats X-irradiated on E12 of gestation has been conducted using self-stimulation through electrodes implanted in the medial forebrain bundle (Michailova, 1966). It appeared that irradiated animals as well as adult controls exhibited practically identical rates of self-stimulation. In controls, the rates were enhanced significantly after administration of 3 mg/kg of amphetamine. In contrast, the same dose changed very little the rates of self-stimulation in exposed rats. Additional doses of amphetamine enhanced locomotion and elicited stereotypies, but did not affect the rates of self-stimulation in prenatally irradiated rats (Michailova, 1966). The effect of non-responsiveness to amphetamine could be attributed to reduced reinforcing properties of dopamine release as is observed in stressed animals (Stamford et al., 1991). Prenatally irradiated rats must have been made intrinsically more sensitive to stress. One might wonder whether this paradoxical blunting of self-stimulation response to amphetamine may not be compared with anhedonia.

Gender effects

Meier (1961) analyzed effects of direct fetal irradiation as compared to irradiation of the mother where the fetuses were partially shielded. It appeared that maze learning was significantly disrupted in males whereas females showed a nonsignificant trend in the same direction. This result suggests that the higher prevalence of abnormality in males, a common finding in neurodevelopmental disorders may be expected among X-irradiated progeny. Meier's study suggests that higher vulnerability of males may be associated with the response of the maternal organism to irradiation. The role of insult to pregnant female remain to be elucidated. Ionizing radiation is known to increase the level of neurotransmitters in the maternal circulation (e.g., serotonin, histamine) which could cross the blood-brain barrier and affect the developing irradiated brain (Cokerham and Prell, 1989). The effects mediated through maternal organisms remain poorly understood.

Delayed effects

An important requirement to any developmental model of schizophrenia is to reproduce the 'delayed incidence effect' (Lipska and Weinberger, this volume), i.e. a cumulative increase of risk to the disorder and ultimately the delayed onset of its symptoms. In general, the presence of "ontogenetic discontinuity" (Spear, 1984) in behavioral manifestations following a neuroteratological insult is a recognizable phenomenon (Weinstock, this volume). The effect of ionizing radiation on the developing brain might also be designated as being "progressive." The signs of embryotoxicity may well appear several weeks postpartum, particularly weaning when the physiological systems of the young are challenged in the independent living. Fetal Sprague-Dawley rats exposed to 0.75 Gy ionizing radiation showed broader base of gait than controls and enhanced activity that was not seen in one month old pups or reached significance until three months after birth (Norton et al., 1991). These rats may develop signs of hyperreactivity which they did not manifest earlier. It is of interest that in rats X-irradiated on E16, circular movements become apparent only after puberty, at about P45 (Goldberg, 1966). Radiation-induced hippocampal damage achieved by postnatal fractionated X-irradiation (P1-16, 13 Gy total) is also known to cause perseverative bouts of turning which becomes more persistent with age (Mickley et al., 1989). In a study conducted by Mintz and Myslobodsky (this volume), Spague-Dawley rats exposed prenatally to γ radiation showed behavioral abnormalities delayed into the period of 'early adulthood' (P55).

Immunological concomitants of prenatal exposure (Schizophrenia and malignancy)

The most common analytic tools in schizophrenia research has been to study experimental animals made behaviorally dysfunctional following administration of centrally active drugs or neurotoxic lesions in the limbic system (McKinney, 1988). We believe we have demonstrated that none have as yet reproduced the specific symptoms of the disorder with the same clarity of the models seen in other somatic maladies. Even the most successful of them stop short of the ability, as Symonds (1937) put it, "to describe a collection of symptoms as belonging to an organic lesion of the kind which one may demonstrate in a glass jar – as one may describe the symptoms of appendicitis or coronary occlusion" (p. 463). The focus is therefore shifting to the examination of somatic disorders which either have unusual affinity to schizophrenia or, by contrast, are less likely to coexist with it (Jeste et al., 1996; Wright, Gill, and Murray, 1993. A case in point, is an unusually low prevalence of rheumatoid arthritis (Allebeck et al., 1985; Eaton et al., 1992) and some forms of cancer (Baldwin, 1979; Mortenson, 1989; Mortenson, 1992, 1994) in schizophrenic patients which could conceivably shed light on the pathophysiology of the disorder itself.

We may reasonably expect to find biological links between genetic predisposition to schizophrenia and the resistance to some medical diseases. For example, a negative association between HLA DR4 and schizophrenia has been observed, and mothers of schizophrenic patients have been reported to have a significantly lower frequency of HLA DR4 than controls (Wright, Gill and Murray, 1993).

A reduced prevalence of lung cancer is particularly striking in view of the high rate of smoking among schizophrenic patients (de Leon, 1996). One might be interested in reproducing a state of higher resistance to lung cancers in laboratory models of schizophrenia.

Alterations of brain asymmetry

The notion (Flor-Henry, 1969) that the "schizophrenic process" is associated with the disruption of development of brain lateralization has evolved in recent years (Taylor and Abrams, 1987; Crow, 1987, 1998). Modeling this anomaly is a challenge for a laboratory model of the disorder (see Carlson et al., this volume). Brain laterality is a multicomponent construct. Its different components (functionally, biochemical and/or anatomical) do not march in step. Likewise, various indices of brain laterality in laboratory animals show no directional uniformity. A number of maneuvers affecting the developing rodent were shown to affect brain laterality as indexed by asymmetry of eye opening, postural imbalance and directionality preference. All were shown to be affected by prenatal exposure to γ radiation. However, one may speculate whether the loss of lateral bias in rats locomotion is a better equivalent of behavioral and emotional ambivalence in schizophrenia and a better functional correlate of reduced morphological hemispheric asymmetry.

CODA

We referred to a number of studies which focused on questions concerning the kind, intensity, and most importantly, the time during developmental history when a traumatic event may affect morbidity in adulthood. However successful in other divisions of medicine, the prevailing mood in psychiatry until very recently did not encourage this approach. In general, the laboratory analysis of pre- and/or neonatal injury in regard to its role in psychopathology is wanting in addressing the two questions of Pasamanick and Knobloch (1966): (1) Why bona fide psychotic patients have limited, if any, history of prenatal abnormalities? and (2) Why numerous individuals with a definite history of prenatal abnormalities do not exhibit psychopathology?

The answers to the first question have been provided by numerous recent studies indicating that such findings are a function of the accuracy of our tools and sampling strategies. The other answer is that neurological sequelae of developmental disturbances could be easily overlooked. Also, they may reflect broad consequences across multiple domains, with limited specific relevance to the pathophysiology of schizophrenia.

The second question also requires two answers. First, there are heritable genetic differences in sensitivity to various stressors, such that identical stressors (whether infectious or traumatic) can have considerable variability in effect. Secondly, in the past the dominant conceptual framework, linking prenatal injury, including embryonic exposure to ionizing radiation, with alteration of higher functions in adulthood was that of exploration of its contribution to a relatively narrow range of cognitive deficits.

Only recently, with the efforts of several groups, has the possibility of embryo- or fetopathology ceased to be considered as merely convenient (and possibly fictitious) way of explaining aberrant behaviors. This communication adds to this trend by exploring the role of embryoneuropathology inflicted by ionizing radiation. Surprisingly, prenatal applications of ionizing radiation have seldom been motivated by neuropsychiatric objectives; the studies examining the role of prenatal damage with the pathophysiology of schizophrenia in mind are practically unknown. We wish to fill this void, in confidence that this technique permits modeling the effects of environmental precipitants, as many have advocated, and allows an emphasis on the time and dose of exposure rather than on the search for the hypothetical culprit.

Given the limited success to date in identifying the specific genetic deficits leading to schizophrenia, our proposed approach has the potential to offer some clues to the role of genes in the pathogenesis of schizophrenia, and their interaction with environmental stressors. There is considerable variability across rat strains in the degree of susceptibility to damage by prenatal irradiation, just as there is variation across strains in propensity for behaviors that are relevant to the schizophrenia. Variability in affiliative behavior can provide an example. If rat strains that show reduced affiliative behavior are less sensitive to the effects of prenatal ionizing radiation in inducing changes in affiliative behavior than controls, then one might suspect that the effect of both genes and ionizing radiation operates through a similar mechanism, such that radiation induced deficits mimic the action of the genes specific to that strain. Alternatively, if strains that are low in affiliative behavior show an increased sensitivity to ionizing radiation, then one might conclude that different mechanisms are involved, particularly if more severe specific deficits are produced by combined action than by either exposure to radiation or by strain differences alone.

Admittedly, the effects accomplished by a single-day prenatal exposure do not give a complete picture of psychopathology we wish to reproduce. One might thus appropriately ask whether any cluster of symptoms following prenatal brain damage forms a coherent symptoms aggregate in a single animal, or whether such symptoms are drawn from a variety of animals exposed on different days of embryogeny. The answer is that such aberrations often represent a cumulative product of several episodes of prenatal exposure on different days. Thus the problem is not in the number of 'schizophrenic' symptoms an animal model would manifest to appear successful, but which symptoms approach those which Kraepelin and Bleuler considered fundamental. Consider such fundamental and specific feature as disturbances in personal contact and rapport. Although this deficit could presumably be reproduced by social isolation, the goal is to achieve a socially deficient animal following pre- or perinatal trauma. Likewise, such a fundamental feature of the disorder as impoverished affect may manifest itself in a diversity of ways which motivates a search for a very limited form of deficit in experimental animals. Yet it is not necessarily a damaging feature for a model based on prenatal injury. It is not realistic to require a model organism to display all of the "textbook" features of schizophrenia when a practicing physician can hardly see them all in a single patient in the psychiatry ward. A parable shared by Hofstadter (1996) about a famous Dublin zookeeper is a case in point. The zookeeper was unusually successful in breeding lion cubs. When asked to share the formula of his achievement, he replied instantly, "Understanding the lions."

- And what is the secret of 'understanding' lions? pressed his interlocutor.

- To bear in mind that every lion is different, - said the zookeeper.

The message is that however gratifying it may be to aim towards developing a single comprehensive model of schizophrenia, no model can be adequate without accurately reflecting that the syndrome does not manifest itself within individuals or families as a single entity, but rather as a set of related states. For now, we may need to continue to formulate confined hypotheses to be tested with partial, but useful, models.

REFERENCES

Akbarian, S., Bunney, W.E., Potkin, S.G., Wigal, S.B., Hagman, J.O., Sandman, C.A., Jones, E.G. (1993a) Altered distribution of nicotinamide-adenine dinucleotide phosphate-diaphorase cells in frontal lobe of schizophrenics implies disturbances of cortical development. Arch Gen Psychiat. 50:169-177.

Akbarian, S., Vinuela, A., Kim, J., Potkin, S.G., Bunney, W.E., Jones, E.G. (1993b) Distorted distribution of nicotinamide-adenine dinucleotide phosphate-diaphorase neurons in temporal lobe of schizophrenics implies anomalous cortical development. Arch Gen Psychiat. 50:178-187.

Allebeck, P., Rodvall, Y., Wistedt, B. (1985) Incidence of rheumatoid arthritis among patients with schizophrenia, affective psychosis and neurosis. Acta Psychiatr Scand. 71:615-9.

Auroux, M. (1997) Behavioral teratogenesis: An extension to the teratogenesis of functions. Biology Of The Neonate. 71: 137-147.

Baldwin, J.A. (1979) Schizophrenia and physical disease. Psychol Med. 9:611-8.

Belichenko, P.V., Sourander, P., Malmgren, K., Nordborg, C., von Essen, C., Rydenhag, B., et al. (1994) Dendritic morphology in epileptogenic cortex from TRPE patients, revealed by intracellular Lucifer Yellow microinjection and confocal laser scanning microscopy. Epilepsy Res. 18:233-47.

Bellinger, D.C., Stiles, K.M., Needleman, H.L. (1992) Low-level lead exposure, intelligence and academic achievement: a long-term follow-up. Pediatrics. 90:855-61.

Benenson, J.F., Philippoussis, M., Leeb, R. (1999) Sex differences in neonates' cuddliness. J Genetic Psychol. 160:332-42.

Benes, F.M. and Bird, E.D. (1987) An analysis of the arrangement of neurons in the cingulate cortex of schizophrenic patients. Arch Gen Psychiat. 44:608-16.

Benes, F.M., McSparren, J., Bird, E.D., SanGiovanni, J.P., Vincent, S.L. (1991) Deficits in small interneurons in prefrontal and cingulate cortices in schizophrenic and schizoaffective patients. Arch Gen Psychiat. 48:996-1001.

Brent, R.L., Beckman, D.A., Jensh, R.P. (1987) Relative radiosensitivity of fetal tissues. Adv Rad Biol. 12:239-56.

Cannon, M., Jones, P., Huttunen, M.O., Tanskanen, A., Huttunen, T., Rabe-Hesketh, S., Murray, R.M. (1999) School performance in Finnish children and later development of schizophrenia: a population-based longitudinal study. Arch Gen Psychiat. 56:457-63.

Clarke, P.G., Cowan, W.M. (1975) Ectopic neurons and aberrant connections during neural development. Proc Natl Acad Sci U S A. 72:4455-8.

Cockerham, L.G., Prell, G.D. (1989) Prenatal radiation risk to the brain. Neurotoxicology. 10: 467-74.

Conrad, A.J., Abebe, T., Austin, R., Forsythe, S., Scheibel, A.B. (1991) Hippocampal pyramidal cell disarray in schizophrenia as a bilateral phenomenon. Arch Gen Psychiat. 48:413-7.

Crow, T.J. (1987) The scope for nongenetic factors in etiology.: the retrovirus/transposon hypothesis. In: Helmchen, H., Henn, F.A., eds. Biological Perspectives of Schizophrenia, Chichester: John Willey and Sons.

Crow, T.J. (1998) Schizophrenia as a transcallosal misconnection syndrome. Schizophr Res. 10:111-4.

De Bellis, M.D., Baum, A.S., Birmaher, B., Keshavan, M.S., Eccard, C.H., Boring, A.M., Jenkins, F.J., Ryan, N.D. (1999) Developmental traumatology part I: biological stress systems. Biol Psychi. 45:1259-70.

De Bellis, M.D., Keshavan, M.S., Clark, D.B., Casey, B.J., Giedd, J.N., Boring, A.M., Frustaci, K., Ryan, N.D. (1999) Developmental traumatology part II: brain development. Biol Psychi. 45:1271-84.

De Leon, J. (1996) Smoking and vulnerability for schizophrenia. Schiz Bull. 22:405-9.

Dobbing, J. and Sands, J. (1979) Comparative aspects of the brain growth spurt. Early Human Develop. 3:79-83.

Donoso, J.A. and Norton, S. (1982) The pyramidal neuron in cerebral cortex following prenatal X-irradiation. Neurotox. 3:72-84.

Eaton, W.W., Hayward, C., Ram, R. (1992) Schizophrenia and rheumatoid arthritis: a review. Schizophr Res. 6:181-92.

EULEP Symposium. (1984) Effects of prenatal irradiation with special emphasis on late effects. Streffer, C., Patric, G., eds. Commission of the European Comunities Publication EUR-8067.

Farmer, A., McGuffin, P., Gottesman I.I. (1990) Problems and pitfalls of the family history positive and negative dichotomy: response to Dalen. Schizophr Bull. 16:367-70.

Fish, B. (1977) Neurobiologic antecedents of schizophrenia in children. Arch Gen Psychiat. 34:1297-313.

Fish, B., Marcus, J., Hans, S.L., Auerbach, J.G., Perdue, S. (1992) Infants at risk for schizophrenia: sequelae of a genetic neurointegrative defect. A review and replication analysis of pandysmaturation in the Jerusalem Infant Development Study. Arch Gen Psychiat. 49:221-35.

Fleming, K., Goldberg, T.E., Binks, S., Randolph, C., Gold, J.M., Weinberger, D.R. (1997) Visuospatial working memory in patients with schizophrenia. Biol Psychiatry. 41:43-9.

Flor-Henry, P. (1969) Psychosis and temporal lobe epilepsy. Epilepsia. 10:363-95.

Fraser, F.C. (1959) Causes of congenital malformations in human beings. J Chron Dis. 10:97-113.

GSF Symposium. (1985) Radiation risks to the developing nervous system. Kriegel, H., ed. Commission of the European Communities Publication EUR-10414.

Goldberg, M.B. (1966) Developmental and functional characteristics of conditioned reflexes in adult rats X-irradiated on day 16 of embryogeny. In: I. Piontkovsky (Ed), Neuroradioembryological Effects. Moscow: Nauka.

Goldberg, T.E., Patterson, K.J., Taqqu, Y., Wilder, K. (1998) Capacity limitations in short-term memory in schizophrenia: tests of competing hypotheses. Psychol Med. 28: 665-73.

Goldschmidt, R. (1935) Zeitschr. fur induktive Abstammungs-und Vererbungslehre. LXIX:46.

Gottesman, I.I. and Bertelsen, A. (1989) Confirming unexpressed genotypes for schizophrenia. Risks in the offspring of Fischer's Danish identical and fraternal discordant twins. Arch Gen Psychi. 46:867-72.

Hicks, S.P. Radiation as an experimental tool in mammalian developmental neurology. Physiol. Rev., 38:337-358, 1958.

Hicks, S.P. and D'Amato, C.J. (1978). Effects of ionizing radiation on developing brain and behavior. In: G. Gottlieb, ed. Studies on the Development of Behavior and the Nervous System. V. 4, Early influences. London: Academic Press.

Hirsch, S.R. and Weinberger, D. (1995) Schizophrenia. London: Blackwell.

Hofstadter, D.R. (1996) Metamagical Themas : Questing for the Essence of Mind and Pattern. New York: Basic Books.

Hollister, J. M., Laing, P., Mednick S.A. (1996) Rhesus incompatibility as a risk factor for schizophrenia in male adults. Arch Gen Psychi. 53:19-24.

Holt, A.B., Renfree, M.B., Cheek, D.B. (1981) Comparative aspects of brain growth: s critical evaluation of mammalian species used in brain growth research with emphasis on the Tamar Wallaby. In: Hetzel, B.S., Smith, R.M., eds. Fetal Brain Disorders - Recent Approaches to the Problem Of Mental Deficiency. Amsterdam: Elsevier.

Huttunen, M.O. and Niskanen, P. (1978) Prenatal loss of father and psychiatric disorders. Arch Gen Psychi. 35:429-31.

Ingraham, L. J. (1995) Family-genetic research and schizotypal personality. In: Raine, A., ed. Schizotypal Personality. Cambridge: Cambridge U. Press.

Ingraham, L. J. (1999) Empirical characterization of the schizophrenia spectrum. In: Maj, M., Sartorius, N., eds. Evidence and Experience in Psychiatry. New York: John Wiley.

Jacob, H. and Beckman, H. (1986) Prenatal developmental disturbances in the limbic cortex in schizophrenics. J Neural Transmis. 65:303-26.

Jeste, D.V., Gladsjo, J.A., Lindamer, L.A., Lacro, J.P. (1996) Medical comorbidity in schizophrenia. Schizophr Bull. 22:413-30.

Kety, S.S., Wender, P.H., Jacobsen, B., Ingraham, L.J., Jansson, L., Faber, B., Kinney, D.K. (1994) Mental illness in the biological and adoptive relatives of schizophrenic adoptees. Replication of the Copenhagen Study in the rest of Denmark. Arch Gen Psychi. 51:442-55

Kim, J.W. and Kirkpatrick, B. (1996) Social isolation in animal model of relevance to neuropsychiatric disorders. Biol Psychiat. 40:918-22.

Kimler, B.F. (1998) Prenatal irradiation: a major concern for the developing brain. Int J Radiat Biol. 73: 423-34.

Kovelman, J.A. and Scheibel, A.B. (1984) A neurohistological correlate of schizophrenia. Biol Psychiat. 19:1601-21.

Lim, K. O., Beal, D.M., Harvey, R.L. Jr., Myers, T., Lane, B., Sullivan, E.V., Faustman, W.O., Pfefferbaum, A. (1995) Brain dysmorphology in adults with congenital rubella plus schizophrenialike symptoms. Biol Psychiatry. 37: 764-76.

Lipska, B.K., Jaskiw, G.E., Weinberger, D.R. (1993) Postpubertal emergence of hyperresponsiveness to stress and to amphetamine after neonatal excitotoxic hippocampal damage: A potential animal model of schizophrenia. Neuropsychopharmacol. 9:67-75.

Lipska, B.K. and Weinberger, D.R. (1993) Delayed effect of neonatal hippocampal damage on haloperidol-induced catalepsy and apomorphin-induced stereotypic behaviors in the rat. Dev Brain Res. 75:213-222.

Matthysse S. (1987) "The middle game" in the genetics of schizophrenia. In H. Helmchen, F.A. Henn, eds. Dahlem Workshop on Biological Perspectives of Schizophrenia. Chichester: Wiley.

McGuffin, P., Farmer, A. E., Gottesman, I. I. (1987) Is there really a split in schizophrenia? The genetic evidence. Br J Psychi. 150:581-92.

McKinney, W.T. (1988) Models of Mental Disorders: A New Comparative Psychiatry. New York: Plenum.

McKinney, W.T. and Bunney, W.E., Jr. (1969) Animal models of depression. Review of evidence: implications for research. Arch Gen Psychi. 21:240-8.

Mednick, S.A. (1970) Breakdown in individuals at high risk for schizophrenia: possible predispositional perinatal factors. Mental Hygiene. 54:50-63.

Mednick, S.A., Machon, R.A., Huttunen, M.O., Bonet, D. (1988) Adult schizophrenia following prenatal exposure to an influenza epidemic. Arch Gen Psychi. 45:171-6.

Meier, G.W. (1961) Prenatal anoxia and irradiation: maternal-fetal relations. Psychol Rep. 9:417-24.

Michailova, N.G. (1966) Effects of amphetamine on self-stimulation in prenatally X-irradiated animal. In: I. Piontkovsky, ed. Neuroradioembryological Effects. Moscow: Nauka.

Mickley, G.A., Ferguson, J.L., Nemeth, T.J., Mulvihill, M.A., Alderks, C.E. (1989) Spontaneous perseverative turning in rats with radiation-induced hippocampal damage. Behav Neurosci. 103:722-30.

Mirsky, A. F., Ingraham, L. J., Kugelmass, S. (1995) Neuropsychological assessment of attention and its pathology in the Israeli cohort. Schiz Bull. 21:193-204.

Mortensen, P.B. (1989) The incidence of cancer in schizophrenic patients. J Epidemiol Community Health. 43:43-7.

Mortensen, P.B. (1992) Neuroleptic medication and reduced risk of prostate cancer in schizophrenic patients. Acta Psychiatr Scand. 85:390-3.

Mortensen, P.B. (1994) The occurrence of cancer in first admitted schizophrenic patients. Schizophr Res. 12:185-94.

Myhrman, A., Rantakallio, P., Isohanni, M., Jones, P., Partanen, U. (1996) Unwantedness of a pregnancy and schizophrenia in the child. Br J Psychi. 169:637-640.

Myslobodsky, M. (1976) Petit Mal Epilepsy. A Search for Precursors of Petit Mal Activity. New York: Academic Press.

Myslobodsky, M., Mintz, M., Kofman, O. (1981) Pharmacologic analysis of the postictal immobility syndrome. Pharmacol Biochem Behav. 15:93-100.

Myslobodsky, M. and Mirsky, A., eds. (1988) Elements of Petit Mal Epilepsy. New York: Lang.

Myslobodsky, M. and Valenstein, E. (1980) Amygdaloid kindling and the GABA system. Epilepsia. 21:163-175.

Nishimura, H. and Sirota, K. (1975) Summary of comparative embryology and teratology. Handbook of Teratology. New York:Plenum.

Norton, S., Kimler, B.F., Mullenix, P.J. (1991) Progressive behavioral changes in rat after exposure to low levels of ionizing radiation in utero. Neurotoxicology and Teratology. 13:181-8.

Ojeda, S.R. and Urbanski, H.F. (1994) Puberty in the rat. In: E. Knobil, J.D. Neill, eds. The Physiology of Reproduction. 2nd ed.

Oppenheim, R.W. and Nunez, R. (1982) Electrical stimulation of hindlimb increases neuronal cell death in chick embryo. Nature. 295:57-59.

Otake, M. and Schull, W.J. (1998) Radiation-related brain damage and growth retardation among the prenatally exposed atomic bomb survivors. Int J Radiat Biol. 74:159-71.

Pasamanick, B. and Knobloch, H. (1966) Retrospective studies on the epidemiology of reproductive casualty: old and new. Merrill-Palmer Quat. 12:7-26.

Pittman, R.H. and Oppenheim, R.W. (1978) Neuromuscular blockade increases motoneuronal survival during normal cell death in chick embryo. Nature. 271:364-6.

Rackic, P. (1988) Defects of migration and the pathogenesis of cortical malformtations. Prog Brain Res. 73: 15-37.

Rugh, R. (1962) Low level of X-irradiation and the early mammalian embryo. Amer. J. Roentgenol. 87:559-566.

Schmajuk, N.A. (1987) Animal model for schizophrenia: The hippocampally lesioned animal. Schiz Bull. 13:317-27.

Schull, W.J., Norton, S., Jensh, R.P. (1990) Ionizing radiation and the developing brain. Neurotoxicol Teratol. 12:249-60.

Shofer, R.J., Pappas, G.D., Purpura, D.P. (1964) Radiation-induced changes in morphological and physiological properties of immature cerebellar cortex. In: T.J. Haley, R.S. Snyder eds. Response of the Nervous System to Ionizing Radiation. Boston:Little Brown.

Spear, L.P. (1984) Age at the time of testing reconsidered in neurobehavioral teratological research. In: Ynai, J. ed. Neurobehavioral Teratology. Amsterdam:Elsevier.

Stevens, J.R. (1973) An anatomy of schizophrenia? Arch Gen Psychiat. 29:177-89.

Stamford, J.A., Muscat, R., OConnor, J.J., Patel, J., Trout, S.J, Wieczorek, W.J, Kruk, Z.L., Willner, P. (1991) Voltammetric evidence that subsensitivity to reward following chronic mild stress is associated with increased release of mesolimbic dopamine. Psychopharmacol. 105: 275-82.

Stein, Z., Kline, J., Kharrazi, M. (1984). What is a teratogen? Epidemiological criteria. In: H. Kalter, ed. Issues and Reviews in Teratology, v.2. New York: Plenum.

Streissguth, A.P., Barr, H.M., Sampson, P.D., Bookstein, F.L. (1994) Prenatal alcohol and offspring development: the first fourteen years. Drug Alcohol Depend. 36:89-99.

Susser, E. and Lin, P. (1996) Schizophrenia after prenatal exposure to the Dutch hunger winter of 1944-1945. Arch Gen Psychi., 53:25-31.

Symonds, C.P. (1937) The assessment of symptoms following head injury. Guys Hospital Gazette. 51:461-468.

Taylor, M.A., Abrams, R. (1987) Cognitive impairment patterns in schizophrenia and affective disorder. J Neurol Neurosurg Psychiatry. 50:895-9.

Walker, E.F. and Lewine, R.J. (1990) The prediction of adult-onset schizophrenia from childhood home movies of patients. Am J Psychi. 147:1052-56.

Wilson, J.G. (1973) Environment and Birth Defects. New York: Academic Press.

Wright, P., Gill, M., Murray, R.M. (1993) Schizophrenia: genetics and the maternal immune response to viral infection. Am J Med Genet. 48:40-46.

17 MODELS OF PSYCHOSES: WHICH ONE, WHEN, AND WHY?

Michael Myslobodsky and Ina Weiner

The term "model" has been colonized by experts and is shared by several disciplines. It is as abused as the overlapping word "paradigm." According to the Webster, a model may be "a structural design," "a miniature representation of something," "an example for imitation or emulation," or "a description or analogy used to help visualize something that cannot be directly observed." Only in some quarters it denotes an original, a standard, a thing copied and thus something superior to the copy (e.g., a model painted by an artist). In the real world, models serve a variety of roles, some committed to their major calling, others rather peripheral to their stated goals, but considered profitable. All appeal to the need of accepting simplified representations as if they were reality. They retreat from its perplexity by offering something less cumbersome, less burdensome technically or ethically, in a word, something *less complex* (Ashby, 1970).

SCOPE

However imperfect, this notion of modeling has been adopted by neuropsychiatry and has become virtually irreplaceable. We use the word to describe an imperfect copy of a thing, a partial and lopsided mock-up of the original. In spite of this disclaimer, animal models of psychological aberrations are seldom greeted with equanimity. But if we hesitate to trust extrapolations from animal experiments in neuropsychiatry, what are the options? Several decades ago, Pribram (1961) pointed out that only two courses are open to us: "We can say, 'Oh well, people are different from animals. Let's forget the whole business'. Or we can search deeply into our understanding (or lack thereof) of what is meant by reward and by punishment, by drive and by attention, by memory processing and learning (p. 569)." Neurosciences took the second path and never looked back. The practice of describing the psychopathological syndromes in the language of neurosciences is thus a relatively new trend. This language ties us snugly with the description of behaviors and mechanisms learned in laboratory animals (e.g., mice, rats, cats) because their breeding, development, behavior, and numerous aspects of brain function, brain neurochemistry and structure have become familiar to us. The price is that we are frequently cautioned that no laboratory animal would ever mimic all the relevant psychopathological responses of humans, and that the results obtained in animal experiments cannot be simply "scaled" to human subjects. And yet, during the past 20 years, the application of new techniques in genetics, behavioral neurosciences, neuroimaging, biochemistry, and psychopharmacology, have contributed more to our understanding of the pathophysiology and etiology of various psychiatric disorders than at any other time in history. Our initial objective has been to focus on these achievements as they are developed by our esteemed crew of contributors, but gradually our summary grew into a more general discussion, revolving, explicitly or implicitly, around the following interrogative outline:

- When is a model needed?
- On what criteria should the human condition be related to its animal model?
- What predictions are afforded by models?
- What problems are likely to emerge when using specific approaches?
- When do we know that a model is successful?
- How quickly and in what manner aberrant features represented in a model should emerge?
- What predictions are possible without the investment into a model?
- What observations are needed for a model to be rejected?

WHY MODELS FAIL IN THE REAL-WORLD PSYCHOPATHOLOGY: GENERAL PRINCIPLES

The Demon of Complexity or on Seeing Part of the Elephant

The issue of complexity has two sources. One is ingrained in the sociology of science which easily questions statements about external reality, but keeps unchallenged reports about the internal world of a patient to which one has privileged epistemic access. Such an asymmetry is integral to our culture in which the "self is worshipped as a sacred object whose privacy ought not to be interfered with" (Fuchs, 1992, p. 23). The other is rooted in the restrictive taboos attributing a different level of complexity to psychopathology as opposed to normal functioning.

The fear of misperceiving the obvious is a corollary of the complexity taboo. It alludes to the limitations inherent in a restricted field of view or an inadequate change in the angle of view when examining a sizable problem whose vastness cannot be grasped *a priori*. The abyss between the simple kinds of behavior represented by models and real-life psychoses suggests that we are more successful when studying vulnerabilities, causes, triggers, and precipitants (McKinney, 1988). A physician looks for combinations of first-order factors that reliably cluster as second- or third-order syndromes, i.e., diseases. This strategy gives a sense of order but carries the risk of uncertainty about the nosological borders. Any continuous measure of symptoms promises to provide a more fine-grained analysis than the dichotomous measure (diagnosis), but makes the reductionistic labor more complex. As Simon (1991, p. 100) put it in the form of Aristotle's paradox, when knowledge increases, localization decreases.

Suspension of Disbelief

A model is often a substitute for a theory inasmuch as it heralds the presence of a theory by stating an argument while withholding the demand to spell out its refutations. In addition, models act like a proof that we are sufficiently advanced in theory to warrant a research effort. In this capacity they set a trap by creating the illusion of an explanation, while begging to suspend disbelief and to hold off criticism. The resistance to animal models in psychopathology derives from a basic inability to suspend the disbelief that they can ever be successful in conveying the understanding of what mental aberrations are.

Models' Mislabeling

The history of modeling is replete with cases when useful models were disregarded simply because they were dispatched with an inaccurate nosological address. A classical case in point is a juvenile monkey confined in a vertical chamber. The monkey showed behavioral aberrations upon reunion with the group members in the form of reduced motility and regressive patterns of social bonding, designated as "contact clinging" (McKinney et al., 1972). Although the model was discussed in the context of depression, the aberrations of social competence and bonding might well be relevant for modeling schizophrenia or the effects of child neglect (Maestripieri and Carroll, 1998). Likewise, helplessness models may be used to model a variety of conditions ranging from schizophrenia to stress-related disorders, or anxiety disorders. Nothing has changed since Marks's (1977) admonition that "learned helplessness" has not produced such cardinal features of severe depression as insomnia, anorexia, guilt, suicidal behavior and ideas, and lasting mood changes.

Tonic immobility is exhibited by a variety of species facing a proximal threat. Such a response presumably minimizes the triggers and cues which could elicit an attack and is of interest because of its high ecological validity (Gullap and Maser, 1977). It is not clear though why this evolutionary adaptation models depression. We wonder whether it would emulate more accurately some virtually disappearing signs of "hysteria" or, perhaps, such controversial construct as atypical depression with its histrionic features, anxiety and phobic symptoms? The same question applies to a variety of behaviors emitted by laboratory animals in response to explicit or implicit threats (e.g., freezing, startle, ultrasonic vocalizations, burying, avoidance/flight) that can be used to model fear, depression, anxiety, impulsivity, and vulnerability to stress. Their clinical worth should be magnified by the demonstration of other behavioral features typical of depression, such as sleep disturbances, loss of sexual drive, and deficient social competence. We still need to develop an animal model of atypical depression which features hyperphagia, weight gain, hypersomnia, and rejection sensitivity, thereby validating the disorder and providing a way of examining the pathophysiology of treatment resistance in depression.

Model Misattribution as a Case for Einheitspsychose

There is always a possibility that different aberrant behaviors share an overlapping pathophysiological territory (e.g., **Geyer** for PPI and **Weiner** for LI), even though a careful comparison shows a range of dissociations between PPI and LI in rats with pre/post-weaning environmental manipulations (**Feldon and colleagues**). For decades, the idea of overlap has been kept on the agenda by the belief that epileptogenicity provides a single explanatory construct for a range of conditions. Epilepsy is indeed capable of mascarading as a variety of syndromes and even emulate such "golden mean" of psychopathology as schizophrenia. **McIntyre and Anisman** indicate that epilepsy is known for the presence of comorbid features, such as cognitive and memory disturbances, anxiety reaction, and depression. Their chapter specifically emphasizes increased impulsivity (and aggression related to impulsivity) in epilepsy which could be studied using chronic repetitive electrical stimulation of the amygdala ("kindling model").

Einat and colleagues argue that amygdala kindling has a sufficient predictive and construct validity to serve as a model of bipolar disorder. Yet it is also a valid model of postictal psychosis associated with medically intractable complex partial seizures (Szabo et al., 1999), and particularly postictal aggression (Myslobodsky and Valenstein, 1980). Predictably, **McIntyre and Anisman** obtain a variety of manifestations which can be interpreted as anxiety-related reactions, such as reduced exploratory locomotion, withdrawal responses, and impulsivity. The invocation of limbic kindling as an explanatory mechanism for psychopathology so far is purely theoretical. Another mechanism which seems attractive as a potential psychotogene, is the progressive amplification of responses to intermittent exposure to a chemical (neural sensitization) discussed by **Robinson**. Similarly to a drug or an environmental toxicant, any endogenous material that normally cannot traverse the blood-brain barrier, may enter the brain under stressful condition and ultimately affect centrally controlled functions (Friedman et. al. 1996). Both the kindling and non-kindling mechanisms of altered excitability provide an interesting perspective on the archaic notion of a unitary psychosis (*Einheitspsychose*), which dominated German psychiatry at the end of the nineteenth century. The concept had comfortably shielded the field from concerns of comorbidity and diagnostic uncertainty contributed by the nosological overlap.

STRATEGIES OF MODELING

Quasi-Emulation Modeling

This approach, however old and naive, is intuitively appealing for it focuses on the necessity to stay in touch with the clinical reality. It may be termed *naturalistic, phenomenological, or composite (syndromological)*. Psychologists designate such models as possessing *"face validity"* whereas McKinney (1988) referred to them as *behavioral similarity models*, which he elevated to the status of "comparative psychiatry."

We are told that to be successful a model should specify an optimal list of features (Myslobodsky and Mirsky, 1988) or as many features as are known about the disease (Bartus, 1988). Such requirements introduce certain shock coefficient into the notion of a model. Models of psychopathology cannot assure of their "purity" at the time when the area is increasingly troubled by the problem of comorbidity. Still, this requirement forces us to make strong predictions regarding presumed relations between pathological signs and modeled variables. This approach is counter to the suggestion that models are useful because we cannot determine the nosological borders, e.g. "Depression is not well defined; for this reason it needs a model" (Miller et al., 1977; p. 111). The latter proposition is so tenuous that nothing solid could come out of it. Unless we have a good idea of what we are looking for, we may be unable to find it. Stated differently, until syndromological requirements are made, a model may prove worthless, no matter how many attractive features it may have.

In general, the reliability of nosological schemata rests on the assumption that relations between the symptoms of the syndrome are pathophysiologically determined. In statistical terms, this means that we should have the ability to "predict" each symptom as though within the context of a regression analysis. Given that human pathology has its own idiosyncrasies this is a difficult proposition for modeling.

The most critical limitation of the emulation approach in modeling is that the semblance of behavioral aberrations in animals to human psychopathology is seldom convincing. Behavioral patterns produced by stimulants (e.g., "ecstasy," amphetamine, cocaine), as opposed to phencyclidine and related drugs (ketamine, MK-801) contribute different aspects of schizophreniform syndrome rather than "schizophrenia" manifestations observed in recreational users. Some aspects of this research have evolved into the analysis of drug-related sensitization (**Robinson**).

Because a gene or a set of genes may have more than a single phenotypic effect whereas virtually identical aberration could be produced by dissimilar genes, the other limitation of the emulation approach is the weak coupling between complex macroscopic systems (behavior) and molecular biology mechanisms. Thus, anxiety-like behaviors in heterozygous GABA-A g2 subunit mice and catechol-*O*-methyltransferase-deficient mice may be dissimilar, thereby highlighting the neurochemical heterogeneity of anxiety disorders (**Holmes and Crawley**). Hopefully, this limitation will be minimized by the successful application of strains and species selected for specific disease-related effects and behaviors, such as the low/high stress sensitive rats (**Lipska and Weinberger**), rats with different turning directionality (**Carlson and colleagues**), or Slow/Fast-kindled strains (**McIntyre and Anisman**). A similar approach has yet to be taken by cognitive models. For example, normal rats might be bred for the magnitude of PP/LI. In a broader sense these selected strains touch on the elusive concept of "mental health" or "normality" of the strains used for modeling. The concept is still unresolved in nomothetic psychology since normality is not easily established in psychometric terms.

Etiologic Models

These are models examining factors, conditions and agents that elicit specific mental aberrations or must be present for a disorder to occur. Given that psychopathology is believed to be of a multifactorial origin, the choice of "causative" factors will vary as a function of the level of scrutiny adopted by a given model. Therefore, any simple etiologic model may require *ex-post-facto* mucking around with several independent or intervening variables in order to attain the intended condition.

Ever since the serendipitous observations by Pavlov and his disciples that dogs exposed to St. Petersburg's flood developed behavioral aberrations, "experimental neuroses" and other conditions were modeled by adding stress to any basic scenario. Stress machinery interacts with so many systems in setting the level of arousal that it is believed to contribute to disorders such as schizophrenia, OCD, anxiety, eating disorders, reduced libido, chronic alcoholism, premenstrual tension and numerous other aberrations. **Weinstock** shows that maternal stress sets in motion a complex machinery of the hypothalamic-pituitary adrenal (HPA) axis such that early environmental experiences in animals leave a permanent impression manifested in their adult physiology. Prenatally stressed rats have higher levels of corticotropin-releasing hormone in the amygdala, fewer hippocampal glucocorticoid receptors and less endogenous opioid and GABA/BDZ (benzodiazepine) inhibitory activity. Early postnatal experience also has apparent long-term effects on organisms' ability to gate out irrelevant or redundant sensory and cognitive information (**Geyer; Weiner; Feldon and colleagues**).

While prolonged perinatal exposure is justifiable ecologically because the impact of damaging factors is by and large continuous, the process of development can presumably be also approximated by a series of threshold effects that could be elicited at certain time-periods when vulnerability is maximal. In this case, however, by missing the maximal vulnerability window one would obtain a meager effect, if any at all, thereby committing an error of attribution when the genuinely damaging factor is misperceived as harmless. An example is shown in **Mintz and Myslobodsky's** chapter on brain reactivity reminiscent of posttraumatic stress disorder (PTSD). The PTSD concept places undue emphasis on the traumatic situation and minimizes the role of constitutional factors and individual predisposition. This concept elevated PTSD to the status of a regular disease by the lay evangelists for its legitimacy (Wilbur, 1990). The potential gain from the neurodevelopmental model is that it directs attention to premorbid factors and mechanisms that may be compromised prior to the traumatic experience. However, **Mintz and Myslobodsky** were able to obtain a syndrome of aberrations reminiscent of PTSD only when animals were exposed to γ irradiation at Day 15 of prenatal development.

A model developed by **Lipska and Weinberger** is the flagship of the armada of schizophrenia models. It is based on neonatal excitotoxic damage to the rat ventral hippocampus, the brain area most consistently implicated in human schizophrenia. Such damage leads to cognitive abnormalities and deficient social interactions at adulthood consistent with some central symptoms of schizophrenia. This model has demonstrated the plausibility of the neurodevelopmental theory of schizophrenia which postulates that this disorder is caused by a subtle defect in cerebral development that disrupts late-maturing, highly evolved neocortical functions, and fully manifests itself only in adult life (Weinberger, 1999). An important feature of this model as well as of some other experimental syndromes is that the clinical signs and aberrations of brain reactivity are not phenotypically apparent until puberty (**Mintz and Myslobodsky**). This, however, does not explain why such delays occur. Any seemingly harmless demographic milestone which eludes identification may do the job. A prototypical case is that of phenylketonuria which can be triggered by any food containing phenylalanine. A variety of diseases appearing at adulthood may be nurtured by an unrecognized or a latent neurodevelopmental disorder. Neurologists are aware of cases when deficient CSF absorption is precipitated following a minor head injury. Even Klippel-Feil abnormality (congenital vertebral fusion of the cervical spine) and a variety of "pediatric" tumors may be asymptomatic until adulthood.

A knockout of a gene encoding an endogenous substance is rapidly becoming a major tool whereby neuroscience immensely magnifies its view. If development can be defined in the spirit of Hebb's (1949) metaphor as an endlessly branching tree, **Miller and colleagues** as well as **Holmes and Crawley** describe the technique of pruning the branch tightly to its shaft by using gene knockout methodology. **Holmes and Crawley** reviewed the feasibility of using rodent emotionality as an animal model for human susceptibility to anxiety and schizophrenia. This tantalizing recent approach demonstrates the multifaceted phenotype of anxiety-like behaviors (associated with deficiencies in either GABA-A, catechol-O-methyltransferase, 5-HT1B receptor, or corticotropin-releasing factor) which may soon be translated into tests of classical and novel therapeutic compounds and delivery systems. The task is not simple. **Holmes and Crawley** caution the reader that a deleted gene of a specific behavior may not lead to the desirable phenotype. Furthermore, it is uncertain how much an acquisition of such a phenotype would depend upon the ability of the brain to compensate for the absence of an "adequate" stressor which causes the deficit. Finally, a specific behavioral abnormality in a mutant mouse may be unjustifiably attributed to the targeted gene switch-off.

Schizophrenia model is an infinitely more difficult target for gene knockout methodology. The disorder is dimensional rather than dichotomous, its various features are not necessarily located on the extremes of a continuum, and its development is influenced by a mixture of genetic and environmental factors. As expected in complex genetics, many studies searching for "genes of schizophrenia" are inconclusive and contradictory. A helpful thread is provided by **Miller and colleagues'** findings on the plasma membrane dopamine transporter (DAT) and the vesicular monoamine transporter (VMAT2) responsible for the packaging of dopamine into small synaptic and dense core vesicles. These are molecular mechanisms which help the cell to live, but may teach us how it dies when this machinery is sabotaged thereby exposing the cell to potential xenobiotics and/or metabolic overload. **Miller and colleagues** hypothesize that the DAT/VMAT2 ratio determines the severity of hyperdopaminergia following the continued excitation of dopamine receptors and sensitization to psychostimulants, as well as the neuron's sensitivity to neurotoxins thereby increasing the likelihood of psychopathology. Would genetic variation in dopamine transporters and the DAT/VMAT2 ratio be useful for predicting psychopathology in general? **Miller and colleagues** suggest that these findings are relevant for examining such diverse conditions as attention deficit hyperactivity disorder, schizophrenia, Parkinson's depression, and dementia. With the tempo of current research the answers will not be long in coming. **Lipska and Weinberger** noticed reduced expression of dopamine transporter in the midbrain neurons of the neonatally lesioned rats (but not in rats with identical lesions inflicted in adulthood). They caution, however, that behavioral hyperresponsiveness may have alternative explanations.

McIntyre and Anisman take the advantage of selective breeding to produce two lines of rats that differ in the time required for low-intensity amygdaloid electrical stimulation to activate maximal seizure. Their Slow kindled rats reach stage-5 seizures following ~45 daily amygdala stimulations, whereas Fast rats need only ~10 sessions to produce a similar effect. These two lines show considerable differences in $GABA_A$ subunit expression in several temporal lobe structures.

The transgenic and knock-out scenarios require in vitro manipulations of cells and embryos for applying retroviral vectors for gene delivery. However, retrovirus-induced perinatal infections are of serious concern as real-life precipitants of latent brain abnormalities. Infected offspring may be born without an apparent defect but develop a psychopathological phenotype later in life. **Pearce** describes developmentally-engineered behavioral aberrations induced by infecting rats intracranially with lymphocyte choriomeningitis virus. The similarities of placentation in mouse and humans suggests the possibility of transplacental transmission of some endogenous retroviruses, and permits to establish causal relationships between the better researched neurochemical changes and immunological events engendered by perinatal viral infections. **Pearce** shows that infections during later stages of embryogeny may cause a variety of milder aberrations which vary as a function of their timing and severity. The offspring will survive but behavioral aberrations may appear as maturation advances. Collectively, behavioral aberrations following such damage are designated as behavioral teratogenesis (Auroux,1997). The notion of experimental behavioral teratology is not a whimsical construct. Although behavioral abnormalities are an expected outcome of an anatomical brain lesion, they may be meager and difficult to prove. So far, behavioral teratology has not been acknowledged on its own right in modeling psychopathology. **Mintz and Myslobodsky** provide a case of behavioral teratology with regard to the capacity of prenatal damage to emulate PTSD.

Pathophysiological Modeling

All etiologic models in the volume have strong pathophysiological claims so as to respond to the requirement of "*construct validity.*" They all rest on the implicit assumption that the term "pathophysiology" describes a broad spectrum of failing steps acting in distinct causal pathways or having distinct role within the same causal pathway. Each step could possibly set the stage for the next process thereby acting as an etiologic factor in its own right. Such a cascade of events may be exerted against any deficient mechanism, i.e., a *locus resistenciae minoris* of old writers. Likewise, an interruption of some steps of the cascade may be of a therapeutic utility. Thus, the division between etiologic and pathophysiological modeling is often arbitrary (**Ingraham and Myslobodsky**).

The pathophysiological approach frequently takes the form of "*risk models*" which identify vulnerabilities; "*interactionists models*" which explore interactions between environmental precipitants and the developmental and risk variables; or various "*genetic models*" which have the benefit of beginning the trail of search from the reproduction of animals with or without specific characteristics or genes. The mechanisms of the pathophysiological caliber may thus be ubiquitous and appear as molecular (genetic liability, metabolic errors), molar (acquired or inborn premorbid defects, malfunctions in various stations in the chain of command of specific functions), behavioral (clinical) and neurochemical phenotypes, as well as environmental risk variables (e.g., nutrition, concurrent stressors, infections, physical or chemical "pollutants"). This historically acquired promiscuity of the term has reduced its appeal and the classical glitter.

Ex-juvantibus Approach

Diagnosis is often not more than an attractive hypothesis, whose correctness is evaluated according to the outcome of drug treatment (assuming that the drug is reasonably selective and specific). Such antiquated diagnosis based on treatment is designated as *Ex-juvantibus* diagnosis. The logic of diagnosis *ex-juvantibus* is identical to what psychologists call *"predictive validity"* and it is commonly used in animal modeling to show that a new model leads to credible therapeutic predictions (Myslobodsky and Mirsky, 1988).

Many of the models in this volume incorporate this approach as an integral aspect of their validity. Thus, it is exemplified by the demonstrations that delayed behavioral aberrations in rats with neonatal hippocampal lesions, as well as disrupted PPI and LI following various pharmacological and physiological manipulations, are reversible with typical (haloperidol) and atypical (clozapine) neuroleptics, implying the proximity of the model to schizophrenia (**Lipska and Weinberger; Geyer; Weiner**). **Einat and colleagues** use anti-depressants to validate models of bipolar disorder. Likewise, hypersensitivity to NMDA antagonists in schizophrenia is employed to test its animal model (**Lipska and Weinberger**). **Holmes and Crawley** raise a related point by showing that the mutant lines need to be tested for the pharmacological specificity of drug candidates. Knockout mice overcome the danger of crudity of *ex-juvantibus* approach by narrowly focusing treatment to specific deficient receptors.

However, *ex-juvantibus* testing is marred by the low-level specificity of drugs, their inherent limitations (delayed response, incomplete efficacy, shallow remissions, and side effects), as well as poorly controlled pharmacokinetic variables. Finally, *ex-juvantibus* diagnosis is determined by the antiquated taxonomic borders so that what we often see is that treatment may be more relevant pathophysiologically than nosologically. As some have observed, the examination of putative therapeutic agents is restricted to those that are antagonistic to the drug used to create models. Such agents are not necessarily most profitable heuristically (**Feldon and colleagues; Ingraham and Myslobodsky; Lipska and Weinberger**); however, some models, e.g., LI, do not require previous drug administration for the detection of putative antipsychotic activity (**Weiner**). In the future, this criterion will probably be jettisoned unless it stands the test of treatment of some "core diagnostic features" (Krueger, 1999) hidden behind the clusters of various psychopathological syndromes.

Markers as Models

Markers are defined as physiological, biochemical, pharmacological, or behavioral responses that reside on a pathophysiological pathway of a disease and have diagnostic utility. They are judged on the criteria of sensitivity (the ability to detect low level of change) and specificity (correspondence to clinical diagnosis). Some "overt" somatomotor or autonomic markers are rather stable even if their specificity is not great. Their benefit is in assisting in prognosis of the disorder and quantifying the disability. The augmentation of the acoustic startle reflex is a popular somatomotor marker of this kind (**Davis and colleagues; Feldon and colleagues; McIntyre and Anisman; Mintz and Myslobodsky**). It signals an inappropriate activation of normal defense reactions to diverse forms of threats, real or imagined. Its potentiation by "anxiety" and "fear" in rats appears to be mediated by the amygdala, so acoustic startle may mark what could be in archaic parlance designated as amygdaloid dysfunction.

Geyer presents a useful and much discussed distinction between the startle response to a stimulus (a pulse) and its alteration by a preceding stimulus (a prepulse). Schizophrenic patients and high schizotypal individuals exhibit deficits in PPI, i.e., the reduction in startle produced by a prepulse stimulus, thereby providing an operational measure of disrupted sensorimotor gating or filtering deficits in these patients that, conceivably, may lead to sensory flooding and cognitive fragmentation. PPI is used for comparing various models of schizophrenia, i.e., those induced by various pharmacological agents in adult rats, or by early developmental insults (neonatally lesioned vs. isolation reared rats), or by targeted gene mutations (**Holmes and Crawley**). Ideally, markers should be selective and specific for distinct clinically diagnosed conditions. However, PPI is also disrupted in other psychiatric disorders such as Huntigton's Disease, obsessive compulsive dissorder, nocturnal enuresis (Ornitz et al., 1992) and Tourette's syndrome (Castellanos et al., 1996). Likewise, LI is potentiated in obsessive compulsive dissorder (Swerdlow et al., 1999). One may hazard a hunch that the specificity of the marker is inversely related to the number of its applications to different disorders. Thus, it appears that we may have markers of specific *dysregulations* rather than clinically *diagnosable* conditions, e.g., PPI disruption may be a marker of deficient central inhibitory mechanisms (Swerdlow et al., 1996). Inasmuch as LI is also disrupted in high schizotypals, it can also be conceived of as a marker. However, its specificity for schizophrenia itself is more limited than to schizotypy, as disrupted LI is found only in some subsets of patients, or only in some states of the disorder, suggesting that it might be a state variable. An alternative implication of this discrepancy is that schizophrenia is a heterogeneous disease, and disrupted LI characterizes only certain subpopulations of ill individuals, whereas persistent LI may be present in other subpopulations (**Weiner**). One would expect that putative markers show unidirectional changes to the same manipulation. Yet they may not necessarily march in step. **Feldon and colleagues** demonstrated that pre-weaning environmental manipulations affect LI and not PPI whereas post-weaning isolation affects PPI and not LI. Also, there was no consistent and predictive relationship between the effect of an environmental manipulation on LI or PPI and its effects on locomotion or behavior in the open field.

Cognitive Models

Cognitive models of psychopathology have their launching platform in some cognitive deficit postulated to characterize the modeled disorder. Examples are inability to ignore irrelevant stimuli, to gate sensory input, or "frontal-like" cognitive deficits as models of schizophrenia (**Weiner**; **Geyer**; **Feldon and colleagues**; **Robbins**) or learned helplessness as a model of depression (**Carlson and colleagues**). **Davis and colleagues** deal with a peculiar aspect of memory disorder, i.e., the tendency of intense trauma to produce vivid memories that last a lifetime. They can be retrieved by stimuli associated with the original traumatic event, and in some individuals may become so intrusive as to preclude normal functioning. Searching for a therapeutic question, how to train memory so that it is able to forget, **Davis and colleagues** take advantage of the observation that extinction does not result in a complete erasure of the original CS-US association. They show that it is not the neutral stimulus alone reinforced by trauma that defines a state of fear. Some emotional and social aberrations may follow due to the overutilization of what Damasio (1996) calls "somatic markers" or musculosceletal and autonomic cues that become coupled to the formerly neutral environmental socio-affective signal.

The strength of the cognitive models is considerably enhanced when they use procedures which can be tested in both rats and humans, in which case they can draw stronger conclusions on the underlying deficit as well as provide technical diagnostic aids in the clinical setting (**Weiner; Geyer; Feldon and colleagues; Robbins**). A functional decomposition of a complex test such as the WCST into simpler components is a particularly powerful technique which allows a more refined analysis of the cognitive deficits in schizophrenia and of the underlying neural substrates of parallel deficits in animals (**Robbins**). However, given that in the laboratory, pharmacological or physiological manipulations are used to produce the cognitive impairment of interest, one of the questions faced by cognitive models is to what extent each impairment produced by such manipulations should be regarded as a variation on the old model, or a new model. According to **Geyer**, "the basic rodent "PPI model" has evolved into at least four distinct "models", differentiated by the manipulations used to mimic the disruption of PPI seen in schizophrenia." One might wonder whether this multiplicity implies the presence of several distinct neural mechanisms which can be manifested in the same cognitive deficit in schizophrenia.

For a "cleaner" cognitive model we might want cognitive alterations which are not produced by a gross anatomical or a neurochemical lesion; one possibility is to utilize variations in some aspects of normal behavior. **Carlson and colleagues** take such an approach, basing their model on "brain laterality" in rodents. They show that dopamine carrying systems project to the prefrontal cortex in a manner that activates them asymmetrically in response to uncontrolled stressors. Moreover, the direction of this activation differs between rats preferentially turning to the left as opposed to those who turn to the right. Right prefrontal activation is associated with depression-like effects, albeit in the left hemisphere model. **McIntyre and Anisman** suggest that the ability to inhibit affective responses too may be laterally controlled. Rarely has a new behavioral tool been so readily embraced and so rapidly advanced to various aspects of brain pathology as this kind of stereotypy (**Carlson and colleagues**). It has become a favorite instrument in the attempts to falsify the concept of aberrant laterality in psychopathology and successfully applied to the understanding of Parkinson's disease, hemineglect, psychopathology, and drug-induced behaviors. The absence of rigid and complex phenomenological requirements could surely account for the enthusiasm for these kinds of models.

Social Network Effects

Genotype-environment interaction issue is invoked when different environmental factors contribute to different effects in individuals with the same genotype or when the same environment contributes to dissimilar effects in individuals with different genotype. Such factors do not need to be harmful. The expression of a gene may be triggered by a benign demographic factor, such as age

(**Lipska and Weinberger**; **Mintz and Myslobodsky**). Social interaction may be another important environmental variable. The latter is a largely ignored aspect of modeling (McKinney, 1988). In the present volume it is represented by pre/post-weaning environmental manipulations in LI and PPI, which are needed to account for the environmental mutability of "deviance" (**Feldon and colleagues**). Some take into account the dependence among individuals or a response to the natural environmental conditions or natural predators (e.g., **McIntyre and Anisman**).

Hippocampus is implicated in exploratory behavior and approach needed for social interaction. **Lipska and Weinberger** showed that rats with neonatal hippocampal lesions tested before puberty already differed from normal controls in social behavior in that they made less social contacts with unfamiliar partners and showed more anxiety. One might wonder how an inability to interact with others would lead to schizophrenia, or alternatively to a variety of posttraumatic stress disorders with manifestations of inhibition and withdrawal, or anxiety in shy individuals. These are tough questions for animal models to tackle. In addition, models testing social behavior typically focus on deficits in social interaction. It would be important to expand the repertoire of these paradigms to include aspects of social interaction in which curiosity, exploration, imitation, and intrinsic motivation are major factors. Imitation phenomena studies by Rizzolatti and Arbib (1998) are particularly intriguing and yet to be explored instruments of social cognitive competence.

METHODOLOGICAL ISSUES

In the past, the prime portion of modeling was an extension of a "Wernicke-styled" attempt to correlate symptoms with lesions and later on, to compare the severity of symptoms with presumed neurotransmitter "disbalances." This cross-sectional concept of psychopathology has significantly decreased in popularity. Lesions are not easy to calibrate. The more severe the damage the more likely that the association between exposure and outcome will be stronger. On the other hand, extensive damage could involve a number of innocent bystanders thereby increasing potential confounds. In addition, lesion models are less concerned with naturalistic, prospective (etiologic) scenarios which are seen following infections, anoxic events, or stressors, nor do they answer the question of how long it takes to develop behavioral deficits and how long it takes to recover. They cannot reproduce the ever increasing "penumbral" tiers of psychopathological conditions which are inflated with every new edition of DSM. Most depressing, even if instructive, is a recent report by De Keyser et al. (1999) of the limitations of animal stroke models in mimicking such a presumably straightforward clinical condition as ischaemic stroke. The difficulty was manifested in clinical trials of several neuroprotective agents which have been proven ineffective in limiting ischaemic brain damage.

Drug administration is a popular alternative for reproducing aberrant behaviors. However, there is an important caveat when using drugs: their effects may differ as a function of age, strain, and sex, and even time of administration. Some specifically alert the reader to the fact that there are significant between-species differences (**Miller and colleagues**; **Holmes and Crawley**; **Einat and colleagues**). The monoaminergic systems of mice and rats may be dissimilar as reflected for example in the remarkable resistance of rats to MPTP (**Miller and**

colleagues). There are still mostly underestimated gender differences in pharmacokinetics and pharmacodynamics for which Rhodes and Rubin (1999) coined the term sexual "diergism" to emphasize differences in responses and vulnerability to pharmaceutic agents that may or may not be recognized on the basis of sexual dimorphism. Drug effects are determined by intrinsic rhythms of various neurotransmitters, enzymes, receptors, and the second messenger systems which make drug responses vary in complicated ways as a function of age, animal species, time of drug administration, and even season of testing (Nagayma, 1999). The optimal time for eliciting maximal drug action ("peak time") may be dissimilar for different drugs. For chlorpromazine, it occurs in the early dark period whereas for haloperidol the peak time is in the early light period. More importantly, various effects of drugs may have dissimilar peak times and differ not only in intensity but in direction or even quality. For example, *l*-norepinephrine given in the early dark period decreases feeding behavior whereas the same dose will increase feeding when given at the end of the light period. Apomorphine elicits stereotypy in the light period but locomotion in the dark period. These and other data on the rhythmicity in drug effects were summarized in a recent review by Nagayma (1999).

Behavioral studies indicate that the effects of psychostimulants are determined by environmental factors (e.g., home vs. novel environment). **Robinson** discusses how environmental context may modulate sensitization to a repeated exposure to amphetamine which takes a form of either context-specific or context-independent sensitization. It has yet to be understood how and under what conditions contextual stimuli may modulate the expression of psychopathological responses.

Individual differences in susceptibility to different manipulations is another factor of concern. **Carlson and colleagues** draw attention to the fact that many individuals experience uncontrollable stressful events, yet relatively few of them become depressed. As an important counterpart of this phenomenon, susceptibility to learned helplessness is a specific behavioral trait that is variably expressed within populations of rats. Any model has to be tested in diverse behavioral conditions. The necessity of complex batteries is exemplified by **McIntyre and Anisman's** demonstration that the greater fear/anxiety manifested by Slow-kindled rats as expressed in their behaviors in fear-potentiation paradigms, augmented startle and vocal signs of distress is not consistent with their somewhat greater initial open-field emergence, and rather active behavior when exposed to the ferret.

Model "Calibration": What Makes One Model Better than Another?

Given that models have an inbuilt systematic error because they either exaggerate or minimize (up to total elimination) the mechanism of illness of interest, they cannot be judged by the accuracy of reproduction, i.e., the degree of "verisimilitude." They can only be expected to manifest a low level of random (unpredictable) errors and be ranked on the scale of precision, i.e., the reproducibility (stability) of observed events. Measurements of stability of composite models (i.e., models based on several obligatory features) cover three aspects: (a) variation of one component within the composite in the same strain; (b) between-component variation in the same strain; (c) variation in different strains (heterogeneity).

The problem of model evaluation resides either in isolating the strategic features of an imputed anomaly or in determining the critical alterations in the degree or the quantity of the measured ("pathological") responses. Both approaches are represented in the volume. The axis of magnitude works handsomely for such disorders as generalized anxiety, posttraumatic stress disorder or impulsivity. The process of picking out the relevant feature is far more complex, as illustrated by the section on model misattribution a few paragraphs above.

An important but seldom discussed problem concerns the way in which various elements of psychopathology can be reproduced in a model. What is aimed at reproduction and how the success of the product is recognized? How are the behavioral aberrations expressed in the model and how do they relate to specific clinical patterns in humans? **Holmes and Crawley** caution us that when a mutation produces a variety of interacting biological actions, there is a danger of false positives, particularly if only a small subset of behavioral tests are conducted. In the latter case, the deduced phenotype may reflect a sensory or motor defect rather than produce a mouse analog of a human psychiatric symptom. By contrast, false negatives arise when a mutation produces subtle effects which could be easily missed if only one or two behavioral tasks within a specific domain are conducted. **Mintz and Myslobodsky** propose two formal criteria for model appraisal, model transfer profile and model intrinsic conformity. They propose that the ratio of adequately transferred features to all diagnostically relevant features is an estimate of model's transfer profile (MTP). The presence of several features of this kind does not invite a nosological commitment, for with a better scrutiny some other, "irrelevant features" may be observed. Model intrinsic conformity (MIC) is defined by the ratio of the planned (relevant) aberrant features (n) to all other aberrant phenomena (Δn) encountered in the model. Although it may seem tautological, it was introduced to define the number of potential confounds a model has. If the list of unplanned features is excessively long we may be at risk for providing a correct answer to the wrong proposition or what is known as a Type II error (Kimball, 1957).

Where Does that Leave Us?

The list of questions which were raised by our crew could surely be lengthened. As our journals are flooded with new neuromodulators and novel mechanisms, the process of classification of models may seem hopeless at times, and we have to be prepared to cope with the never-ending stream of candidates. Although this volume shows that considerable progress has been made, the major task of objective assessment of experimental models of psychopathology is still ahead of us. Even though each step adds a little to the understanding of factors contributing to "brain vulnerabilities" and prepares us to anticipate possible errors, we are still tentative about the picture we wish to reproduce. Among problems that hinder the analyses there are a few that are shared by many groups. These are:

- The paucity of specific inclusion or exclusion criteria for a laboratory syndrome that are clear and measurable, and allow for the genetic search in phenotypically homogenous groups.
- Dearth of longitudinal data on the syndromal stability of psychopathology models based on standardized diagnostic procedures (stability over time).

- Scarcity of relationships between abnormal behaviors with specific somatic or immunological features co-morbid or incompatible with psychopathology.

- Difficulties in using methodologies and measurement techniques standardized in neurological models (e.g., norm-referenced scores for differentiating optimal vs. suboptimal performance; acceptable concurrent and predictive validity).

To a degree, these problems will be mitigated by collaborative multicenter studies which will foster comparisons of models proposed for similar purposes and ultimately will tend to reduce the often extreme methodological variations between laboratories. Other problems are inherited from the discipline itself and they are with us because the acceptance of models has been so rapid and total. Thus, the conviction that *"Nomen est numen"* (naming is knowing) exerts a lasting and intoxicating effect of virtual reality in psychiatry. Small surprise that the tendency to name a model after specific disease dies hard. At their best, models reproduce the "worst-case" scenarios so to speak, such as epilepsy, infarction, or coma. Likewise, such signs as fear, panic, anxiety, or vulnerability to stress, reduced drives, difficulties in social interaction or mating are among those which are more easy to agree upon and to reproduce in laboratory animals. They would not get psychiatrists' hair up so much as, perhaps, calling an animal a "schizophrenic."

There is another problem which is frequently overlooked in discussions on modeling. In the most common case, model is not so much a part of a specific psychopathological concept as the psychopathological concept is part (and only one part) of research spurred by modeling efforts. An inherent interest in the created phenomenon perpetuates its analysis irrespective of the reasons the model had been designed for. This style of research is a nemesis of psychologists who are frequently blamed for spending too much time on the interim results leading into diverse directions rather than responding more forcefully to the needs of practice. Because of their complexity and resistance to reductionistic efforts, cognitive models are most zealously perpetuating their object. The rotation model is a good case in point. The refreshing certainty and simplicity of animal laterality based on rotation was predictably blurred with the advancement of our knowledge of the surprising multiplicity of directionality biases. Initially seeming as simple as one can dream of, the model of the circling rodent has become not only an instrument of analysis but an area of active research of rotation itself. Another familiar example is that of startle which has become an area of a complex and exciting research. In a longer run, this tendency could make cognitive models trotting behind the novel paradigms of contemporary psychiatry. The latter is armed with functional and spectroscopic magnetic resonance imaging, positron emission tomography, magnetoencephalography, and other advanced techniques which allow to localize and quantify the disturbances of various brain regions of the human brain.

Pearce rightly points out that models are multifunctional and not sufficiently restrictive. Table 1 captures the essential argument we wish to make: The conception of what is a "model" depends upon one's perspective or intentions to exploit its specific functions; the term cannot be monopolized since a model is always a composite of virtues and sins. In psychopathology, models attract by their ability to "objectify subjectivity:" they overcome (or rather ignore) the ontological problem of assuming what a rat tends to assume. We offer no proof for this view and state it as a widely held sentiment of many workers in the field. The editorial by Parent and Cicchetti (1998) summarizes our ambivalence about models most eloquently: "Models in science tend to reassure and appease researchers who do not like to wander alone in the universe of knowledge. However, models may have a perverse effect, such as the selective neglect of data that do not fit into the model (modellus deformans disease)" (p. 202). Modellus deformans disease remains so prevalent because, to paraphrase Leopold Kroneker (1823-1891), God made psychoses; their models is the work of man.

Table 1. Models defined by their functions

Explicative	presents a list of essential components and interactions
Inferential	invites inferences of the possible casual relationships within the model components and input-output interactions
Connotive	serves to denote veracity, establish "likeness"
Communicative	allows to signal implied solutions, thereby facilitating crosstalk within- and between-professional groups
Referential	alludes to prior experience and knowledge (e.g. comparative, developmental, biochemical)
Reductionistic	shortens the list of conditions/mechanisms eliciting a disorder
Interpretative	shifts arguments (e.g., from ecological to causal); when observations are made on populations (ecological level) the model will bolster causal interpretations
Managing	helps organizing inferences, predictions, corollaries, and implications
Counseling	exposes the range of effects relevant for public health
Metaphoric	legitimizes metaphoric arguments when translating psychopathology in the language of animals behaviors, "objectify subjectivity"
Gambling	conveys premature assurance of success
Evasive	exports the analysis hampered by limitations or ethical problems into the domain of biology, mathematics, computer science, etc.

The present volume reflects the limited interest in models which emulate either the presence of somatic comorbidity or its unusually low prevalence in psychotic patients. The fecundity disadvantage in schizophrenia, leukocytosis and neutrophilia accompanying severe depression, particularly noticeable in males (Maes et al., 1992), and perilabial herpes which is reactivated with the onset of affective episode and terminated by lithium (Rybakowski, 1999, for review) are certainly worth reproducing experimentally. An opposite example is the reduced risk of rheumatoid arthritis (Allebeck et al., 1985; Eaton et al., 1992), relative resistance to prostaglandins mediated pain and inflammation (Marchand et al., 1969), absence of niacin skin flush (Ward et al., 1998), or low rates of some forms of cancer (Baldwin, 1979), particularly, reduced prevalence of lung cancer, in patients with schizophrenia (who are known for their avid appetite for smoking). Perhaps, in this context, the finding by **McIntyre and Anisman** deserves a special mention. Their observations of the robust difference of *in vivo* NA release in the amygdala to a cytokine (interleukin-1b) in their Fast and Slow-kindled lines may suggest that immune profiles may covary as a function of brain epileptogenicity.

Holmes and Crawley, Miller and colleagues, Lipska and Weinberger, and **Robinson** give us hope that some clues to psychopathology will be pursued molecularly. The sentiment among our young scientists is that molecular biology research is the only type of scientific research worth doing. Indeed, without transgenic and knockout models we are learning something about the brain and its aberrations but infinitely less about the functions of neurons and neuronal systems. However, although molecular genetic modeling is certainly promising, it will have bleak prospects without a firm pathophysiological foundation. The most humbling and potentially most lasting hurdle in a search for the genetic foundation of psychopathology is the multifactorial character of psychoses. The genetic strategies may not produce a "strong" model of major psychoses because the inherited susceptibility for psychopathology is expected to be explained by multiple genes of small effect as well as uncertain intervening variables. Though we may soon understand how cocaine interacts with the plasma membrane dopamine transporter (**Miller and colleagues**), it is clear that the whole gamut of addictive behavior and its variability cannot be reduced to such mechanisms. A good example is a form of experience-dependent plasticity modeled by repeated administration of drugs that is seen in a variety of structures (**Robinson**).

Data from some laboratories (**Carlson and colleagues; McIntyre and Anisman**) suggest that if the control of stress-related behaviors, receptor changes induced by stress, drug intake, impulsive behaviors, drug self-administration, and the development of addictive strategies is lateralized (as they seem to be), they will not be detected in (bilateral) knockout animals. Such data prompt us to realize that psychiatry is in the domain of gray where the various mechanisms and disorders we model shade one into another. The descriptions of psychoses overlap at times so significantly that some entries in the DSM look as group portraits or morphs with patently shared features rather than unitary disorders. We have learned this all along from the clinic. Almost any final diagnostic closure gets in the way of knowing the patient and Taylor (1978) was doubtful that an honest psychiatric diagnosis could ever be a single-word verdict. Still, maybe we do not need to diversify animal models so as to adhere to the contemporary nosological catalogue before the heterogeneity we see is given a proper neurochemical or molecular genetic descriptor.

The Achilles' Heel of Modeling

To remain within the familiar ontological frame of reference, our models must be evaluated by a parallel taxonomy of syndromes or certain aberrations of animal behaviors. Alternatively, all psychopathology syndromes should be rephrased in terms of deficient behavioral responses and basic functions (e.g., orienting reflex, memory, mood, emotion, motivation, fear, self-protection, and social affiliation; Cummings, 1999). We have to learn how these responses vary as a function of lesion parameters (e.g., nature of damaging agent, size and location of lesion) as well as host-related factors (e.g., genetic liability, developmental factors, age at lesion, gender, brain laterality, co-morbidity) and, perhaps, context-dependent modulation of responsiveness (**Robinson**). The parallel taxonomy will not solve our ontological problem but will make the language of neuronal systems, neurotransmitters, receptors, and genes more relevant to the clinical syndromes. This is because the genes may not confer specific overall susceptibility. Rather, they might affect certain aspects of the disorder which could only be revealed by modeling specific behaviors or specific mechanisms. Ultimately, the level of complexity of such language may diminish our dependence on experimenting with mammals. The examples are mounting that the cellular anatomy, cell lineage, neuronal wiring, and genomic sequence of such inexpensive organisms as parasitic worms may give us valuable insights into drug mechanisms and behavior. Indeed, biological models rest on the Darwinian notion of the presence of man in amoebae, emulating restricted aspects of reality and providing phenotypic homologues on a limited scale. Though the amoebas and nematodes are not particularly cognitive creatures, they appear to use similar genes for similar developmental purposes to those of mammals. They might certainly provide an exciting shortcut at least to pharmacotherapy of psychoses (e.g., Schaeffer et al., 1994); they could also serve us well by reducing our penchant to measure animal behaviors by the standards of human psychopathology, the Achilles'* heel of modeling. This tempts us to conclude that in a longer run, the behaviors of bacteria, insects and worms may turn out to be the fittest models of "psychopathology" in their quest to survive.

FOOTNOTE

*This relates to the Ancient Greek hero, the seventh son of Neried Thetis and Peleus, who though virtually immortal had a meager neurodevelopmental anomaly, in his heel. Ultimately, this small defect had sealed his fate during the Trojan War.

REFERENCES

Allebeck, P., Rodvall, Y., Wistedt, B. (1985) Incidence of rheumatoid arthritis among patients with schizophrenia, affective psychosis and neurosis. Acta Psychiatr Scand 71:615-619.

Ashby, W.R. (1970) Analysis of the system to be modeled. In: Stogdill, R.M. (ed.), The process of model-building in the behavioral sciences. (pp 94-114). Columbus: Ohio state University.

Auroux, M. (1997) Behavioral teratogenesis: an extension to the teratogenesis of functions. Biol Neonate, 71:137-147.

Baldwin, J. A., (1979) Schizophrenia and physical disease. Psychol. Med. 9: 611-618.

Bartus, R.T. (1988) The need for common perspectives in the development and use of animal models for age-related cognitive and neurodegenerative disorders. Neurobiol Aging, 9:445-451.

Castellanos, F.X., Fine, E.J., Kaysen, D. et al. (1996) Sensorimotor gating in boys with Tourette's syndrome and ADHD: preliminary results. Biol. Psychiat., 39:33-41.

Cummings, J.L. (1999) Principles of neuropsychiatry: Towards a neuropsychiatric epistemology. Neurocase, 5: 181-188.

Damasio, A.R. (1996) The somatic marker hypothesis and the possible functions of the prefrontal cortex. Phil. Trans. Royal Soc. Series B., 351: 1413-1420.

De Keyser, J., Sulter, G., Luiten, P.G. (1999) Clinical trials with neuroprotective drugs in acute ischaemic stroke: are we doing the right thing? TINS, 22: 535-540.

Eaton, W. W., Hayward, C., Ram, R. (1992) Schizophrenia and rheumatoid arthritis: a review. Schizophr Res 6: 181-192.

Friedman A, Kaufer D, Shemer J, Hendler I, Soreq H, Turkaspa I. (1996) Pyridostigmine brain penetration under stress enhances neuronal excitability and induces early immediate transcriptional response. Nature Medicine 2: 1382-1385.

Fuchs, S. (1992) The professional quest for truth. A social theory of science and knowledge. State University of New York Press: Albany.

Gullap, Jr. G.G. and Maser, J.D. (1977) Tonic immobility: evolutionary underpinnings of human catalepsy and catatonia. In: Maser, J.D., and Seligman, M.E.P. (Eds.), Psychopathology: Experimental models. San Francisco: Freeman and Co., pp 334-357.

Hebb, D.O. (1949) The organization of behavior. New York: Wiley.

Kimball, A.W. (1957) Errors of the third kind in statistical consulting. J Amer Stat Assoc 52:133-142.

Krueger, R. F. (1999) The structure of common mental disorders. Arch Gen Psychiatry 56:921-926.

Maes, M., Vanderplanken, M., Stevens, W.J., Peeters, D., Declerck, L.S, Bridts, Ch., Schotte, C., Cosyns, P. (1992) Leukocytosis, monocytosis and neutrophilia - hallmarks of severe depression. J. Psychiat. Res., 26: 125-134.

Maestripieri, D. and Carroll, K.A. (1998) Child abuse and neglect: Usefulness of the animal data. Psychol Bull, 123: 211-223.

Marchand, W.E., Sarota, B., Marble, H.C., Leavy, T.M., burbank, C.B., and Bellinger, M.J. (1969) Occurrence of painless acute surgical disorders in psychotic patients. New Engl J.Med., 260-580.

Marks, I. (1977) Clinical phenomena in search of laboratory models. In: Maser, J.D. and Seligman, M.E.P. (Eds.), Psychopathology: Experimental models. San Francisco: Freeman and Co., pp 174-213.

McKinney, W. T., Jr., Suomi S. J. and Harlow H. F., (1972) Vertical-chamber confinement of juvenile-age rhesus monkeys. A study in experimental psychopathology, Arch Gen Psychiatry. 26: 223-228.

McKinney, W.T. (1988) Models of mental disorderrs. A new comparative psychiatry. New York: Plenum Medical Book Company.

Miller, W.R, Rosellini, R.A, Seligman, M.E.P. (1977) Learned helplessnes and depression. In: Maser, J.D. and Seligman, M.E.P. (Eds.), Psychopathology: Experimental models. San Francisco: Freeman and Co., pp 105-130.

Myslobodsky, M., and Mirsky A.F. (1988) Update on Petit Mal: The case for heterogeneity. In: Myslobodsky M., and Mirsky, A.F (eds), Elements of Petit Mall Epilepsy. Peter Lang: New York.

Myslobodsky, M. and Valenstein, E. (1980) Amygdaloid kindling and the GABA system. Epilepsia 21:163-175.

Nagayma, H. (1999) Influences of biological rhythms on the effects of psychotropic drugs. Psychosomatic Med., 61:618-628.

Ornitz, E.M., Hanna, G.L., de Traversay, J. (1992) Prestimulation-induced startle modulation in attention-deficit hyperactivity disorder and nocturnal enuresis. Psychophysiology, 29:437-451.

Parent, A. and Ciccetti, F. (1998) The current model of basal ganglia organization under scrutiny. Mov Dis, 13: 1999-202.

Pribram, K. H. (1961) Implications for systemic studies of behavior. In: D. E. Sheer, Electrical stimulation of the brain. Austin: Texas University Press, pp. 563-574.

Rhodes, M. E. and Rubin, R. T. (1999) Functional sex differences ('sexual diergism') of central nervous system cholinergic systems, vasopressin, and hypothalamo-pituitary-adrenal axis activity in mammals: a selective review. Behav Brain Res. 30:135-152.

Rizzolatti, G. and Arbib, M.A. (1998) Language within our grasp. TINs, 21: 188-194.

Rybakowski, J.K. (1999) The effect of lithium on the immune system. Human Psychopharmacology, Clinical and Exp., 14: 345-353

Schaeffer, J.M., Bergstrom, A.R., Frazier, E.G., Underwood, D. (1994) Nematocidal activity of MK-801 analogs and related drugs. Structure-activity relationships. Biochem Pharmacol. 48(2):411-418.

Simon, J.C. (1991) Regularities and singularities in line images. In: Watt, R.J. (Ed.), Pattern recognition by man and machine. CRC Press, Inc.: Boca Raton, pp. 98-106.

Swerdlow, N.R., Braff, D.L., Hartston, H., Perry, W., Geyer, M.A. (1996) Latent inhibition in schizophrenia. Schiz Res. 20: 91-103.

Swerdlow, N.R., Hartston, H. J., Hartman, P. L. (1999) Enhanced visual latent inhibition in obsessive-compulsive disorder. Biol Psychiatry 45:482-488.

Szabo, C. A., Wyllie, E., Dolske, M. et al. (1999) Epilepsy surgery in children with pervasive developmental disorder. Pediatr Neurol. 20: 349-353.

Taylor, S. (1978) Psychiatry and natural history. British Medical Journal, 2:1754-1758.

Ward, P., Sutherland, J., Glen, E., Glen, A.I., Horrobin, D.F. (1998) Niacin skin flush in schizophrenia: a preliminary report. Schizophrenia Res., 29:296-275.

Weinberger, D. R. (1999) Cell biology of the hippocampal formation in schizophrenia. Biol Psychiat. 45:395-402.

Wilbur, J.S. (1990) PTSD in DSM-III: A case in the politics of diagnosis and disease. Social Problems, 37:294-310.

INDEX